Nutrition Essentials and Easy Recipes for Adults 50+

PLANT-POWERED SENIORS

Brenda Davis, RD, Vesanto Melina, MS, RD,
and Charlyn Black, MD, ScD

Health Communications, Inc.
Mt. Pleasant, South Carolina

www.hcibooks.com

Library of Congress Cataloging-in-Publication Data
is available through the Library of Congress

ISBN-13: 978-07573-2616-5 (Paperback)
ISBN-10: 07573-2616-1 (Paperback)
ISBN-13: 978-07573-2617-2 (ePub)
ISBN-10: 07573-2617-X (ePub)

Publisher: Health Communications, Inc.
1240 Winnowing Way, Suite 100
Mt. Pleasant, SC 29466

Cover, interior design, and formatting by Larissa Hise Henoch
Color photos by Janis Nicolay Photography

Praise for **PLANT-POWERED SENIORS**

"Plant-predominant eating promotes health at every stage of life, but nutrient requirements for optimal health do change with age and chronic conditions. In *Plant-Powered Seniors*, decades of scientific expertise are distilled into an authoritative, practical, and inspiring guide for getting the best of health—for yourself, and the planet too—in our golden years. Comprehensive and detailed, yet so easy to digest—this landmark resource deserves a place in every home and every health-care professional's library."

—**David L. Katz, MD, MPH,** author, with Mark Bittman, of *How to Eat*, past president, American College of Lifestyle Medicine

"I spent years pulling people out of burning buildings, but Brenda, Vesanto, and Charlyn are doing something even more impressive—they're pulling seniors back from the brink of a bad diet. *Plant-Powered Seniors* is the real deal: science-backed, practical, and proof that the best years of your life might just be ahead. All you have to do is eat your plants. Keep it plant strong!"

—**Rip Esselstyn,** founder, Plant Strong Foods, author of *Engine 2 Diet*

"*Plant-Powered Seniors* does something I've never seen before: a truly comprehensive, science-backed guide written specifically to help older adults flourish on a plant-powered diet. Drawing on the authors' combined century-plus of expertise in nutrition, clinical practice, and public health, they address everything from chronic disease prevention and nutrient optimization to navigating social situations, stocking a plant-powered pantry, and cooking meals that are as delicious as they are nourishing. This book is a gift to the millions of seniors who deserve better guidance, and anyone who loves them."

—**Ocean Robbins,** Food Revolution Network, author of *31-Day Food Revolution*

"As clinicians and researchers who have spent our careers studying how lifestyle shapes the aging brain, we're heartened by how rigorous and honest this book is. The authors don't oversell—they distinguish prevention from management, respect the evidence, and give older adults a clear, practical path to protect their brains and bodies. This is the rare guide that is both scientifically sound and genuinely usable. We recommend it wholeheartedly."

—**Dean Sherzai, MD, PhD, MPH, MAS,** and **Ayesha Sherzai, MD, MAS,** The Brain Docs, authors of *The Alzheimer's Solution*

"*Plant-Powered Seniors* is the definitive guide to healthy aging on a plant-based diet. The authors bring together a wealth of expertise to deliver practical, evidence-based guidance on everything from protein and bone health to cognitive function and chronic disease prevention. This book fills a critical gap and belongs on the shelf of every health-conscious older adult."

—**Neal D. Barnard, MD, FACC,** president, Physicians Committee for Responsible Medicine, adjunct professor, George Washington University School of Medicine

"*Plant-Powered Seniors* is an outstanding example of evidence-based nutrition at its best. It combines decades of expertise with the latest science to create a practical, comprehensive guide to healthy aging. This book empowers readers to embrace a lifestyle that supports personal health and the health of our planet."

—Dr. Shireen Kassam, MD, PhD, DipIBLM, haematologist, lifestyle medicine physician, director of Plant-Based Health Professionals UK

"Getting older is inevitable. Getting old is optional. *Plant-Powered Seniors* shows exactly how a plant-powered lifestyle can help us stay active, independent, and full of life for years to come. If you're over fifty—or hope to be someday—this book is essential reading."

—Chef AJ, author of *The Secrets to Ultimate Weight Loss* and *Unprocessed*

"*Plant-Powered Seniors* offers something precious: hope grounded in science. With wisdom, warmth, and decades of experience, Davis, Melina, and Black show that growing older need not mean surrendering health, vitality, or independence. Filled with practical guidance, delicious recipes, and evidence-based nutrition insights, this inspiring book empowers readers to nourish themselves for longer, stronger, and more fulfilling lives. A valuable gift for aging loved ones—and for yourself."

—Dr. Michael Klaper, author of *Moving Medicine Forward*

"*Plant-Powered Seniors* is an authoritative and much-needed resource for healthy aging. Grounded in sound science and decades of clinical experience, it provides practical guidance for meeting the nutritional needs of older adults while maximizing the health benefits of plant-based eating. This comprehensive guide is an invaluable resource for both consumers and health professionals."

—Joan Sabaté, MD, DrPH, professor of nutrition and epidemiology, Loma Linda University

"If I could place one plant-based nutrition book into the hands of every older adult, *Plant-Powered Seniors* would be at the top of the list. Thoughtful, comprehensive, and deeply inspiring, this book is a landmark contribution to the fields of plant-based nutrition, longevity, and healthspan."

—Julieanna (Hever) Risse, MS, RD, CPT, The Healthspan Dietitian, author of *The Healthspan Solution* and *Plant-Based Nutrition (Idiot's Guides)*

"I can think of no one better suited to write *Plant-Powered Seniors* than Brenda Davis, Vesanto Melina, and Charlyn Black. Between them, they bring decades of clinical and research experience, making a complex topic feel simple and digestible. They present a compelling case for how a plant-based diet can help us age healthfully and tools needed to make the shift as easy as possible."

—Dr Matthew Nagra, ND

"*Plant-Powered Seniors* provides clear, evidence-based guidance on plant-based eating. Presented with warmth, wisdom and a thoughtful focus on the realities of aging, this comprehensive resource offers practical solutions for thriving on a plant-based diet. For anyone looking to shift their diet toward one that optimizes health, compassion, and sustainability, this is an essential resource."

—Virginia Messina, MPH, RD, co-author of *Vegan for Life* and *Never Too Late to Go Vegan*

CONTENTS

CHAPTER 1

PLANT-POWERED AGING

Chapter at a Glance

Welcome to healthy, plant-powered living. In this chapter, you'll learn how dietary choices influence health outcomes and how this guide can support your journey at every step:

- Discover how being powered by plants supports brain, heart, metabolic, and digestive health, and how it can help you embrace other health-promoting habits.
- Learn what "plant-based" means across the spectrum (from flexitarian to plant-exclusive) and why diet quality matters.
- See how this book will guide you, step-by-step, toward a plant-powered lifestyle tailored to your needs.

Maria's Story: A Turning Point

For Maria, the idea of removing meat, poultry, and other animal products from her diet was not something she had ever considered, until the day she was diagnosed with hypertension and prediabetes. Her physician, a lifestyle medicine enthusiast, provided a few handouts and encouraged her to attend a community screening of a documentary, *Forks Over Knives*, a film that explores how a whole-food, plant-based diet can prevent and, in some cases, even reverse chronic disease. Maria felt skeptical but decided there was no harm in going.

It was a crisp January evening as Maria approached the venue, a quiet stillness settling around her. The day had felt long, but stepping inside, she was met with a gentle hum of activity in the cozy main hall. Conversations flowed easily, and there was a welcoming sense that she could simply listen and take things in.

As the film unfolded, it struck a nerve. For months, Maria had felt powerless, her health slipping further out of reach. But here were real people reclaiming their lives, supported by credible experts and compelling scientific evidence. By the time the credits rolled, something inside her shifted. Maria realized her health story wasn't over. It was hers to rewrite.

After the screening, Maria engaged in a lively conversation with other attendees. She felt inspired by the people who shared their own health transformations and newfound energy from adopting a plant-based diet. This strengthened her resolve to regain control of her health. What began as a casual evening out had unexpectedly become a turning point in her life.

A Fresh Start at Any Age

Perhaps you can relate to Maria's story. Whether it's a health challenge, a moment of doubt, or simply the desire for change, the path to better health often begins with a single step.

Aging isn't just about adding years, it's about adding wisdom and capability. The foods we choose today shape how we move, think, and engage tomorrow. Imagine waking with energy, enjoying meals that nourish body and spirit, and maintaining the independence to do the things you love.

We're not just health professionals, we're seniors ourselves. Collectively, we have spent more than a century living, teaching, and thriving on plant-based diets. Two of us are registered dietitians, one is a physician and professor in public health, and all of us have lived through decades of evolving nutrition trends, personal health transformations, and countless shared meals with loved ones. We've seen and felt what works, and what doesn't. You can feel confident that the guidance in this book is grounded in both scientific expertise and real-life experience.

The plant-powered lifestyles we have adopted and share in this book are not a recent craze but proven and enduring ways of eating that promote health, support vitality, and nurture joy in living.

This book is more than recipes and advice. It is a blueprint for thriving in your senior years—supported by science, enriched by personal stories, and grounded in practical strategies that you can use every day. Together, let's make the years ahead not just longer but stronger, brighter, and more fulfilling.

Plant-Based or Plant-Powered: What's the Difference?

You may already be familiar with the term *plant-based*, which refers to dietary patterns that prioritize plant foods to meet our nutritional needs. The scientific support for these diets is substantial and continues to grow. Later in this chapter, you'll learn about various eating patterns that fall under the plant-based umbrella.

In this book, we also use the term *plant-powered* to capture the energy, vitality, and wide-ranging benefits that come from embracing a diet centered on plant foods, especially those in their whole or minimally processed forms. Why "powered" by plants?

- **Plants are the original source of energy for nearly all life on Earth.** Through photosynthesis, plants convert sunlight into glucose, the foundational fuel for most living organisms, and release the oxygen we need to survive. Unlike animals, plants don't just consume energy; they create it. When we eat plants, we tap into that solar-powered life force directly.
- **Plants reconnect us to nature and traditional food wisdom.** Whole plant foods bring us closer to the sun-driven energy that sustains life, and to the simpler, less processed eating patterns of earlier generations—patterns often associated with vitality and longevity.
- **Plant foods fuel every pillar of healthy living.** A plant-powered diet supports more than physical health, it enhances energy, mood, sleep, and resilience. This vitality can empower other lifestyle choices, from being active and well-rested to managing stress and avoiding harmful substances—all of which promote healthier aging. We explore these pillars more fully in Chapter 7.

Why Plant-Based Eating for Elders

Embracing a plant-based diet is one of the most powerful steps older adults can take to enhance well-being, prevent or manage chronic disease, and enjoy food that is both delicious and nourishing. The benefits extend far beyond numbers on a medical chart—they touch nearly every aspect of daily life, from mental clarity and physical vitality to digestion, independence, and joy.

- **Sharpen your mind.** Plant-based diets supply "premium fuel" for the brain. Antioxidants, anti-inflammatory compounds, and healthy plant fats protect memory, support focus, and reduce the risk of dementia.
- **Maintain a healthy weight with ease.** As we age, our metabolisms typically slow down and we need fewer calories to maintain a healthy weight. Whole plant foods are naturally nutrient dense yet low in calorie density, which means you can enjoy generous portions without feeling deprived. Filling your plate with beans, grains, vegetables, and fruits makes it easier to maintain a healthy weight, support mobility, and feel satisfied, all while avoiding the frustration of fad diets.
- **Lower chronic disease risk.** Plant-powered eating serves as a protective shield against some of the most common health conditions associated with aging. Diets rich in legumes, whole grains, vegetables, fruits, nuts, and seeds consistently reduce the risk of heart disease, type 2 diabetes, hypertension, and certain cancers. For many, these diets also reduce cholesterol and improve blood sugar control, sometimes allowing for a reduction in medication. (Note: For more information on how plant-based eating patterns can help to prevent or treat a wide variety of medical conditions, see Chapter 4.)
- **Support healthy digestion.** While animal products contain no dietary fiber, plant foods are packed with it. Fiber keeps bowels regular, helps prevent constipation, and feeds a thriving and health-supportive gut microbiome—the community of bacteria that influences everything from our immunity to our mood. Paired with adequate water and regular activity, fiber is one of the most underrated keys to aging comfortably and energetically.

Taken together, these benefits do more than improve lab results. They enhance the quality of daily life, supporting strength, independence, and a more meaningful engagement with the world. Plant-based eating is not simply about avoiding disease; it is about building resilience and vitality for the years ahead.

Embracing Aging, Impoving Overall Well-Being

One thing we know is that age does not dictate health. How we age is strongly influenced by the lifestyle choices we make. While the body naturally changes as we age, how we embrace those changes can shape our overall well-being.

Aging presents a unique opportunity for self-reflection, growth, and prioritizing what truly matters, such as maintaining a healthy body and mind. With a thoughtful approach to nutrition, exercise, and self-care, many older adults find themselves in better health than they were in their younger years.

The wisdom, resilience, and experience gained over time can also lead to a deeper understanding of personal needs, allowing us to make informed decisions that support vitality and longevity. Aging can be a time of renewal, not decline. It is an opportunity to invest in our health and enjoy the richness of life in every stage.

You're Not Too Old, and It's Not Too Late

You may wonder if adopting a healthy diet at this stage of life is worth it. You may think it's too late to make a difference or that changing the way you eat will be too difficult. The truth is, it's never too late, and even small steps can make a big difference.

It may ease your mind to know that this doesn't have to be an overnight transformation. In fact, a gradual transition is often the most comfortable and sustainable approach. Moving step-by-step allows your taste preferences, daily routines, and even your digestive system time to adjust to a more plant-forward way of eating. And even if you only add more healthy plant foods to your diet, you will begin to notice a difference in how you feel. If you're wondering how to begin, we'll give you tips and walk you through it in Chapter 3, "Designing a Plant-Powered Diet That Work for You."

Plant-Based Diets Are Protective

Studies have shown that individuals who eat plant-based diets have a lower risk of chronic diseases such as heart disease, type 2 diabetes, hypertension, and cancer. High-quality plant-based diets can provide effective management and, in some cases, even drive these conditions into remission.

That's because whole plant foods are key sources of dietary components that afford protection. Plant foods have the highest nutrient density (the most nutrients per calorie) and the lowest calorie density (the fewest calories per gram).

You may think that you need animal protein, but you actually don't. In fact, when you replace animal protein with plant protein, your risk of disease and death is typically reduced. In addition, protein-rich plant foods are low in dietary components linked with increased health risks, such as saturated fat, trans-fatty acids, refined carbohydrates, pro-oxidants, and pro-inflammatory compounds.

There is broad agreement within the scientific community that people who center their diets on plant-based foods are at a health advantage. This was perhaps most eloquently stated by Dr. David Katz, one of the world's most respected leaders in health and nutrition. In a peer-reviewed article titled "Can We Say What Diet Is Best for

Health?" he sums up by writing: *"A diet of minimally processed foods close to nature, predominantly plants, is decisively associated with health promotion and disease prevention."*

Plant-Based Diets and the Planet

While the health advantages of plant-based eating patterns are undeniable, the advantages beyond human health may be even more compelling. Plant-based diets offer advantages for the planet and the animals with whom we share it. Dietary changes that favorably impact climate and planetary health help us as we strive to leave a viable planet for our children, grandchildren, and future generations. A landmark study in the *Proceedings of the National Academy of Sciences* (PNAS) modeled the health and climate impacts of different global diet scenarios by 2050. It found that shifting toward more plant-based diets could reduce food-related greenhouse gas (GHG) emissions by about 29 percent and lower the total number of deaths globally (in that year) by 6 to 10 percent. In even more transformative scenarios, such as universal adoption of a vegan diet, the researchers projected up to 8.1 million fewer deaths per year by 2050, alongside a reduction of up to 70 percent in food-related GHG emissions compared with a "business-as-usual" dietary trajectory. In other words, dietary changes can not only reduce food-related GHG emissions globally, but also significantly reduce the number of premature deaths from chronic conditions such as heart disease, stroke, and certain cancers worldwide.

Another recent U.S.-based study compared popular diet types in terms of kilograms of CO_2 equivalents per 1,000 kcal of food. The results are shown in Figure 1.1.

Figure 1.1: Carbon Footprints of Popular Diets

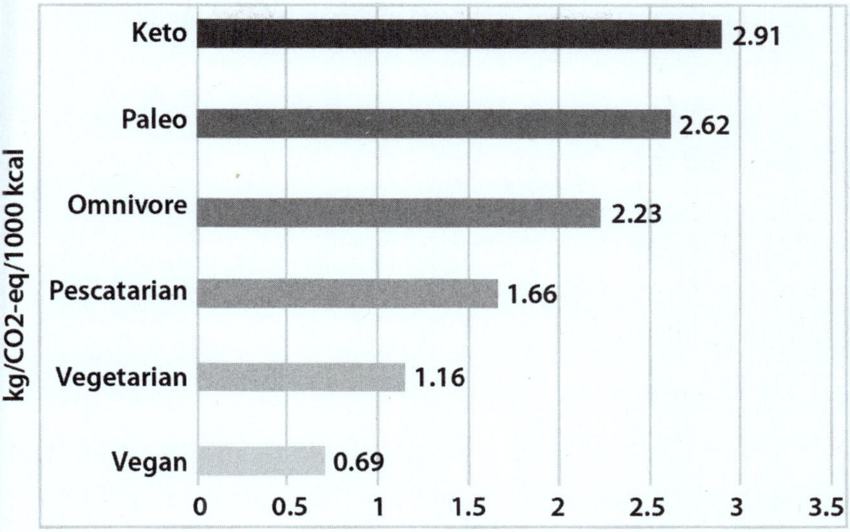

As you can see, the carbon footprint of a keto diet was about 4.2 times higher than a vegan diet, and an omnivorous (nonvegetarian) diet was about 3.2 times higher. By shifting what we eat today, we help ensure a healthier, more livable world for many generations to come.

Eating more plant-based foods and reducing animal-product consumption is one of the most effective levers available for cutting our food system carbon footprint. As the landmark 2019 EAT-Lancet Commission Report succinctly stated: *"Food is the single strongest lever to optimize human health and environmental sustainability on Earth."*

Vote with Your Fork for a Kinder World

By adopting a plant-based diet, individuals can align their values of compassion with their everyday actions, transforming the simple act of eating into a meaningful expression of empathy for animals, people, and the planet.

Today's reality for food animals is starkly different from the idyllic, storybook scenes of cows grazing in open fields, chickens roaming freely, and pigs lounging in the sun. Much of modern animal agriculture is dominated by factory farming, a system designed for maximum efficiency and profit, at the expense of animal welfare, environmental sustainability, and public health.

Plant-based diets eliminate or reduce reliance on animal products, sparing animals from factory farming practices associated with confinement, stress, and inhumane treatment. It's a simple way to vote with our fork for a kinder world.

Whether you are enjoying a colorful veggie stir-fry, trying a new lentil recipe, or simply incorporating more plant-based foods and fewer animal products, these choices can create a positive change. Many people find that eating more plant-based meals not only benefits their health but also brings a sense of peace, knowing their food choices reflect their values of kindness and compassion.

Perhaps the most extraordinary aspect of plant-based eating is that it recognizes the deep connections among our health, the environment, and the well-being of animals. As we grow older and wiser, we can see the world through this wider lens, and our choices gain even greater meaning.

Imagine Your Next Decade

Whether you are just beginning your plant-based journey or have been thriving on this path and are keeping up with the latest research, there is always a next step. This book will provide the guidance, evidence, and encouragement you need to move forward with confidence.

Sometimes people say, "*You can't teach an old dog new tricks.*" However, the lived experiences of countless older adults tell a very different story. Change is absolutely possible at any age, especially when you see the potential for more energy, fewer medications, greater independence, and a life filled with purpose.

Take a moment to reflect on what the years ahead may hold. Which of these futures would you choose? In your later years:

- Would you prefer to
  a) be healthy and vigorous, walking in the forest, playing with grandchildren, exploring new places, or
  b) face years dependent on caregivers, medications, and medical interventions?
- Would you like your final decades to be
  a) a time of sharing wisdom, enjoying books and films, and connecting with friends and family, or
  b) years marked by memory loss, declining function, and frequent doctor's visits?
- For your children and grandchildren, would you rather
  a) be part of the solution to climate change, or
  b) contribute to environmental challenges such as wildfires, floods, and rising temperatures?

If you chose the first option in each scenario, this book will give you tremendous support in achieving your goals!

What Exactly Is a Plant-Based Diet?

Now that you see and understand the big picture of plant-based and plant-powered eating, let us clarify what we mean by the word *diet*. While many people associate this word with a time-limited period of food deprivation, chronic hunger, and intense cravings for the foods we love, weight loss diets are just one diet category.

Actually, the word *diet* has a much broader definition, encompassing all aspects of what and how we eat on a regular basis. It originates from the Greek word *diata,* meaning "way of life."

Sometimes, we use *diet* to refer to our general eating habits, such as plant-based, paleo, or Western-style diets. We also use the word to refer to cultural, religious, or ethical eating patterns such as vegetarian, kosher, or halal diets. Also included are special diets, such as low-sodium or gluten-free diets, which are used to treat specific medical conditions.

It's important to keep in mind that when we use the term *plant-based diet,* we are not referring to a restrictive weight loss diet but rather a pattern or way of eating. Simply stated, a plant-based diet is one in which plant foods predominate. There is a broad *spectrum* of dietary patterns that meet the plant-based definition (see Figure 1.2).

Figure 1.2 Plant-Based Dietary Spectrum

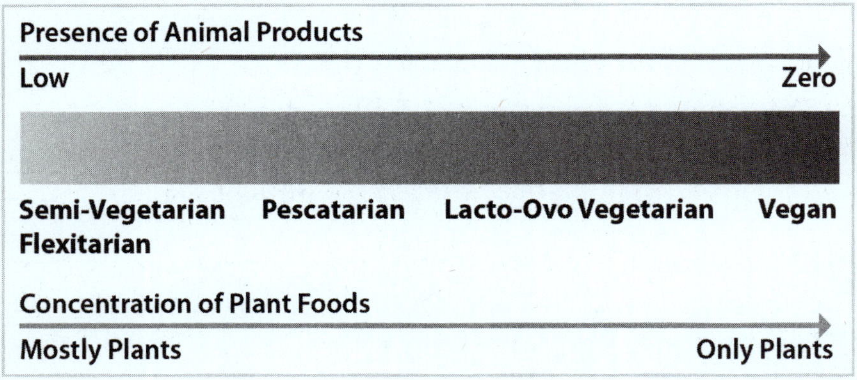

At the left end of the spectrum are semi-vegetarian or flexitarian diets (these include small amounts of animal products such as meat, poultry, fish, dairy, and eggs). At the right end are plant-exclusive or vegan diets (these include plant foods and exclude all animal products).

Between these are pescatarian diets (vegetarian or vegan diets plus fish; no meat or poultry) and lacto-ovo-vegetarian diets (plant foods plus dairy and eggs; no meat, poultry, or fish).

There are many variations within these realms, such as raw vegan diets (which consist of at least 75 percent uncooked food by weight) and very low-fat vegan diets (which contain no more than 10 to 15 percent of calories from fat and no added oils).

While there is no precise definition of a plant-based diet, the term is generally used to describe a dietary pattern in which plant foods form the foundation of the diet and provide the majority of calories and nutrients. Table 1.1 provides a summary of plant-based diet definitions, as well as definitions for related diets.

Table 1.1 Plant-Based and Related Diet Definitions

Diet Type	Definition
Plant-based	Plant foods form the foundation of the diet May be vegan, vegetarian, pescatarian, or semi-vegetarian
Whole-food, plant-based (WFPB)	Plant-based with predominantly whole or minimally processed plant foods May be SOS-free (free of added salt, oil, and sugar)
Vegan	Plant-exclusive or 100% plant-based Zero animal products
Raw vegan	Vegan with at least 75% uncooked foods
Lacto-ovo vegetarian	Free of meat, poultry, and fish; includes eggs and dairy
Lacto-vegetarian	Free of meat, poultry, fish, and eggs; includes dairy
Ovo-vegetarian	Free of meat, poultry, fish, and dairy; includes eggs
Pescatarian	Vegetarian or vegan plus fish
Semi-vegetarian or Flexitarian	Plant-predominant diets that include small amounts of animal products

Another important consideration when comparing various types of plant-based diets is diet quality. Diet quality is a function of many factors, including diversity, nutritional adequacy, and the degree of food processing. High-quality diets include a wide variety of nutritious, unprocessed or minimally processed foods such as vegetables, fruits, legumes, whole grains, nuts, and seeds.

Such diets are associated with a low risk of chronic diseases such as heart disease, hypertension, type 2 diabetes, and several cancers. In Chapter 3, we delve into the details of diet quality, and in Chapter 5, we examine the finer points of nutritional adequacy.

How This Book Will Help You

Plant-Powered Seniors is a comprehensive guide designed specifically for older adults who are transitioning to or fine-tuning a plant-based lifestyle. What sets this book apart is its accessibility and practicality as we navigate our later years, when many of our nutritional needs change. Written by experts with a deep understanding of the health needs and challenges associated with aging, we provide research-backed insights into how a plant-based diet can enhance vitality, support the management of chronic diseases, and promote overall well-being.

In this opening chapter, we've explored the basics of plant-based eating—what it is and why it matters. In the chapters that follow, we go deeper into how to adopt this new way of eating. You'll learn how food choices support healthy aging, and how diet quality makes a difference. We will explore the unique nutritional needs of older adults and offer practical strategies to ensure that you get all the nutrients your body needs.

You'll also find tools to navigate the food system with confidence: how to shop, interpret food labels, and identify healthy, affordable options. We'll provide guidance on creating personalized, culturally relevant, and budget-friendly plant-based meal plans, along with a guide to supplements. For those managing specific health challenges, you'll learn how to adjust menus to optimize outcomes.

Because food is never just about nutrients, we also address the emotional and social aspects of switching to a new diet. You'll learn strategies to help you embrace new habits, stay connected with friends and family, and enjoy social events, dining out, and travel, all while honoring your new plant-powered lifestyle. For those living in shared environments, we offer practical tips to make plant-forward eating realistic and enjoyable.

Ultimately, we link the benefits of plant-based eating with other pillars of a longevity-promoting lifestyle, including staying physically active, managing stress, fostering strong social connections, and a sense of higher purpose or meaning.

To help you succeed, we'll encourage you to take small, manageable steps toward mastering the art of plant-based cooking. To make this easier, we've included simple, affordable, nutritious, and tasty recipes designed to inspire and support your thriving lifestyle.

We are delighted that you are joining us on this journey. Together, we will explore how food can be a powerful ally in aging, improving longevity and the quality of your life!

KEY TAKEAWAYS:

Well-designed plant-based diets can improve longevity and health, and reduce the risk of chronic diseases.

High-quality plant-based patterns include a variety of whole plant foods such as vegetables, fruits, legumes, whole grains, nuts, and seeds, and minimize the intake of low-nutrient, heavily processed foods and animal products.

Adding more healthy plant foods to your diet or transitioning to a plant-based pattern can be done at your own pace, either gradually over many months or rapidly over a few days or weeks.

Plant-based diets bring benefits that make it easier to adopt other lifestyle changes, such as being physically active, getting a good night's sleep, and avoiding risky substances, all of which help to support healthy aging.

Plant-based lifestyles also are more ecologically sustainable and kind to animals.

Next Stop: The Big Picture

Embracing a plant-powered lifestyle protects your brain, heart, metabolism, and more. But how exactly do our everyday food choices shape our long-term health?

In the next chapter, we'll take a closer look at dietary patterns and the science behind what makes some eating styles more beneficial than others. You'll discover how plant-powered diets compare to other common approaches, and how the quality of your food choices can make all the difference as you age.

CHAPTER 2

DIETARY PATTERNS, DIET QUALITY, AND HEALTH

This Chapter at a Glance

In this chapter, we explore how eating habits—including dietary patterns and food quality—affect health, energy, and disease risk as we age. We address key questions such as:

- What are dietary patterns, and why do they matter?
- Which dietary patterns are most healthful—or harmful?
- How do plant-based diets compare with other patterns?
- What defines a high- or low-quality diet?
- What is food processing, and how does it affect health?
- How can we ensure our diets support healthy aging?

Maria's Story: Coming Home to Health

Growing up in an Italian family, Maria's diet was rooted in the Mediterranean tradition, rich in fresh vegetables and fruits, beans, whole grains, nuts, and olive oil. But during college, the lure of convenience foods and the pull of social eating gradually shifted her toward a more typical Western diet, high in processed foods, added sugars, and unhealthy fats.

Decades later, facing hypertension and prediabetes, Maria's healthcare provider suggested she consider adopting a plant-based approach. Initially, she was intimidated by the idea of making such a drastic change. But with the help of a plant-based diet support group, Maria began to reconnect with the flavors of her roots, swapping processed fare for vibrant salads, hearty soups, legume-based dishes, and vegetable-rich tomato sauces reminiscent of her family's table.

The cooking skills she'd learned as a child, like preparing lentil stews or tasty wraps, became her greatest allies. This shift not only improved her diet quality but also transformed her relationship with food, paving the way to better health and a renewed sense of well-being.

Dietary Patterns for Health and Longevity

People everywhere are living longer than ever before. Life expectancy in the United States now exceeds eighty years for women and seventy-five years for men—a remarkable achievement! But as our lifespans grow, it's worth asking ourselves an important question: What do we want those extra years to look like?

Do we want to spend them feeling strong, mobile, and connected or tied to medications, medical devices, and doctor's appointments? While living longer is a common goal, living well is what makes those years fulfilling and joyful.

That's where the concept of health span comes in: the years of life spent in good health, with the energy, freedom, and independence to do the things we love, whether that's gardening, dancing, traveling, caring for others, or simply enjoying a good meal with friends. Supporting a longer health span means investing in quality of life, not just quantity of years.

A Life Reclaimed: The Ikaria Story of Stamatis Moraitis

Consider the story of Stamatis Moraitis, a Greek war veteran who returned to his homeland of Ikaria, Greece, after being diagnosed with terminal lung cancer in his mid-sixties. Having lived in the United States for more than thirty years, he had built a good life, raising three children who were now grown and independent.

When his doctors told him he had only six to nine months to live, he chose to go home to Ikaria, a small island in the Aegean Sea known as one of the world's five Blue Zones, which include Okinawa in Japan, Sardinia in Italy (the Ogliastra region), the Nicoya Peninsula in Costa Rica, Ikaria in Greece, and Loma Linda in California. These are regions where people have lived longer, healthier lives than almost anywhere else on Earth.

The term *Blue Zones* was coined by Dan Buettner, a National Geographic Fellow who worked with a team of scientists and demographers to identify pockets of exceptional longevity around the world. Early researchers marked these regions with blue circles on a map as they tracked unusually high numbers of people living into their nineties and hundreds—giving rise to the now widely used term. What made these regions so remarkable was a shared pattern of everyday living. Across Okinawa, Sardinia, the Nicoya Peninsula, Ikaria, and Loma Linda, people tended to eat mostly plant-based. Rather than being sedentary, they moved naturally throughout the day; they also maintained strong family and social connections; managed stress through daily rituals; and they had a clear sense of purpose. In other words, longevity in these regions was driven by environments and cultures that made healthy living the default.

Once home, Stamatis slipped naturally back into the traditional Ikarian way of life. He tended a garden, ate the foods he grew, walked the hills each day, and reconnected with lifelong friends. He expected to grow weaker with time, but the opposite happened. His strength returned, his energy improved, and months turned into years. Remarkably, he lived to the age of *ninety-nine,* cancer-free and thriving until the very end.

Of course, no one story proves that diet and lifestyle alone can cure disease, and, of course, medical interventions can be very effective. But Stamatis's experience reminds us that the foundations of health are far more powerful than we may realize.

These foundations, or the six pillars of healthy living, encompass nutrition, regular physical activity, adequate sleep, effective stress management, strong social connections, and freedom from addictive habits. We'll explore each of these in greater depth in Chapter 7.

Aging and Chronic Disease: How Lifestyle Shapes Longevity

Aging is closely linked to our risk of chronic diseases, also known as noncommunicable diseases. These include heart disease, high blood pressure, diabetes, cancer, and conditions such as Alzheimer's disease. Chronic diseases account for about 74 percent of deaths worldwide, and evidence suggests that up to 80 percent of these conditions may be preventable. They not only shorten lifespan but also reduce *health span.*

The story of Stamatis Moraitis highlights a crucial truth: While longevity is influenced by genetics, it's even more profoundly shaped by lifestyle. According to the U.S. Burden of Disease Collaborators (*JAMA* 2018), the leading causes of preventable death and disability in the United States are measurable, modifiable, and often driven by lifestyle.

At the very top of the list is dietary risk. In fact, an unhealthy diet contributes to more deaths than tobacco, inactivity, or alcohol. Poor dietary habits—too many sugary drinks, red and processed meats, highly processed foods, and too few protective fruits, vegetables, legumes, whole grains, and nuts—top the list of health threats in the United States.

Here's How the Top Ten Risk Factors for Premature Death and Disability Stack Up:

1. Dietary risks
2. Tobacco use
3. High blood pressure
4. High body mass index (BMI)
5. High fasting blood sugar
6. High total cholesterol
7. Impaired kidney function
8. Alcohol and drug use
9. Air pollution
10. Low physical activity

This is a powerful call to action. While we often focus on treating disease after it appears, the most impactful strategy is to prevent disease by targeting the root causes, and that starts with the food on our plates.

The Power of the Blue Zones

The good news is that many of the lifestyle factors that support longevity are within our control as demonstrated by populations living in the Blue Zones. Across these regions, daily life is structured in ways that naturally promote health and resilience. Common patterns include:

- Plant-rich dietary patterns
- Daily movement such as walking, gardening, and manual work
- Strong social connections and effective stress management
- A clear sense of purpose—referred to as *ikigai* in Okinawa and *plan de vida* in the Nicoya Peninsula

Researchers studying these populations have further distilled these patterns into nine interconnected lifestyle characteristics—often referred to as the Power 9. In essence, these reflect how environments and cultures shape everyday behaviors that support long-term health.

1. A predominantly whole-food, plant-based way of eating, centered on legumes, whole grains, vegetables, fruits, nuts, and seeds
2. Regular, low-intensity physical activity embedded into daily routines rather than relying on structured exercise alone
3. A strong sense of purpose that provides direction and meaning in daily life
4. Daily practices that help manage stress, such as rest, reflection, prayer, or social connection
5. Eating patterns that emphasize moderation, including stopping before feeling overly full
6. In some regions, modest and social consumption of alcohol, typically with meals and within a cultural context that discourages excess

7. A deep prioritization of family, including care for older adults and intergenerational connection
8. Participation in supportive communities, often faith-based or culturally rooted, that reinforce healthy behaviors
9. Close social networks that encourage and sustain positive lifestyle choices

These factors do not operate in isolation. They are reinforced by environments that favor minimally processed foods, regular movement, social cohesion, and low exposure to harmful habits such as smoking or substance misuse.

Together, these patterns create a powerful foundation for flourishing as we age—one that not only extends lifespan but also preserves independence, vitality, and quality of life. By intentionally shaping our own environments and daily routines, we can begin to create "mini Blue Zones" wherever we live.

Dietary Patterns in Health and Disease and Why They Matter

The foundations of the healthy lifestyles in the Blue Zones are dietary patterns. These refer to the ways we eat over time, including the types of foods and drinks we choose, how often we consume them, and how these foods interact and complement one another. You might think of your dietary pattern as your *"food personality."*

Many factors shape our eating patterns, including culture and family traditions, peer groups, access to food, financial security, time pressures, education and nutrition knowledge, personal preferences, allergies or intolerances, health conditions, schedules, ethical beliefs, how we spend time with others, and even our emotional state.

Nutrient Dense Versus Empty Calorie Dietary Patterns

Dietary patterns play a critical role in determining our overall health and risk of chronic disease. Diverse, nutrient-dense dietary patterns, based primarily on whole or minimally processed plant foods, help regulate body weight, strengthen immunity, and reduce inflammation, oxidative stress, and metabolic dysfunction. This, in turn, lowers our risk of lifestyle-related diseases.

Conversely, poor dietary patterns, characterized by high consumption of heavily processed foods, red meat, added sugars, unhealthy fats, and refined grains, are associated with obesity, chronic inflammation, oxidative stress, insulin resistance, and unhealthy gut microbiome. These raise the risk of chronic diseases such as cardiovascular disease, hypertension, type 2 diabetes, and cancer.

Which Dietary Patterns Are the Most Healthful?

Healthy eating isn't about strict rules or one "perfect" way to eat. It's about creating a pattern that nourishes your body, suits your lifestyle, and supports your long-term health.

A healthy dietary pattern includes a variety of nutrient-rich foods in the right amounts to meet your body's needs without exceeding your energy (calorie) requirements. It provides a good balance of macronutrients (protein, carbohydrates, and fat), micronutrients (vitamins and minerals), and phytochemicals (protective plant compounds). Plant foods form the foundation of the diet, along with generous amounts of fiber. May be vegan, vegetarian, pescatarian, or semi-vegetarian.

As we age, our calorie needs often decrease, but our need for specific nutrients, especially protein, calcium, vitamin B_{12}, and vitamin D, may actually increase. This means that eating a nutrient-dense diet—one that delivers more nutrition for every calorie—becomes even more critical.

Plant-Based Dietary Patterns

Decades of research have highlighted several dietary patterns that are associated with better health, longer life, and lower rates of chronic disease. Although they may differ in the finer points, they are all predominantly plant-based, emphasizing whole foods and minimizing highly processed options.

1. DASH (Dietary Approaches to Stop Hypertension) Diet

Originally designed to help lower blood pressure, the DASH diet focuses on whole plant foods, such as vegetables, fruits, legumes, whole grains, nuts, and seeds. It optionally includes moderate amounts of dairy and small portions of lean fish or skinless poultry. It minimizes red and processed meats and limits foods high in added salt, sugar, and saturated fat.

Key benefits: DASH diets are proven to reduce blood pressure and improve heart health.

2. Mediterranean Diet

This diet draws inspiration from the traditional eating patterns of countries bordering the Mediterranean Sea. It emphasizes vegetables, fruits, legumes, whole grains, nuts, seeds, and olive oil, includes moderate amounts of fish, poultry, dairy products, and wine, and limits red meat and highly processed foods. This way of eating has been associated with lower risks of heart disease, stroke, type 2 diabetes, and cognitive decline.

Key benefits: Mediterranean diets enhance longevity and provide cardiovascular protection.

3. Plant-Based, Vegetarian, and Vegan Diets

These dietary patterns are either plant-predominant or plant-exclusive. When well-planned, with an emphasis on whole plant foods, including vegetables, fruits, legumes, whole grains, nuts, and seeds, these diets support a healthy body weight, lower cholesterol and blood pressure, and reduce the risk of chronic diseases, such as heart disease and type 2 diabetes.

When plant-based diets are not well planned and include ultra-processed foods (such as refined grains, fried snacks, or sugary beverages) as a significant portion of the diet, this type of eating can increase the risk of disease although it does reduce animal suffering and our carbon footprint.

Key benefits: Well-planned plant-based diets support disease prevention, environmental sustainability, and animal welfare.

Which Dietary Patterns Are the Most Harmful?

Dietary patterns that are low in fiber and whole plant foods and high in nutritionally depleted, ultra-processed foods are consistently linked to poorer health outcomes. These diets tend to promote chronic inflammation, metabolic dysfunction, and nutrient deficiencies. The most common harmful dietary patterns include:

1. The Standard American Diet and Other "Western Diets"

The Standard American Diet (SAD) is one example of a broader Western dietary pattern—a style of eating common in industrialized nations but rapidly spreading globally. Characterized by a heavy reliance on processed and ultra-processed foods, red and processed meats, refined grains, added sugars, fried foods, and fast food, this dietary pattern is short on fiber-rich plant foods such as vegetables, fruits, legumes, whole grains, nuts, and seeds.

Western dietary patterns, including SAD diets, are strongly linked to obesity, type 2 diabetes, cardiovascular disease, certain cancers, dementia, and other chronic conditions. As these eating habits continue to displace traditional diets, they contribute to rising rates of preventable disease worldwide. (Note: In our discussions throughout this book, we generally refer to Western dietary patterns as SAD).

Key drawbacks: The hallmark of Western-style diets, including SAD, is excess—too much sugar, saturated fat, salt, refined carbohydrates, and calories, and too little of the whole plant foods that protect health. This imbalance promotes chronic inflammation, metabolic dysfunction, nutrient deficiencies, and accelerated aging.

2. Very Low-Carbohydrate and Ketogenic Diets

Very low-carbohydrate diets typically restrict carbohydrate intake to 10 to 20 percent of total daily calories. These include ketogenic diets (high in fat and moderate in protein) and carnivore diets, which are almost entirely animal based and extremely high in protein.

While these approaches can lead to short-term weight loss and temporary improvements in blood sugar control, they often fall short in important dietary components, particularly fiber, antioxidants, phytochemicals, and several vitamins and minerals. Because carbohydrate-rich whole plant foods, such as fruits, vegetables, legumes, and whole grains, are primary sources of these protective factors, long-term adherence to such diets may increase the risk of cardiovascular disease, impair gut microbiome diversity, and lead to side effects such as constipation, fatigue, bad breath (due to ketosis), and low mood. In addition, many very low–carbohydrate and ketogenic diets are high in saturated fat, which is associated with increased cardiometabolic risk. Emerging research also raises questions about the sustainability and the safety of very low–carbohydrate diets over the long term, especially in older adults.

Key drawbacks: When carbohydrate restriction crowds out whole plant foods, it sacrifices long-term health for short-term results.

Bringing It All Together

A powerful and well-documented connection exists between certain dietary patterns, chronic disease risk, cognitive function, and overall well-being. For most individuals, a whole-food, plant-predominant or plant-exclusive diet offers the strongest protection. The fiber, phytochemicals, and complex carbohydrates in plant foods provide sustained energy, support brain function, and protect against chronic disease.

However, it's important to remember that not all plant-based diets are automatically healthy. Diets centered on nutritionally depleted, ultra-processed foods, even if they are entirely plant-based, can harm health just as much as Western-style eating patterns.

FOOD FOR THOUGHT

Regardless of whether you eat mostly plants or exclusively plants, it's the quality of the foods you choose that determines their impact on your health. Whole, minimally processed plant foods remain the foundation of every health-promoting dietary pattern.

Quality Matters in Plant-Based Diets!

George thought that vegan diets were practically foolproof. For nearly a decade, he proudly identified as a vegan. He avoided all animal products, participated in discussions about ethical eating, and advocated for sustainability. But there was one problem: He rarely cooked.

Most of his meals came from boxes and bags, such as frozen plant-based nuggets and burgers, dairy-free mac and cheese, granola bars, and sweet soy lattes. If it was vegan, it was fair game. He never gave much thought to fiber, variety, or nutrient density. After all, he was eating plant-based, which meant he was healthy, right?

That illusion was shattered during a routine medical checkup. His doctor studied the lab results with a concerned look. "George, your blood pressure is elevated, and so are your cholesterol and triglycerides." George's heart sank. "That can't be right," he protested. "I'm vegan. I don't even eat cholesterol."

His doctor, who practiced lifestyle medicine, smiled gently. "Plant-based doesn't automatically mean healthy. Diet quality matters. If most of your foods are refined, deep fried, sugary, or highly processed, they can cause the same health problems as a Western diet."

The message landed. George looked online for ideas about healthy and easy vegan meals and decided to make a simple plant-based bowl for dinner (an example of this dish can be found in the recipe on page 304, the Multicolored Bowl). That afternoon, he shopped for some precut vegetables, a few cans of beans, a can of corn, and some salsa, and when he came home, he cooked up some quinoa. That evening, instead of microwaving another processed meal, he was able to easily put together a healthy dish that tasted great and was very satisfying. He was surprised and pleased about how easy it could be, and it was the beginning of a healthier chapter.

What Does Diet Quality Mean?

Diet quality refers to the extent to which an overall eating pattern supports health, prevents chronic disease, and provides the body with all the essential nutrients it needs. It's shaped by several factors, including the diversity of foods we eat, their sources, and the degree of processing they undergo.

High-Quality Diets Share Several Key Features:

- **Predominantly plant-based:** High-quality diets are centered around a wide variety of plant foods. If animal products are included, they play a small, complementary role. This approach aligns with global patterns of longevity, such as those observed in *Blue Zones*, and is reinforced by the EAT-Lancet 2.0 report (2025), which outlines a framework for healthy, sustainable, and equitable diets. It reaffirms that predominantly plant-based eating remains a key lever for both human and planetary health.

- **Unprocessed or minimally processed:** These diets prioritize foods in their most natural or least altered forms, such as fresh, frozen, and lightly cooked vegetables, intact whole grains, legumes, fruits, plain tofu, and raw or dry-roasted nuts. These foods retain their nutritional integrity and are rich in fiber, micronutrients, and phytochemicals.
- **Low in nutritionally poor, ultra-processed foods:** High-quality diets limit foods that are heavily processed; high in added sugars, sodium, refined oils, and artificial additives; and low in nutritional value. Frequent consumption of these products is strongly linked to chronic disease risk and displacement of more healthful options.
- **Nutritionally adequate and balanced:** A high-quality diet meets energy and nutrient needs without consistent excess or deficiency. It incorporates a wide range of nutrient-dense, mostly plant-based foods and, when needed, uses fortified foods or supplements to fill potential gaps.
- **Include a diversity of plant foods:** Several studies have shown that people who eat thirty or more different plants per week (including vegetables, fruits, nuts, seeds, herbs, spices, whole grains, and fermented foods such as sauerkraut and miso) have been shown to maximize gut microbiome diversity, which improves immunity, reduces inflammation, and lowers chronic disease risk.
- **Culturally relevant and enjoyable:** These diets are not only health-promoting but also practical, enjoyable, and adaptable.

When eating patterns align with cultural traditions, values, and individual preferences, they are far more likely to be maintained over time, making them both effective and sustainable.

Healthy eating patterns that reflect these principles are consistently associated with reduced risk of premature death, better immune and cognitive function, improved metabolic health, and lower incidence of chronic diseases such as heart disease, type 2 diabetes, cancer, and dementia.

How Researchers Measure Diet Quality

How do scientists determine whether a person's eating habits support long-term health? One common approach is to use standardized scoring systems that assess overall diet quality based on what people regularly eat. Here are four of the most widely used diet quality indices:

Healthy Eating Index (HEI): This score looks at how closely someone's diet follows the U.S. Dietary Guidelines. Higher scores reflect more vegetables, fruits, whole grains, and plant proteins, and less salt, sugar, and saturated fat. People with higher HEI scores tend to live longer and have lower risk of chronic diseases.

Mediterranean Diet Score (MDS): This reflects how well someone follows a Mediterranean eating pattern, rich in vegetables, fruits, whole grains, legumes, nuts, seeds, and olive oil, with limited red meat. Higher scores are linked to lower risks of heart disease, diabetes, cancer, and cognitive decline.

Plant-Based Diet Index (PDI): This measure helps distinguish between wholesome plant foods (such as whole grains, beans, vegetables, fruits, nuts, and seeds) and less healthful ones (such as sugary cereals, white bread, and ultra-processed snacks). Higher scores for whole-food plant eating predict better heart and metabolic health.

Planetary Health Diet Index (PHDI): This score considers both human health and environmental sustainability. Diets high in whole plant foods and low in red or processed meat receive higher scores and are linked to longer life and a smaller environmental footprint.

Across all of these measures, the conclusion is consistent: Eating more vegetables, fruits, legumes (beans, peas, lentils), whole grains, nuts, and seeds, and fewer highly processed foods, sugary drinks, red and processed meat, supports better health at every age.

How Food Processing Can Impact Diet Quality

When it comes to adopting a high-quality diet and making smart, healthy choices, it's important to understand that not all processed foods are created equal. Researchers often use a system called NOVA to group foods by how much they've been processed, from unprocessed (e.g., fresh fruits and vegetables) and minimally processed (e.g., frozen fruits and vegetables) to moderately processed (e.g., canned fruits and vegetables with added salt, sugar, or fat) and ultra-processed (like packaged snacks, sodas, and many frozen meals).

Why does this matter?

Large studies show that eating too many ultra-processed foods is linked to a higher risk of heart disease, diabetes, obesity, cancer, poor sleep, depression, and even early death. But here's where it gets tricky. The NOVA system doesn't reflect a food's nutritional value. For example:

- Fortified plant-based milks or plant-based meat alternatives may be labeled ultra-processed, but they help to fill nutrition gaps for many people.
- Meanwhile, red meat may be considered "unprocessed" even if it comes from animals raised on highly processed feed, with antibiotics and additives.

That's why it's important to look at both how processed a food is and the food's nutritional value. Does it nourish your body or just fill your stomach?

Some processing can improve nutrition and safety, like freezing vegetables at their peak or enriching foods with key nutrients. Other foods, especially ultra-processed snacks high in sugar, salt, or unhealthy fats, can harm your health if eaten regularly.

- Focus on whole or minimally processed foods most of the time: vegetables, fruits, beans, whole grains, nuts, and seeds.
- When choosing more processed items, look for nutrient-dense options with ingredients that you recognize. You don't need to avoid all processed foods, just choose wisely.

A Closer Look at Food Processing

Understanding food quality is one thing; putting it into practice is another. It is reassuring to know that you don't have to overhaul everything overnight. Small, steady improvements can make a big difference, especially in maintaining energy, strength, and independence as we age.

Table 2.1 offers everyday examples to help you visualize how the same food can range from unprocessed to ultra-processed, depending on how it's prepared and packaged. This table is not about perfection; it's a guide to help you move toward a diet where unprocessed and minimally processed foods make up the foundation. Think of it as a tool for making more informed choices in the grocery store, in the kitchen, and on your plate.

Table 2.1 Food Processing: Everyday Examples

Food	**Unprocessed** *(Foods in their natural state or with basic preparation needed to make them edible)*	**Minimally Processed** *(Slightly altered for safety or convenience but nutritionally intact)*	**Moderately Processed** *(Includes added salt, sugar, or oils but retains some whole-food qualities)*	**Ultra-Processed** *(Industrially processed, heavily refined foods that contain artificial additives)*
Apples	Fresh whole apple	Sliced apples Unsweetened applesauce	Sweetened applesauce	Apple fritter Apple turnover Apple pie
Peanuts	Raw peanuts in the shell	Dry roasted peanuts Natural peanut butter	Peanut butter with added oils/sugar Salted, roasted peanuts	Peanut butter candy bars Peanut butter ice cream
Corn	Fresh corn on the cob, cooked	Frozen corn Canned corn (no added salt)	Canned creamed corn Corn tortillas with preservatives	Corn chips Corn syrup Corn puffs
Oats	Whole oat groats, cooked	Steel-cut oats Rolled oats	Instant flavored oatmeal with added sugar	Oat-based sugary granola bars Oat cereals with added sugars and artificial flavors

Food	Unprocessed	Minimally Processed	Moderately Processed	Ultra-Processed
Chickpeas	Boiled chick-peas	Canned chickpeas (no added salt)	Hummus with added oil and salt	Chickpea chips Fried chick-peas with flavorings
Potatoes	Fresh, steamed potatoes	Frozen plain potato chunks Prewashed chopped potatoes	Hash brown potatoes	Potato chips
Brown Rice	Brown rice, cooked	Quick cooking or parboiled, plain brown rice	Brown rice cakes Plain puffed brown rice	Brown rice cakes with flavoring Puffed brown rice with sugar coating

Here Are Five Simple, Practical Ways to Use the Food Processing Framework in Everyday Life:

1. **Make small upgrades when you shop.** Compare labels and choose items with more fiber and less added fat, sugar, or salt. For example, choose an unsweetened, calcium-fortified soy milk instead of a sweetened version, canned beans with no added salt instead of regular canned beans, or fresh whole grain bread with simple ingredients over white bread.
2. **Use lightly processed foods to make life easier.** You don't have to cook from scratch every day. Convenient, healthy options include frozen vegetables, canned beans, lentils, or chickpeas, low-sodium soups, seasoned tofu, and veggie burgers made from whole-plant foods.

3. **Check the ingredient list.** Look for familiar items on ingredient lists. Ingredients like oats, chickpeas, or almonds are great, but skip products with long lists lists of unfamiliar stabilizers, additives, and artificial colors or flavors.
4. **Let helpful processing work in your favor.** Some processing can help to make food safer, more digestible, or even more nutritious. For example, fermented foods like tempeh support gut health, pasteurized fortified nondairy milks provide extra calcium and vitamins B_{12} and D, and nutritious smoothies can serve as a highly digestible protein source and a way to incorporate more fruits and nutritious greens into your diet.
5. **Zoom out and see the big picture.** Enjoying an occasional treat won't derail your progress. It's your overall pattern that counts. If most of your meals come from whole or minimally processed foods, there's plenty of room for flexibility and joy in your diet.

FOOD FOR THOUGHT

A healthy diet is only effective if it works for you, not just nutritionally, but also in daily life. Choosing mostly unprocessed or minimally processed foods and making thoughtful choices within each category allows you to nourish your body, support healthy aging, and enjoy your meals in a way that's both sustainable and satisfying.

KEY TAKEAWAYS

Diet quality matters more than any single food or nutrient. The most health-supportive eating patterns prioritize whole or minimally processed plant foods, reduce reliance on ultra-processed products, and are sustainable over time.

The degree of food processing influences health, but it's not the only factor. Nutritional quality, ingredient composition, and how a food supports or undermines dietary patterns also matter. Some processed and even ultra-processed foods can contribute positively when chosen thoughtfully.

Not all plant-based diets are created equal. A diet based on whole grains, legumes, vegetables, fruits, nuts, and seeds is protective while a plant-based diet high in refined and ultra-processed foods may still increase disease risk.

Healthy eating is about patterns, not perfection. A high-quality diet is one you can enjoy and maintain. Small, steady shifts in food choices can make a meaningful difference in health and longevity.

The Power on Your Plate

As we've seen, the quality of our eating pattern has a profound impact on how we age—from reducing disease risk to preserving energy and vitality. But how do we turn that knowledge into everyday meals?

What does a high-quality, plant-based diet actually look like in practice? In the next chapter, we'll break it down with simple tools, practical examples, and visual guidance to help you confidently build a balanced, nourishing plate, every single day.

CHAPTER 3

DESIGNING A PLANT-POWERED DIET THAT WORKS FOR YOU

This Chapter at a Glance

In this chapter, you'll gain the tools and guidance to build balanced, plant-based meals that support strength, energy, and long-term health. Whether you prefer simple meals or enjoy cooking from scratch, you'll learn how to nourish yourself with confidence and ease.

You will:

- Get to know Your Plant-Powered Day, a visual guide to the five core food groups and essential add-ons for healthy aging.
- Learn how much to eat from each group, and which foods offer key nutrients like calcium, protein, and omega-3s.
- See how it all comes together through sample menus tailored to a variety of needs and preferences.

Maria's Story: Nourishing with Intention

Now in her early seventies, Maria had settled comfortably into her plant-based lifestyle. Her blood pressure was stable, her energy had returned, and she felt lighter on her feet. But not everything was easy. Since her husband passed away three years ago, cooking for one wasn't the same.

She found herself nibbling on toast and tea, especially on days when her arthritis flared or her energy dipped. Some evenings, the thought of chopping vegetables and cleaning dishes felt overwhelming. "I know what I *should* be eating, but sometimes it just feels like too much."

One chilly Sunday, her daughter dropped by with a warm lentil, tomato, and kale soup. It was fragrant with herbs and bubbling with flavor. "I made a double batch," she said, smiling. "I thought you might like a few freezer portions."

As Maria savored her first bite, she felt more than just full; she felt cared for. That simple gesture reminded her that nourishing herself didn't need to be elaborate. It just needed a little planning, some familiar flavors, and a few go-to recipes that made her feel good.

In the weeks that followed, Maria began setting aside time each Sunday to prepare a couple of simple meals, such as hearty soups, dinner bowls, and one-pot stews she could portion and freeze. She discovered that eating well in her seventies wasn't about perfection; it was about small acts of self-care. A stocked pantry, a bit of prep, and the comforting smell of something wholesome cooking made all the difference.

As Maria quickly learned, good nutrition in later life doesn't have to be complicated, it just needs to be intentional. A few simple strategies, supportive habits, and a handful of nourishing recipes can make healthy eating both doable and deeply satisfying.

Laying the Foundation for Healthy Eating

Eating well is one of the most powerful ways to support healthy aging. Yet many older adults face unique challenges that can make it harder to prepare and enjoy balanced meals. Changes in appetite, low energy, reduced social connection, limited mobility, unfamiliarity with plant-based cooking, or a tight budget can all play a role.

The good news? Eating well doesn't have to be complicated or costly. With a few simple tools and a bit of planning, a plant-based diet can be deeply nourishing, practical, and enjoyable—fueling your energy, resilience, and well-being at every stage of life.

In this chapter, we introduce a visual guide to building balanced meals, enhancing our daily food intake, and making meal planning intuitive and flexible.

Figure 3.1 Your Plant-Powered Day (page 42) depicts five core food groups: vegetables, fruits, grains, legumes, and nuts and seeds, together with the recommended number of servings that a healthy plant-powered senior should strive to eat in a day. (For weight loss, you can reduce amounts from the Grains group.) It also highlights especially nutrient-dense choices, such as foods rich in calcium and protein, that are important for maintaining strength, bone health, and vitality as we age.

In addition to the core food groups, Your Plant-Powered Day includes a category of essential Add-ons, which are nutrients that require special attention, even in a varied, well-planned plant-based diet. These include vitamin B_{12}, vitamin D, iodine, and omega-3 fatty acids. While plant-based diets are naturally rich in many vitamins, minerals, and protective compounds, these specific nutrients can be more difficult to obtain in sufficient amounts without some intentional choices.

Figure 3.1 Your Plant-Powered Day (also shown in color insert)

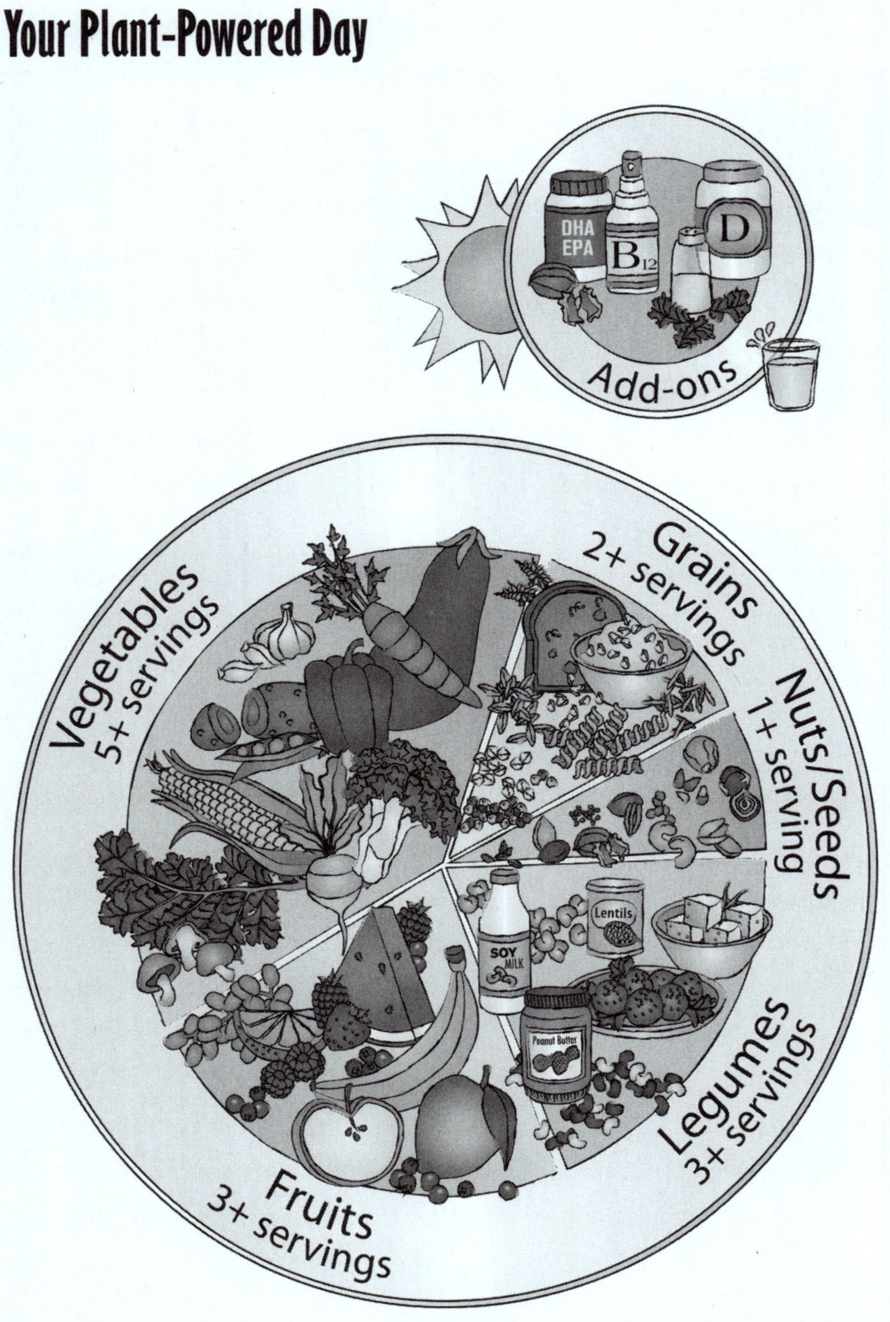

Table 3.1 Your Plant-Based Day: A Daily Guide to Major Food Groups. This table provides this information in a different format. It includes serving sizes and a focus on calcium-rich and protein-rich choices, and how to incorporate them into meals. (Also shown in color insert)

FOOD GROUP *(Suggested Number of Servings *)*	**FOODS INCLUDED** Serving Sizes*	**CALCIUM-RICH CHOICES** Within Each Food Group**	**PROTEIN-RICH CHOICES** (Grams of Protein per Serving)
Vegetables *(5 or more servings)* Choose a rainbow of colors!	½ cup raw or cooked vegetables 1 cup raw leafy vegetables ½ cup pure vegetable juice	Bok choy, broccoli, collard greens, kale, mustard greens, napa cabbage, or okra** Calcium-fortified tomato or vegetable juice	Fresh peas (4 g) Hubbard squash (3 g) Spinach, cooked (2.7 g) Corn (2.4 g)
Fruits *(3 or more servings)* Go for variety!	1 medium fruit ½ cup fruit or pure fruit juice ¼ cup dried fruit	Dried figs Oranges Calcium-fortified 100% fruit juice	Guava, durian, mango (2 g) Avocado (1.5 g)
Legumes *(3 or more servings)* Include with meals and snacks.	½ cup cooked beans, peas, lentils, tofu, or tempeh 1 cup peas or sprouted lentils or peas 1 cup soy or pea milk ¼ cup peanuts 2 tbsp peanut butter 2 oz veggie meat	Calcium-fortified soy or pea milk Soy or pea-based yogurt Edamame, soybeans, black beans, or white beans Calcium-set tofu	Tofu or tempeh (10–20 g) Soybeans, cooked (17 g) Veggie meat (15 g) Edamame (11 g) Peanuts (10 g) Adzuki beans, lentils, split peas (9 g) Other beans (7–8 g)

FOOD GROUP *(Suggested Number of Servings *)*	**FOODS INCLUDED** Serving Sizes*	**CALCIUM-RICH CHOICES** Within Each Food Group**	**PROTEIN-RICH CHOICES** (Grams of Protein per Serving)
Grains *(2 or more servings)* Choose mostly whole grains.	3 oz seitan ½ cup cooked grain pasta ½ cup sprouted grains 1 oz ready-to-eat cereal, bread, flatbread, or crackers	Calcium-fortified oat milk Calcium-fortified cereal Calcium-fortified tortilla	Seitan (16 g) Amaranth, kamut, spelt, or wheat (5 g) Quinoa (4 g) Pasta (4–5 g) Other grains (2–3 g)
Nuts & Seeds *(1 or more servings)* Include an omega-3-rich choice.	¼ cup nuts or seeds 2 tbsp nut or seed butter	Calcium-fortified nut or seed milk Almonds, almond butter Chia seeds Sesame seeds, tahini	Hempseeds (14 g) Hemp hearts (13 g) Pumpkin seeds (10 g) Almonds (8 g) Chia or sunflower seeds (7 g) Nut or seed butter (6–7 g) Most other nuts or seeds (5–6 g)

*This is a general guide. Serving sizes and numbers of servings can be adjusted to suit appetites and activity levels.

**Note that there are calcium-rich choices within each food group. Beet greens, spinach, and Swiss chard contain calcium, but because the calcium is poorly absorbed from these greens (due to high oxalate content), they are not listed.

Table 3.2 Your Plant-Based Day: A Guide to Add-Ons (Other Essentials). This table explains each of the essential add-ons in more detail, including how to build them into your routine through fortified foods, sunlight, supplements, or targeted food sources. Hydration is also addressed in this section, with water featured as the optimal beverage to support digestion, circulation, and energy.

Nutrient	Getting Enough	Notes
Omega-3 fatty acids	Include at least one of the following daily: • 1 tbsp ground flaxseeds or chia seeds • 2 tbsp hempseeds • 3 tbsp chopped walnuts • 1 tsp flaxseed oil	Each example provides about 2 g alpha-linolenic acid (ALA), which exceeds the RDA* for both men and women. A microalgae-based supplement of 500–1500 mg DHA/EPA daily is also recommended, depending on body size and omega-3 status. (see page 63).
Vitamin B_{12}	Include at least one of the following: • Ages 65+ or taking metformin—take a daily supplement providing 500–1,000 mcg of vitamin B_{12}. • Under age 65, take a supplement that provides at least 1,000 mcg of vitamin B_{12} two to three times a week.	Have B_{12} status checked using lab tests (see page 143).
Vitamin D	Take a supplement, eat fortified foods, get daily sunlight exposure, or use a combination of these. 25–50 mcg (1,000–2,000 IU) or more may be needed for seniors to reach optimal serum 25-hydroxy vitamin D levels (which can be determined by a lab test); (see page 151).	As we age, our skin becomes less efficient at producing vitamin D from sunlight. However, spending a short time outdoors—such as exposing the face and forearms to warm sunlight between 10 AM and 3 PM for 10 to 30 minutes—may still support vitamin D production. Do not overexpose the skin and protect it if you stay outside for extended periods.

Nutrient	Getting Enough	Notes
Iodine	Take a multivitamin with iodine, use iodine drops, or consume about ½ teaspoon of iodized salt daily to ensure the RDA* of 150 mcg of iodine. Sea vegetables, such as kelp, can also be sources of iodine, though the iodine content can vary widely and even reach toxic levels (above the safe Upper Limit of 1100 mcg/day).	Iodine in seaweed varies widely, and its levels are less reliable than those in supplements and iodized salt. For approximate amounts of dried, flaked seaweed to provide ~150 mcg of iodine, consume: • Kelp flakes—1/20 tsp • Arame flakes—1/8 tsp • Wakame flakes—¼ tsp flakes • Dulse—¾ tsp • Nori—4 full-sized nori sheets
Water	The healthiest beverage to consume is water. Keep a glass or bottle of water nearby and drink it throughout the day. Aim to drink 6 to 8 cups of water every day.	Staying well hydrated is crucial for seniors, as it may slow down the aging process and prevent or delay chronic disease.

*RDA = Recommended Dietary Allowance

To help bring all this to life, later in this chapter you'll also find three sample menus tailored to different needs and preferences—from quick, no-fuss meals to more creative or culinary options—so you can see how everything might fit into a realistic, enjoyable day of plant-based eating.

Feeling a bit overwhelmed? It's important to think of bringing more plants into your diet as a journey rather than a destination, and we'll guide you every step of the way. At the end of this chapter, we provide advice about getting started with a plant-based diet as well as some tips for making the transition. We're here to help you build confidence in moving your plant-powered lifestyle forward, one meal at a time.

Building a Balanced, Nutrient-Packed Plate

Eating well isn't just about getting enough calories; it's about making every bite count. To support healthy aging, we need to pack our meals with the nutrients and phytochemicals that keep our bodies strong and resilient.

One of the best ways to do this is to include a wide variety of plant foods every day (see Figure 3.1, page 42). Here's a simple way to put it into practice:

- **Colorful Vegetables and Fruits**
  Choose an assortment of vegetables, with an emphasis on dark greens and other nonstarchy vegetables. Select a variety of fruits, including berries and citrus. Each color group brings unique antioxidants and phytochemicals that support health.
- **Protein-Rich Legumes (or Other Plant Proteins)**
  Feature protein-rich foods such as lentils, beans, split peas, tofu, tempeh, edamame, peanut butter, and plant-based meat alternatives. If you include small amounts of animal products, such as dairy, eggs, fish, or chicken, these would also fall into this category.
- **Whole or Minimally Processed Grains**
  Focus on whole or minimally processed options. The most nutritious choices include intact grains (such as barley, quinoa, or brown rice), broken grains (such as bulgur or steel-cut oats), and rolled grains (such as old-fashioned oats). If you're aiming for weight loss, you can reduce the quantity from this group.
- **Healthy Fats: A Sprinkling of Nuts or Seeds**
  Top it all off with a small handful of nuts or seeds for healthy fats, micronutrients, and a satisfying crunch. Flax, chia, hemp,

and walnuts are notable sources of omega-3 fatty acids. Healthy fats help boost the absorption of fat-soluble nutrients.

- **Primary Beverage: Water**
  Drink water with your meals and throughout the day to stay well hydrated. Proper hydration supports digestion, brain function, and energy metabolism, which are especially important as we age.
- **Other Add-ons: Omega-3 Fatty Acids, Vitamin B_{12}, Vitamin D, and Iodine**
  Some nutrients, such as vitamin B_{12}, vitamin D, iodine, and omega-3s, can be challenging to obtain in sufficient amounts from a plant-based diet alone, especially for older adults. Ensure reliable intake through a combination of supplements, fortified foods, and whole foods (such as seaweed for iodine and UV-exposed mushrooms for vitamin D).

How to Make Mushrooms Even Healthier by Boosting Vitamin D

Mushrooms are one of the few plant foods that can provide vitamin D. Like human skin, mushrooms contain a compound called ergosterol, which converts to vitamin D_2 when exposed to ultraviolet (UV) light.

Some commercially available mushrooms are intentionally exposed to UV light after harvest to increase their vitamin D content. These are often labeled "vitamin D mushrooms" and can provide meaningful amounts of vitamin D in a single serving.

You can also boost the vitamin D content of fresh mushrooms yourself using sunlight:

- Place whole or sliced mushrooms gill-side up (underside exposed).
- Set them in direct sunlight, ideally between late morning and early afternoon.
- Leave them for about fifteen to sixty minutes (longer exposure can increase vitamin D further).
- Most of the vitamin D formed remains stable for about five to seven days when mushrooms are stored in the refrigerator. Store them in a paper bag or breathable container.

The vitamin D content can vary depending on the type of mushroom, sunlight intensity, and exposure time, but UV-exposed mushrooms generally provide approximately 10–25 mcg (400–1,000 IU) of vitamin D per 100 grams (about 1 cup).

Because vitamin D_2 from mushrooms can help contribute to overall vitamin D intake, UV-exposed mushrooms can be a helpful addition, especially for those following plant-based diets. However, depending on individual needs, additional sources such as fortified foods or supplements may still be important.

Menus for Different Eating Styles

The following sample menus offer practical, real-life examples of how to meet your nutritional needs with a variety of plant-based meals, no matter your cooking style or daily routine. Each menu provides a balanced selection of foods that, when paired with reliable sources of "add-ons" (vitamin B_{12}, vitamin D, iodine, and long-chain omega-3s), can support optimal health in older adulthood.

Table 3.4 highlights three menu styles tailored to suit a variety of preferences, energy levels, and time constraints. Each includes nourishing examples for breakfast, lunch, and dinner:

1. **Super Simple Menu:** Ideal for those seeking quick, no-fuss meals with minimal preparation. This menu is especially helpful for individuals living alone or anyone who prefers convenience without compromising nutrition.
2. **Traditional Homemade Menu:** Designed for those who enjoy spending some time in the kitchen and appreciate familiar, comforting meals. Perfect for couples or individuals who value home-cooked flavors without overly complex steps.
3. **Gourmet and Entertaining Menu:** Created for those who find joy in cooking or love sharing food with others. These meals require a bit more time and are well suited for special occasions or for impressing guests with flavorful, plant-based dishes.

These menus are meant to inspire, not prescribe. Feel free to mix and match elements based on your mood, schedule, or energy level. Prefer smaller meals? Simply divide a full meal into smaller portions or enjoy leftovers as a snack later in the day. Corresponding recipes can be found in Chapter 9.

Table 3.3 What Is Your Eating Style?

Type of Eating Style	Breakfast	Lunch	Dinner
Super Simple: Short prep time	Loaded Overnight Oats (page 250) or Quick Oats with toppings (page 251) OR Power-Packed Blueberry Smoothie (page 258)	Middle Eastern Red Lentil Tomato Kale Soup (page 282) Whole grain crackers Peanut butter Carrot sticks Fresh orange	Mediterranean Hummus Wrap (or other wrap (page 287) Grapes OR other fruit OR Easy Chocolate Pudding (page 312)
Traditional Homemade: Moderate prep time	Old Fashioned Rolled Oats or Steel-Cut Oats with toppings (page 252)	Full-Meal Salad with colorful vegetables and fruits, 1–2 protein options, and starchy additions (page 262) Tahini-Balsamic Dressing or other dressing (pages 271–273) Fresh apple	The Multicolored Bowl (page 304) OR Marvelous Mushroom Ragout (page 307) Creamy Chia Pudding (page 314) Simple Stewed Fruit (page 316)
Foodie/Gourmet: Longer prep time	Golden Scrambled Tofu (page 256) with toast OR Nondairy yogurt parfait with fruit, seeds, granola	White Bean and Mushroom Soup (page 284) Rainbow Quinoa Salad with chickpeas (page 267) Fresh pear	Tofu Cacciatore (page 309) Steamed broccoli Baked potato Nutty Date Cookies (page 328) OR Cranberry Pecan Muffins (page 320) Fruit

Getting Started with a Plant-Based Diet

If you grew up eating a Standard American or Western Diet, shifting to a more plant-based way of eating might seem daunting at first. But change doesn't have to be drastic to be effective. In fact, the most lasting results often come from small, steady steps. With a bit of planning and curiosity, you can discover delicious new foods that support your energy, health, and well-being, without feeling overwhelmed.

- **Start Small and Build Gradually**
  Begin by adding one or two plant-based meals per week. As you find dishes you enjoy, increase their frequency. Some people find it helpful to focus on just one meal at a time, like swapping out their usual breakfast or lunch. (You'll find plenty of meal ideas and inspiration in Chapter 9.)
- **Try Plant-Based Days**
  Consider designating a day or two each week as entirely plant-based, such as *Meatless Mondays*. This can be a fun and low-pressure way to explore new meals.
- **Explore and Experiment**
  Enjoy trying new recipes, whether from this book or trusted online sources. You don't have to give up your favorite meals; try adapting them with plant-based alternatives. For example, use veggie ground round instead of beef in chili, or swap tofu for chicken in stir-fries. Explore dishes from cultures where plant-based eating is already the norm, as they can offer incredible flavor and inspiration.
- **Stock Up on Staples**
  Keeping your kitchen well stocked with nutritious, long-lasting ingredients makes creating healthy meals easier. Choose fruits and vegetables that last (like apples, oranges, carrots, and broccoli), along with frozen items such as berries, green peas, and

spinach. Canned beans and chickpeas, whole grains (like oats, brown rice, and quinoa), and unsalted nuts and seeds are great to have on hand. Plant-based essentials like tofu, tempeh, fortified nondairy milk, and vegan nut- or seed-based cheese round out your toolkit. Over time, you will come to know what you will need to have on hand to create some of your favorite plant-based meals.

- **Keep Some Fresh Favorites**
  In addition to staples, keep some fresh greens and seasonal produce in your fridge. A handful of leafy greens or a few fresh herbs can really elevate a meal.
- **Cook Once, Eat Many Times**
  If you have a freezer, batch cooking can be a game changer, especially for those living alone. Make a big pot of soup, stew, or casserole, and freeze portions for later. Invest in glass containers with lids that can withstand temperature changes. Label them clearly so they're easy to grab when time or energy is low. Some people enjoy meal-prepping once a week to set themselves up for success all week long.
- **Find a Food Buddy**
  Transitioning is easier (and more fun) with support. A friend, family member, or neighbor who's also curious about healthy eating can be a wonderful source of encouragement. Try shopping together, swapping recipes, or even sharing meals. Search for "online plant-based cooking club" to share even more ideas and have fun cooking together.

Practical Steps for a Plant-Powered Transition

These practical strategies can help you build a plant-powered way of eating at your own pace—without overwhelm.

Begin with One Meal a Day

Start with a single plant-based meal—breakfast or lunch is often easiest. Once that feels routine, build from there.

Increase Fiber Gradually

Plant-based diets are naturally rich in fiber, which supports gut health. However, a sudden increase can cause temporary bloating or discomfort. A gradual approach allows your gut microbiome time to adapt:

- Start with smaller portions of beans and lentils (e.g., a few spoonfuls added to a salad, soup, or grain dish).
- Replace refined grains (white pasta, white rice, baked goods) with whole grains slowly—one change at a time.
- Introduce raw vegetables and salads gradually.
- Increase fiber-rich foods steadily over several weeks.

Support Digestion

Mild digestive changes are common at first—but they are typically temporary and often a sign of beneficial changes in the gut. Simple practices can help:

- Drink plenty of fluids.
- Chew thoroughly and eat slowly.
- Start with easier-to-digest options like lentils, split peas, tofu, tempeh, plant-based meat alternatives, and smoothies.
- Use blended forms of legumes—soups, hummus, and spreads—to help improve tolerance.

Build Simple, Repeatable Meals

You don't need complicated recipes to get started. Think simple, familiar, and satisfying:

- Overnight oats with nuts, seeds, and fruit
- Smoothies with fruit, greens, and soy milk or soft tofu
- Beans or lentils with rice and vegetables
- Whole grain toast with nut butter and banana, or hummus and tomato

A Practical Approach: Start with Simple Swaps

Transitioning to a plant-powered lifestyle at any age is about progress —not perfection. There's no need to overhaul your entire kitchen overnight. One of the most effective ways to begin is to make small, high-impact "swaps" in your usual meals. This approach keeps your routine familiar while substantially increasing your intake of fiber, antioxidants, and nutrient-dense whole foods.

The Breakfast Swap

Instead of eggs and bacon, try a bowl of oats topped with walnuts and berries (pages 250–252), Golden Scrambled Tofu (page 256), Cashew French Toast (page 255), or whole grain toast with peanut or nut butter and fruit.

Replace cow's milk with unsweetened soy, almond, or oat milk in your smoothies, coffee, tea, cereal, puddings, and cooking. For bone health, choose plant milks fortified with calcium and vitamin D. Try unsweetened plant-based yogurts, and if you enjoy cheese, explore the growing variety of flavorful nut-based alternatives.

The Protein Swap

Once or twice a week (or more often), replace the meat in your favorite dishes with legumes. Try Easy Minestrone Soup (page 277), Tofu Cacciatore (page 309), or Easy Peasy Chili (page 297). To support digestive comfort, begin with smaller portions, choose well-cooked legumes, and start with lentils or split peas, which are often better tolerated.

Plant-based meat alternatives can also be a helpful bridge—they are familiar, convenient, and typically well tolerated. Over time, incorporate more whole or minimally processed options such as beans, lentils, tofu, and tempeh.

The "Crowding Out" Method

Focus on what you add rather than what you remove. Fill half your plate with colorful vegetables, and you'll naturally reduce your intake of animal products and processed foods—without feeling deprived.

A Final Thought

While your best results will come from adopting several of these strategies, even small changes can make a meaningful difference in how you feel and in your long-term health.

Remember: Transitioning to a plant-based diet is a journey, not a destination. Be kind to yourself, stay curious, and enjoy the process of discovering new foods and flavors. Celebrate every positive change, no matter how small. With time, what once felt unfamiliar can become second nature, and even joyful.

KEY TAKEAWAYS

Balance is the foundation of healthy eating. A nutritious plant-based day includes five core food groups: vegetables, fruits, legumes, whole grains, and nuts/seeds, along with key "add-ons" such as vitamin B_{12}, vitamin D, iodine, and omega-3s, with water as the primary beverage. Aim to include at least four of the five food groups from Figure 3.1 at every meal.

Plant-based eating works for every lifestyle. Whether your style is fast and easy, traditional and homemade, or gourmet and adventurous, there are delicious, balanced options for you. It's all about choosing nutrient-dense foods that fit your preferences, schedule, and energy level.

Simple planning makes a big difference. Stocking your kitchen with versatile staples, prepping a few meals ahead of time, and keeping nutritious frozen and canned foods on hand can make healthy eating feel effortless, especially when time or energy is limited.

Start small, build gradually. Transitioning to a plant-based diet doesn't have to happen overnight. Begin with one plant-based meal or day each week or try easy swaps in your favorite recipes. With each step, you'll gain skills, confidence, and momentum.

Every positive change counts. Whether you cook every day or only occasionally, every nourishing choice supports your energy, health span, and overall well-being. Be kind to yourself, enjoy the process, and celebrate progress over perfection.

Connecting the Plate to Prevention

Now you're ready to take the next step: understanding how your choices influence your long-term health. In the next chapter, we explore some of the most common health conditions affecting older adults, and how plant-based nutrition can play a powerful role in both prevention and management.

CHAPTER 4

FINE-TUNING YOUR DIET FOR CHRONIC HEALTH CONDITIONS

Chapter at a Glance

In this chapter, we'll explore some of the most common health conditions that affect older adults, examine their causes, risk factors, and approaches to management. You'll learn how a plant-based diet can serve as a powerful, evidence-based tool, not just for one condition, but for nearly all of them.

While factors like genetics and aging are beyond our control, many lifestyle choices we make every day, including the foods we eat, how we move, how we sleep, and how we connect, can significantly influence our risk and resilience. In the pages ahead, you'll find targeted guidance and practical strategies for fifteen of the most common conditions we face with aging.

Maria's Story: Standing Strong

Before Maria began to invest in her health and longevity, terms like *oxidative stress* and *chronic inflammation* didn't register. But after attending a community seminar on nutrition and aging, she began to understand how these factors could shape her own health journey.

Yes, her blood pressure had improved and her energy was up since adopting a plant-based diet, but a recent bone density scan revealed early signs of osteoporosis. At first, the news felt like a setback. But Maria had learned to view these moments not as failures but as invitations to fine-tune her approach to health.

With help from a plant-based dietitian, she began adding calcium-rich leafy greens, tofu, tahini, and fortified plant milks to her meals. She also committed to short daily walks and simple resistance exercises with light weights. "I may be in my seventies," she said, "but I'm not done taking care of my body." Her story is a reminder that living with chronic conditions doesn't mean surrendering to decline. It means adapting with intention, leaning on evidence-based guidance, and using food as a powerful tool for healing and resilience.

A Unified Approach to Aging and Health

As we age, the risk of developing chronic conditions increases. Unfortunately, health challenges rarely occur in isolation. Many chronic conditions develop side by side, sharing common roots. In the pages that follow, we examine fifteen of the conditions most commonly associated with aging:

1. Arthritis (page 62)
2. Autoimmune conditions (page 66)
3. Cancer (page 69)
4. Coronary artery disease (page 74)
5. Cognitive impairment and dementia (page 76)

6. Diabetes, prediabetes, and metabolic syndrome (page 81)
7. Frailty and being underweight (page 86)
8. Gout (page 90)
9. Hypertension (page 93)
10. Macular degeneration and cataracts (page 97)
11. Osteoporosis and osteopenia (page 101)
12. Overweight and obesity (page 105)
13. Respiratory disorders (page 108)
14. Sarcopenia (page 111)
15. Stroke (page 114)

Many people assume that each of these illnesses requires a separate diet plan, with its own set of complex rules.

But what if one dietary pattern could cut across all of them, offering broad protection, reducing risk, and even playing a role in treatment? That's exactly what a whole-food, plant-based diet has consistently been shown to do.

The same dietary approach that lowers blood pressure and improves insulin sensitivity can help prevent type 2 diabetes. The same nutrients that support heart health also benefit the brain and reduce cancer risk.

That's because many chronic conditions share common underlying drivers:

- Chronic inflammation (persistent, low-grade activation of the immune system, which damages tissues)
- Oxidative stress (an imbalance between harmful free radicals and the body's antioxidant defenses)
- Dysbiosis (an unhealthy gut microbiome)
- Lipotoxicity (the buildup of fat in organs where it doesn't belong)

Each of these factors is directly influenced by what we eat. In the pages that follow, we take a closer look at individual chronic conditions, exploring how they develop, how they impact quality of life, and how a plant-based diet can play a key role in prevention, symptom management, and even reversal.

1. Arthritis

What Is Arthritis?

Arthritis refers to inflammation in one or more joints, causing pain, stiffness, swelling, and reduced mobility. It can make everyday activities, like walking, dressing, or preparing meals, more difficult. The two most common forms are:

- **Osteoarthritis (OA):** A "wear and tear" condition in which cartilage in the joints gradually breaks down. Without this cushioning, bones may rub against one another, leading to pain and loss of movement.
- **Rheumatoid arthritis (RA):** An autoimmune disease in which the body's immune system mistakenly attacks healthy joint tissue, causing inflammation, pain, and long-term joint damage.

How Does Aging Affect Risk?

As we age, our risk of developing arthritis increases, especially for osteoarthritis, the most common form. In fact, about half of adults over age sixty-five, and nearly 80 percent of those over seventy-five, are affected. Rheumatoid arthritis, while less common, still impacts around 2 to 3 percent of adults over sixty, with women being more frequently affected than men.

Although joint pain, muscle weakness, and changes in bone density often occur with age, arthritis is not an inevitable part of getting older. Diet and lifestyle choices play a powerful role in reducing risk, easing symptoms, and maintaining joint health and mobility.

Can Plant-Based Diets Help?

Yes, a well-planned plant-based diet can reduce inflammation, support a healthy weight, and improve joint function, all of which are important in managing arthritis. Many whole plant foods contain anti-inflammatory compounds. Good examples include:

- **Leafy greens** (e.g., kale and collards) are rich in antioxidants and vitamin K.
- **Berries** are packed with flavonoids and vitamin C.
- **Turmeric,** particularly its active compound curcumin, has been shown in some studies to help reduce joint pain and stiffness when taken consistently.

These foods work together to calm the immune system and reduce the kind of chronic inflammation that contributes to joint damage.

What Key Nutritional Factors Support Joint Health?

As you age, supporting joint health through good nutrition becomes even more important. Specific nutrients and other dietary components have been shown to reduce inflammation, strengthen surrounding muscles, and promote overall joint function. Key examples include:

- **Omega-3 Fatty Acids.** These healthy fats have anti-inflammatory properties that can help reduce joint pain and morning stiffness, especially in RA. Good plant sources of omega-3s (ALA) include flaxseeds, chia seeds, hempseeds, and walnuts. Consider algae-based long-chain omega-3 supplements (DHA/EPA) if you have an inflammatory form of arthritis, as the body's conversion of ALA to long-chain omega-3s is limited. Although the effectiveness of DHA/EPA varies, clinical studies suggest therapeutic benefits for rheumatoid arthritis with 2.5–3 grams (2,500–3,000 mg) daily.

- **Vitamin D.** This vitamin helps the body absorb calcium and may reduce inflammation. Since vitamin D deficiency is common in older adults, many people benefit from a supplement, especially those who live in northern climates or have limited sun exposure. A simple blood test can check your serum vitamin D levels.
- **Protein.** Getting enough protein is key to maintaining muscle strength and supporting the joints. An intake of at least 1.0–1.2 g/kg/day for older adults is recommended to maintain muscle and joint integrity. Emphasize legumes, soy foods, nuts, seeds, and whole grains.
- **Prebiotics and fiber.** A healthy gut microbiome plays a vital role in immune regulation, especially in autoimmune conditions like RA. Whole-plant foods rich in fiber help feed beneficial gut bacteria and may reduce inflammation.

What About Trigger Foods?

Some individuals with RA notice that their symptoms worsen after eating certain foods, though triggers can vary widely from person to person. For example, nightshade vegetables (such as tomatoes, potatoes, eggplant, and peppers) contain a natural compound called solanine, which, in theory, may contribute to inflammation or exacerbate joint pain in sensitive individuals, possibly through its effects on gut or immune function. However, clinical studies have not confirmed a consistent link between nightshades and arthritis symptoms. Still, some people report relief after avoiding them.

In other cases, eliminating foods like meat, dairy, or wheat has been associated with reduced joint pain, less inflammation, and modest weight loss, particularly in people with RA. If you suspect that specific foods may be affecting your symptoms, consider keeping a food and symptom journal and discussing patterns with your healthcare provider or a registered dietitian. Personalized dietary changes may offer valuable support alongside conventional RA treatment.

What Other Lifestyle Factors Are Important?

Exercise is one of the best ways to support joint health and manage arthritis symptoms.

- **Low-impact activities**, like swimming, tai chi, cycling, and walking, help maintain flexibility, reduce stiffness, and improve mood and sleep.
- **Strength training**, even using light resistance bands or bodyweight exercises, such as squats, push-ups, planks, or lunges, can support joint function and reduce falls.

If you're carrying extra weight, losing just 5 to 10 percent of your body weight can significantly relieve pressure on your knees and hips and may help reduce inflammation throughout the body.

3 KEY TAKEAWAYS

1. Enjoy colorful, anti-inflammatory plant foods, especially leafy greens, berries, seeds, and spices like turmeric.
2. Ensure adequate intakes of key nutrients such as protein, vitamin D, and omega-3s, from plant sources or supplements.
3. Incorporate low-impact activities into your daily life that protect your joints and support strength.

2. Autoimmune Conditions

What Are Autoimmune Conditions?

Autoimmune conditions are diseases in which the body's immune system, which is responsible for defending us against infections, mistakenly attacks its own healthy tissues. Instead of targeting viruses or harmful bacteria, the immune system turns against cells in the joints, skin, thyroid, intestines, or other organs. This misdirected immune activity leads to chronic inflammation and, over time, tissue damage and disrupted function.

Autoimmune conditions that are common in older adults include:

- Lupus (SLE)
- Multiple sclerosis (MS)
- Graves' disease (thyroid)
- Crohn's disease, and ulcerative colitis (gut)
- RA and type 1 diabetes

As we age, the immune system can gradually lose its ability to defend against threats while inappropriate inflammatory responses become more common. This can contribute to both the development and progression of autoimmune conditions.

Can a Plant-Based Diet Help?

Yes, a plant-based diet rich in whole, minimally processed foods can support the immune system, reduce inflammation, and improve overall well-being. Your Plant-Powered Day on page 42 provides a perfect starting point. The foods featured on this plate work together to nourish the body, support immune balance, and reduce inflammation. For example:

- Colorful fruits and vegetables provide antioxidants and phytochemicals that can protect tissues from inflammatory damage.

- Whole grains, legumes, nuts, seeds, and vegetables contain fiber, which feeds beneficial gut bacteria. A healthy gut microbiome is vital for immune balance.
- Fermented and cultured plant foods, such as kimchi, sauerkraut, or cultured nondairy yogurts, as well as probiotics, may help modulate immunity and reduce gut permeability (often called "leaky gut"), which is associated with several autoimmune conditions.

In contrast, diets high in ultra-processed foods, red and processed meats, refined grains, and sugary drinks, typical of Standard American Diets (SAD), are linked to increased inflammation and may worsen autoimmune disease risk and severity.

What Key Nutrients Support Immune Health?

A strong immune system effectively identifies and eliminates pathogens while maintaining balance to prevent overreaction. It needs the right nutrients to function at its best, especially as we age. Here are three key players that help keep immunity resilient and inflammation in check:

- **Vitamin D.** This vitamin helps regulate immune activity and reduces excessive inflammation. Many autoimmune diseases are associated with vitamin D deficiency, and older adults may have decreased ability to synthesize this vitamin from sun exposure. Experts often recommend 1,000–2,000 IU (25–50 mcg) per day, but the optimal dose is best determined by a serum 25(OH)D test.
- **Vitamin B_{12}.** Essential for nerve health and DNA repair, vitamin B_{12} is a nutrient to pay close attention to for all seniors. Since B_{12} is produced by microorganisms and is not found in plant foods, daily supplementation is critical on a plant-based diet.

- **Omega-3 Fatty Acids.** These fatty acids reduce pro-inflammatory cytokines and support immune regulation. DHA and EPA, especially at doses of 500–1,500 mg/day, may offer benefits beyond those of ALA in plant foods. Some people with active inflammation may benefit from higher doses.

What About Food Triggers and Sensitivities?

For some individuals, certain foods can worsen symptoms. These may include dairy, eggs, gluten or wheat, soy foods, nightshade vegetables (e.g., tomatoes, potatoes, eggplant, peppers), yeast, citrus, or undercooked beans. Everyone is different, and food sensitivities are highly individual. A healthy food for one person can be problematic for another.

How Can I Identify Trigger Foods?

Detecting food sensitivities is not a simple task! Since we typically eat more than one food at a time, and often a beverage along with it, it can be difficult to pinpoint which item or items are the culprits. A reaction can occur immediately or as long as several hours after eating an offending food. Also, the body may not react the same way every time. Tracking symptoms and food intake is a practical way to start. Here's one approach:

- **Step 1.** Eliminate all suspected trigger foods for at least three to four days and monitor symptoms.
- **Step 2.** Reintroduce each food one at a time, in normal portions, every forty-eight hours, observing for reactions.
- **Step 3.** Keep a detailed diary of symptoms and food intake to help connect patterns.

If you suspect multiple food triggers, a short-term "Few Foods" elimination diet can help. For two weeks, eat only a small group of low-reactivity foods (e.g., well-cooked lentils, rice, sweet potatoes, squash, and pears). Then, reintroduce new foods every two to three days to identify problematic ones. This process should be done with the guidance of a dietitian or knowledgeable healthcare provider.

Do Other Lifestyle Factors Matter?

Yes! Many people find that unusual stress has led to their autoimmune condition. Not only can chronic stress trigger flares, but the daily challenges of living with an autoimmune condition can increase your emotional burden. Mindfulness practices, deep breathing, yoga, gentle movement, and social connection all play a role in calming the nervous system. Engaging in creative, meaningful activities can also help to restore emotional balance.

3 KEY TAKEAWAYS

1. A well-designed plant-based diet supports immune balance, reduces inflammation, and fosters gut health—key factors in preventing and managing autoimmune disease.
2. Be sure to get adequate vitamins D and B_{12} and omega-3s. Consider algae-based DHA/EPA.
3. If symptoms persist, explore individual food sensitivities through careful elimination and reintroduction under professional guidance.

3. Cancer

What Is Cancer?

Cancer refers to a group of diseases characterized by uncontrolled cell growth, which can spread to other parts of the body. Healthy cells may become precancerous when their DNA, the genetic blueprint that governs cell division, is damaged.

This damage can result from chronic inflammation, certain infections, tobacco smoke, alcohol, environmental toxins (including pesticides), ultraviolet radiation, or even prolonged psychological stress. Fortunately, the body is equipped with natural defenses. The immune system, including T cells and natural killer (NK) cells, can often detect and eliminate abnormal cells before they become harmful. However, this surveillance system tends to weaken with age, increasing vulnerability.

How Does Aging Impact Risk?

As we age, our ability to repair DNA declines, and immune surveillance becomes less efficient, making it harder to eliminate cells that could turn cancerous. Prostate cancer is the most common cancer in men over sixty-five, while breast cancer is common in postmenopausal women. Colorectal cancer risk rises with age and is strongly linked to diet and lifestyle. Lung cancer is associated with smoking history but can also arise from occupational or environmental exposures. Bladder cancer, more common in men, is linked to inflammation and carcinogens that pass through the urinary system.

Can a Plant-Based Diet Help?

Yes. Decades of research support the role of a whole-food, plant-based diet in cancer prevention and survivorship. According to the World Cancer Research Fund and the American Institute for Cancer Research, well-planned plant-centered diets are associated with lower cancer risk, slower disease progression, and improved survival, particularly in breast, prostate, and colorectal cancers. These benefits are likely due to the synergistic effects of fiber, phytochemicals, antioxidants, and anti-inflammatory compounds found across a variety of whole-plant foods, including:

- **Vegetables and fruits** provide vitamins C and E, folate, carotenoids, and a wide array of phytochemicals that help neutralize free radicals, protect DNA, reduce inflammation, and regulate cell growth.
- **Whole grains and legumes** are rich in dietary fiber, promoting healthy gut microbiota and supporting regular elimination, both of which are linked to a reduced risk of colorectal and other gastrointestinal cancers.
- **Soyfoods** (e.g., tofu, tempeh, soy milk, and edamame) are rich in isoflavones, plant compounds that may protect against hormone-related cancers such as breast and prostate cancer.
- **Cruciferous vegetables** (e.g., broccoli, kale, cabbage, Brussels sprouts) contain glucosinolates, which break down into bioactive compounds like sulforaphane and indole-3-carbinol, agents known to support detoxification and inhibit cancer cell growth.
- **Berries** are packed with anthocyanins and other polyphenols that exhibit antioxidant, anti-inflammatory, and anti-proliferative effects.
- **Mushrooms,** particularly varieties like shiitake, maitake, and turkey tail, contain beta-glucans and other compounds that enhance immune surveillance and may suppress tumor development.
- **Flaxseeds,** the richest dietary source of lignans, have weak estrogenic and anti-estrogenic properties and may protect against breast cancer.

- **Green tea** is rich in catechins, particularly epigallocatechin gallate (EGCG), which is capable of inhibiting cancer cell growth and promoting cancer cell death.

What Foods Increase Cancer Risk?

Certain foods can increase cancer risk by promoting inflammation, oxidative stress, and DNA damage.

- Processed meats, including bacon, ham, sausages, wieners, and deli meats, are classified as carcinogenic to humans (Group 1) by the World Health Organization. Red meat (such as beef, pork, and lamb) is classified as probably carcinogenic (Group 2A). High intake of these meats is associated with increased risk of breast, colorectal, and gastric cancers. When cooked at high temperatures (e.g., frying, roasting, grilling), they form heterocyclic amines (HCAs) and polycyclic aromatic hydrocarbons (PAHs), which are linked to colorectal and pancreatic cancers. Heme iron, found in red meat, can trigger oxidative reactions that damage cells.
- Alcohol, even in small amounts, is known to increase the risk of at least seven types of cancer: breast, colorectal, liver, oral cavity, pharynx (throat), larynx (voice box), and esophagus. Alcohol is metabolized into acetaldehyde, a toxic compound that damages DNA, impairs repair mechanisms, and increases absorption of other carcinogens into cells.

What Other Lifestyle Choices Provide Protection Against Cancer?

Maintaining a physically active lifestyle is one of the most effective ways of reducing cancer risk. Extensive population studies have shown that regular exercise is associated with a lower incidence of several cancers, including those of the bladder, breast, colon, endometrium, kidney, stomach, and esophagus.

Physical activity also plays a role in reducing the risk of cancer recurrence and improving survival outcomes. In tandem with movement, maintaining a healthy body weight is critically important. Excess body fat promotes chronic inflammation, alters levels of hormones such as estrogen and insulin, and impairs immune surveillance, which makes it harder for the body to detect and destroy abnormal cells before they become cancerous. Together, regular physical activity and weight management form a cornerstone of cancer prevention and survivorship.

3 KEY TAKEAWAYS

1. A whole-food, plant-based diet, rich in vegetables, fruits, legumes, whole grains, and fiber, is associated with reduced cancer risk, slower disease progression, and improved survival outcomes.

2. Limiting processed and red meats, avoiding alcohol, and minimizing high-temperature cooking methods can lower cancer risk by reducing oxidative stress, inflammation, and DNA damage.

3. Regular physical activity and achieving or maintaining a healthy body weight reduce the risk of several cancers, improve immune function, and support long-term survivorship.

4. Coronary Artery Disease

What Is Coronary Artery Disease?

Coronary artery disease (CAD) is a common condition characterized by the buildup of plaque lining the arteries that supply blood to our hearts. Plaque is composed of cholesterol, fatty substances, waste from cells, calcium, and a clotting material. Plaque can narrow and reduce blood flow and even block arteries, leading to chest pain (angina), heart attacks, or even sudden death.

How Common Is CAD?

CAD is the most common heart disease in America, affecting approximately 20 million adults, or about 7 percent of the adult population. With age, CAD becomes more prevalent, impacting approximately 20 percent of American seniors ages sixty-five and older. Although men have a relatively high risk earlier in life, more women than men ultimately die of CAD each year, partly because women often experience less typical symptoms and delay seeking care.

What Diet and Lifestyle Factors Increase Our Risk of CAD?

A diet high in saturated fats, processed foods, red and processed meats, sugar, and salt contributes directly to artery-clogging plaque. Smoking, physical inactivity, obesity, diabetes, high blood pressure, high cholesterol, and chronic stress will also significantly elevate our risk.

Do Plant-Based Diets Provide Protection?

Research consistently shows that plant-based diets, rich in vegetables, fruits, whole grains, legumes, nuts, and seeds, can substantially reduce the risk of CAD. Studies indicate that plant-based eaters have an approximately 30 percent lower risk of developing CAD compared to those consuming typical Western diets. These diets reduce inflammation, improve cholesterol profiles, and help maintain healthy blood pressure.

Plant-based diets not only help prevent CAD but can also aid in its treatment. Groundbreaking research by Dr. Dean Ornish, published back in 1990, was the first to demonstrate that comprehensive lifestyle changes, including a low-fat, plant-based diet, could reverse CAD by decreasing arterial plaque buildup, improving blood flow, and reducing symptoms. A large body of subsequent research has confirmed and expanded upon these findings.

What Other Lifestyle Factors Help Prevent or Manage CAD?

Regular physical activity, such as walking, swimming, and yoga, improves heart health.

Quitting smoking significantly reduces heart attack risk. Managing stress through mindfulness, meditation, or hobbies helps control blood pressure.

Regular medical checkups can monitor blood pressure and cholesterol, screen for diabetes, and inspire us to adopt or maintain health-supportive practices!

3 KEY TAKEAWAYS

1. CAD is widespread among seniors but is largely preventable and manageable.
2. A well-planned plant-based diet significantly lowers our risk of developing CAD and can even reverse it.
3. Regular exercise, smoking cessation, and stress management further protect our hearts.

5. Cognitive Impairment and Dementia in Older Adults

What Is Cognitive Impairment? Is It the Same as Dementia?

As we age, it's normal to have occasional memory slips, like forgetting where we put our keys. However, cognitive impairment refers to a measurable decline in thinking skills, including memory, decision-making, and attention. It exists on a spectrum, from mild lapses to severe dysfunction.

- Mild cognitive impairment (MCI) is an intermediate stage between normal aging and dementia. Individuals with MCI may notice memory lapses or slower processing but can still carry out daily activities independently.
- Dementia is more advanced. It involves significant disruptions in memory, reasoning, language, and the ability to perform everyday tasks. The most common types include Alzheimer's disease, vascular dementia, and Lewy body dementia. For example, someone with MCI may forget the name of an old classmate while someone with dementia may forget the name of a close family member.

Does Aging Increase the Risk of Cognitive Decline?

Yes. As we age, several changes make us more vulnerable to memory loss and cognitive decline. Blood flow to the brain gradually decreases, oxidative damage and inflammation become more pronounced, and neuroplasticity—the brain's ability to adapt, form new connections, and repair itself—declines. These age-related shifts can affect memory, learning, and decision-making.

However, cognitive decline is not an inevitable part of aging. Lifestyle also plays a significant role. In fact, strong evidence shows that nutrition, physical activity, restorative sleep, and stress management can help preserve brain function and reduce the risk of dementia, even in later life.

Can a Plant-Based Diet Help Protect the Brain?

A growing body of research suggests that well-planned plant-based diets, especially those rich in antioxidants, polyphenols, fiber, and anti-inflammatory compounds, may support brain health and are associated in some studies with slower cognitive decline and reduced dementia risk. However, the overall evidence is still evolving. Some studies report benefits while others show neutral or less favorable outcomes. For example, findings from the Adventist Health Study-2 reported that among vegetarians—including vegans and pescatarians—there was a tendency toward higher rates of dementia compared with nonvegetarians. These findings underscore the importance of ensuring adequate intake of key nutrients that support cognitive function, such as vitamin B_{12}, vitamin D, iodine, zinc, and long-chain omega-3 fatty acids.

Several dietary patterns have shown a benefit, including:

- The Mediterranean diet
- The DASH (Dietary Approaches to Stop Hypertension) diet
- The MIND (Mediterranean-DASH Intervention for Neurodegenerative Delay) diet

The MIND diet, designed specifically for brain health, emphasizes leafy greens, berries, nuts, legumes, whole grains, and olive oil while minimizing red meat, dairy, fried foods, and sweets. While not entirely plant-based, it is strongly plant-forward and can be readily adapted to an exclusively plant-based lifestyle.

Importantly, plant-based diets vary widely in quality. Diets centered on whole, minimally processed plant foods appear most protective, whereas those high in refined grains, added sugars, and ultra-processed foods may not confer the same benefits. As with any dietary pattern, ensuring adequate intake of key nutrients—such as vitamin B_{12}, vitamin D, omega-3 fatty acids, iodine, and zinc—is essential for supporting optimal cognitive function.

What Foods Matter Most?

What we put on our plates each day can have a massive impact on how well our brains age. Certain foods nourish and protect the brain, helping to preserve memory, focus, and mental clarity as the years go by. A brain-supportive diet includes:

- Antioxidant-rich plants, especially berries, dark leafy greens, turmeric, and green tea, to reduce oxidative stress
- Omega-3 fatty acids, which support brain structure and function:
    - ALA (from flax, chia, hemp, and walnuts) offers some benefit for brain health.
    - DHA and EPA (from algae-based supplements) support healthy cognitive aging by contributing to neuronal structure, inflammation regulation, and communication between brain cells. While the body can convert ALA into EPA and DHA, this process is inefficient, making direct sources a more reliable way to support omega-3 status.
- Vitamins B_{12} and D are essential for brain and nerve health, and often are low without supplementation.
- Minimal intake of ultra-processed foods, which dominate the Standard American Diet, is critical. These foods are linked to inflammation and increased risk of cognitive decline.

What Other Lifestyle Factors Support Brain Health?

What's good for the heart is also good for the brain. Regular physical activity improves circulation and stimulates the release of brain-derived neurotrophic factor (BDNF), a molecule that protects neurons and encourages the growth of new brain cells.

Mental stimulation, such as reading, learning new skills, or playing strategy games, helps build and maintain cognitive reserve, making the brain more resilient over time. Getting quality sleep is essential, as it allows the brain to clear waste products and consolidate memories. Finally, staying socially connected and managing stress through techniques like mindfulness, deep breathing, or meaningful engagement supports emotional well-being and long-term cognitive health.

How Do Genetics Affect Risk?

While genetics can influence the risk of dementia, it accounts for less than 5 to 10 percent of all cases. The majority of cognitive decline is associated with modifiable lifestyle factors, not inherited traits.

That said, one of the most well-recognized genetic risk factors for late-onset Alzheimer's disease is the apolipoprotein E (ApoE) gene—specifically the ApoE4 allele. Carrying one or two copies of ApoE4 can increase the likelihood of developing Alzheimer's, but it is not a guarantee.

The encouraging news is that lifestyle choices can significantly influence brain health, even for those with a genetic predisposition. Protective strategies include following a plant-predominant, nutrient-rich diet, engaging in regular physical activity, not smoking, limiting alcohol intake, and prioritizing restorative sleep and stress reduction. These evidence-based strategies may not only delay the onset of cognitive decline but can also slow its progression, supporting long-term brain health regardless of genetic background.

3 KEY TAKEAWAYS

1. Cognitive decline is influenced by age, lifestyle, and genetics, but lifestyle is the most powerful factor affecting long term brain health.
2. A whole food, plant-forward diet, along with essential nutrients like vitamin B_{12}, vitamin D, iodine, zinc, and omega-3s, helps preserve memory and thinking skills.
3. Staying physically active, mentally engaged, and well-rested supports long-term cognitive health and reduces the risk of dementia.

6. Diabetes, Prediabetes, and Metabolic Syndrome

What Are Diabetes, Prediabetes, and Metabolic Syndrome?

Diabetes is a condition in which the body has difficulty regulating blood sugar (glucose) levels. There are several types, each with distinct causes:

- **Type 1 diabetes** is an autoimmune condition in which the body's immune system attacks the insulin-producing cells of the pancreas, resulting in little or no insulin production.
- **Type 2 diabetes (T2D)** is a disease of insulin resistance, in which the body still produces insulin, but the cells do not respond to it effectively. Over time, insulin production also declines.
- **Gestational diabetes** is a form of diabetes that occurs during pregnancy, usually resolving after delivery, but increasing the long-term risk of developing type 2 diabetes.

- **Prediabetes** is a condition where blood sugar levels and insulin resistance are elevated but not high enough to meet the criteria for a type 2 diabetes diagnosis.
- **Metabolic syndrome** is a cluster of risk factors that occur together, increasing the risk for type 2 diabetes, heart disease, and stroke. It is diagnosed when a person has at least three out of the following five markers:
    - High blood pressure
    - Excess abdominal weight (increased waist circumference)
    - Elevated triglycerides
    - Low HDL ("good") cholesterol
    - Elevated fasting blood sugar

What's the Difference Between Prediabetes and Metabolic Syndrome?

While distinct, prediabetes and metabolic syndrome frequently overlap. Both involve insulin resistance and elevated blood sugar, and both significantly increase the risk of type 2 diabetes, cardiovascular disease, and stroke. About a third of American adults have metabolic syndrome while about 50 percent have either prediabetes (38 percent) or diabetes (12 percent).

If you have prediabetes, it's important to assess for metabolic syndrome, as having both conditions indicates a higher level of metabolic dysfunction. The good news is that the same evidence-based lifestyle strategies, such as eating a whole-food, plant-based diet, staying physically active, and achieving a healthy weight, can reverse metabolic syndrome and reduce the risk of progression.

What Type of Diabetes Is Most Common and How Many of Us Are Affected?

Type 2 diabetes accounts for approximately 90 percent of all diabetes cases in most regions of the world. In the United States, more than half of all adults have either prediabetes or type 2 diabetes.

The good news is that both conditions are strongly influenced by lifestyle. Prediabetes can often be reversed, and type 2 diabetes can often be driven into remission through healthy, sustainable changes, such as adopting a plant-based diet, engaging in regular physical activity, and reducing body fat stores.

What Factors Increase the Risk of Type 2 Diabetes and Prediabetes?

While age and family history do contribute to risk, they are not the primary drivers of type 2 diabetes. The most significant factors relate to lifestyle and body composition, including:

- **Overconsumption of calories** leading to excess body fat, particularly visceral fat around the organs and fat in the liver, pancreas, and muscle tissue, which interferes with insulin signaling.
- **Poor-quality diets,** especially those high in red and processed meats, saturated fats, refined carbohydrates, added sugars, and ultra-processed foods, drive inflammation and metabolic dysfunction.
- **Physical inactivity,** reduces glucose uptake, promotes fat accumulation in muscle and liver tissue, and contributes to insulin resistance.

These factors create a metabolic environment that promotes insulin resistance, chronic low-grade inflammation, and elevated blood sugar levels, increasing the risk of both prediabetes and type 2 diabetes.

Do Plant-Based Diets Reduce Risk and Help with Treatment?

Yes. A growing body of research shows that whole-food, plant-based diets can significantly reduce the risk of type 2 diabetes. For example, in the Adventist Health Study-2, vegans had a 62 percent lower risk of developing diabetes compared with similar, health-conscious nonvegetarians while lacto-ovo vegetarians and pescatarians had 38 percent and 21 percent lower risks, respectively. For those already diagnosed, this way of eating can support weight loss, improve blood sugar control, reduce the risk of complications, and in many cases, even lead to remission.

Well-designed plant-based diets improve insulin sensitivity, reduce inflammation, enhance gut health, and help lower harmful fat deposits in the liver, pancreas, and muscle tissue. These improvements contribute to better blood glucose control and often reduce the need for medication. For those adopting a more plant-based diet, it is important to work with your healthcare provider to manage your decreasing need for treatment.

What Diet Strategies Are Most Effective for Treatment?

When it comes to managing, or even reversing, type 2 diabetes, reducing excess fat in and around vital organs, particularly the liver, pancreas, and skeletal muscles, is key. This internal fat interferes with insulin's ability to function properly.

Evidence shows that losing at least 15 kg (about 33 pounds) significantly increases the chance of diabetes remission. In one major study, 86 percent of participants who reached this target experienced full reversal of their condition. But remission isn't just about weight loss; it's also about improving the quality of what you eat. A whole-food, plant-based diet can help you do both.

Here are some of the most effective, evidence-based strategies:

- **Fill your plate with low-energy-dense foods.** Choose foods that provide fewer calories per bite, such as vegetables, fruits, and broth-based soups, to increase satiety while naturally reducing calorie intake, without having to restrict the volume of food you eat.

- **Eat a wide variety of colorful, high-fiber foods.** A diet based on vegetables, fruits, legumes, whole grains, nuts, and seeds supports insulin sensitivity, reduces inflammation, and promotes a healthier gut microbiome.
- **Minimize saturated fat, especially from animal sources.** Saturated fats, such as palmitic acid (found in red meat, cheese, butter, and tropical oils such as palm oil, palm kernel oil, and coconut oil), can impair insulin signaling and metabolic function.
- **Avoid ultra-processed and refined foods.** These foods are linked to increased insulin resistance and inflammation. Stick to whole, minimally processed choices whenever possible (pages 32–36).
- **Use oils sparingly and enjoy nuts and seeds in moderation.** While some plant oils may have neutral or even beneficial effects, they are calorie-dense and easy to overconsume, which may hinder fat loss—particularly around vital organs. Nuts and seeds, by contrast, are whole foods rich in healthy fats, fiber, plant protein, and essential micronutrients. They have a low glycemic impact and may improve metabolic markers when consumed in modest portions, such as a small handful daily or the use of sesame tahini in a dressing (page 271).
- **Avoid red and processed meats.** These foods are associated with poorer metabolic outcomes, increased insulin resistance, and higher risk of developing type 2 diabetes.
- **Ensure nutritional adequacy.** For those following a plant-based diet, supplementing with vitamin B_{12} and vitamin D is essential for long-term health and balance.

Should Carbohydrates Be Minimized?

Not necessarily. That said, both the quality and quantity of carbohydrate intake play critical roles in metabolic health and weight management. For individuals aiming to lose weight or improve insulin sensitivity, moderating total carbohydrate intake while enhancing the quality of carbohydrates consumed can be very beneficial.

Refined carbohydrates, including white bread, sugary cereals, pastries, and sweetened beverages, are rapidly absorbed, nutrient-poor, and promote glycemic volatility. These should be minimized. In contrast, high-fiber, minimally processed carbohydrate sources, such as legumes, intact whole grains (e.g., oats, barley), starchy vegetables (e.g., winter squash), and fruits, are digested more slowly, promote satiety, and contribute to better glycemic control.

Ultimately, the goal is not to eliminate carbohydrates but to prioritize high-quality, unrefined sources and consume them in portions aligned with individual energy requirements and metabolic goals. Even nutrient-dense carbohydrate sources can contribute to excess caloric intake when consumed in large quantities, particularly among individuals with insulin resistance or sedentary lifestyles.

What Other Lifestyle Factors Are Important?

While diet is foundational, other lifestyle habits are also critical in preventing and managing type 2 diabetes. Regular physical activity is one of the most effective tools for improving insulin sensitivity and lowering blood sugar. Even a brief fifteen- to twenty-minute walk after meals can significantly reduce post-meal glucose spikes. In addition to movement, getting adequate sleep, managing stress, avoiding smoking, and maintaining strong social connections all support better metabolic health and long-term outcomes.

3 KEY TAKEAWAYS

1. Prediabetes and type 2 diabetes are largely preventable and often reversible with a healthy diet, daily physical activity, stress management, and good sleep.

2. Eating a whole-food, plant-based diet rich in vegetables, fruits, legumes, whole grains, nuts, and seeds improves insulin function, supports weight loss, and reduces complications.

3. Minimizing intake of ultra-processed foods, red and processed meats, and added fats is an effective strategy for treating diabetes and achieving long-term blood sugar control.

7. Frailty and Being Underweight

What Is frailty?

Frailty is a complex, age-related condition marked by increased vulnerability to stressors, such as infections, injuries, or hospitalization. It often includes symptoms like muscle weakness, fatigue, slowed walking, weight loss, and low physical activity. Frailty can make everyday tasks, like climbing stairs or carrying groceries, more difficult. This raises the risk of falls, disability, and loss of independence.

While frailty often overlaps with sarcopenia (age-related muscle loss), it also reflects broader physiological decline involving nutrition, energy metabolism, and resilience. Being underweight, typically defined as having a body mass index (BMI) below 18.5, frequently accompanies frailty and further contributes to weakness and poor health outcomes. In older adults, even a BMI under 22 may be associated with increased risk of mortality or functional decline.

The good news? Frailty is not an inevitable consequence of aging. With thoughtful diet and lifestyle strategies, strength, mobility, and vitality can be maintained.

What Increases the Risk of Frailty and Being Underweight?

Frailty and underweight become more common with age due to factors like chronic illness, poor appetite, reduced intake of calories, protein and other nutrients, depression, and social isolation. Without adequate nutrition and activity, older adults lose not only muscle mass but also energy reserves and functional resilience. Medical conditions such as heart disease, diabetes, and osteoporosis can further contribute to frailty risk.

Do Plant-Based Diets Increase the Risk?

Poorly planned plant-based diets can increase the risk of frailty and unintended weight loss, particularly if they are low in calories, high-quality protein, or essential nutrients such as vitamin B_{12}, vitamin D, calcium, and omega-3 fatty acids. Diets that rely heavily on refined grains and ultra-processed foods, or that lack dietary variety, may accelerate muscle loss and impair functional recovery in older adults.

However, research consistently shows that well-planned, nutrient-dense plant-based diets can fully support muscle strength, physical resilience, and healthy longevity. A recent systematic review found a 45 percent lower risk of frailty among those with the highest adherence to a plant-based Mediterranean dietary pattern. In another large cohort study of women, replacing just 5 percent of calories from animal protein with plant protein was associated with a 42 percent reduction in frailty risk.

Can Plant-Based Diets Help Reverse or Prevent Frailty?

Yes. A well-planned, nutrient-dense, and energy-adequate plant-based diet can help prevent or reverse frailty by supporting muscle strength, energy, and resilience. The goal is to consume enough calories, spread protein intake throughout the day, and include a variety of protein-rich plant foods, such as legumes, tofu, tempeh, nuts, seeds, and whole grains. It's also essential to ensure adequate intake of nutrients like calcium, vitamin D, vitamin B_{12}, and omega-3 fatty acids, which may require fortified foods or supplements, particularly for older adults.

What Foods Best Support Strength and Resilience?

Specific plant-based foods provide the nutrients and energy older adults need to maintain muscle, prevent frailty, and promote resilience. These include:

- **Protein-rich foods.** Lentils, tofu, tempeh, quinoa, beans, nuts, seeds, and protein-rich plant milks provide high-quality protein to maintain muscle mass and support energy needs. Protein powders can be added to smoothies. (See page 127.)
- **Calcium-rich foods.** Fortified plant milks, calcium-set tofu, low-oxalate leafy greens like kale and bok choy, and seeds such as chia and sesame provide the calcium needed to protect bone strength and reduce fracture risk.
- **Vitamin D-fortified foods and mushrooms.** Fortified plant milks and cereals, as well as UV-exposed mushrooms (see page 49), can help support vitamin D status and improve calcium absorption. Supplements and/or safe sunlight exposure are often needed, particularly in older adults.

- **Foods rich in healthy fats.** Avocados, olives, nut butters, and seeds provide energy-dense calories that aid in nutrient absorption and help prevent unintended weight loss.
- **Sources of plant-based omega-3s.** Flaxseeds, chia seeds, hempseeds, walnuts, and algae-based DHA/EPA supplements support brain, nerve, and muscle function.

Do People with Frailty Need More Protein?

Yes. Older adults with, or at risk for, frailty typically require higher daily protein intakes than younger adults to support muscle maintenance, strength, and recovery. Without sufficient protein, it becomes much harder to preserve lean body mass, especially when appetite is reduced or weight loss is occurring. Aim for at least 1.2 to 1.5 grams of protein per kilogram of healthy body weight per day. For example, a person whose healthy weight is 150 pounds (68 kg) would need about 82 to 102 grams of protein daily. Distributing protein across meals, rather than concentrating it in one sitting, helps maximize muscle protein synthesis.

What Other Lifestyle Factors Matter?

While nutrition is essential, movement and connection are also important. Engaging in regular physical activity, especially resistance training, helps maintain strength and balance. Simple practices like walking, yoga, and light stretching can make a big difference. Staying socially connected, through community programs, friends, or family, can also boost appetite, mental well-being, and motivation to keep active and well.

3 KEY TAKEAWAYS

1. Frailty and underweight are not inevitable parts of aging. A well-balanced plant-based diet can help preserve physical strength, prevent unintentional weight loss, and support healthy aging.
2. Adequate intake of protein, calories, and key nutrients, especially vitamin B_{12}, vitamin D, calcium, and omega-3s, is essential for preventing and managing frailty on a plant-based diet.
3. Regular physical activity and social connection play vital roles in maintaining mobility, building resilience, supporting mental health, and enhancing overall quality of life.

8. Gout

What Is Gout?

Gout is a painful form of inflammatory arthritis caused by excess uric acid in the bloodstream. Uric acid is a waste product formed when the body breaks down purines—naturally occurring compounds found in many foods and in human cells. When uric acid levels become too high, it can form sharp crystals in the joints, most commonly the big toe, ankles, or knees, leading to sudden episodes of pain, swelling, redness, and heat. These flares may last several days and can recur more often and more severely over time if left untreated.

What Increases the Risk of Gout?

While genetics and age play a role, the greatest contributors are lifestyle related. Risk increases if you are overweight or obese, have type 2 diabetes, metabolic syndrome, kidney disease or hypertension, and are taking certain medications (e.g., diuretics). Diet is also a key player:

- Foods high in animal-based purines, such as red meat, organ meats, and shellfish, raise uric acid levels.
- Alcohol, especially beer and liquor, and sugar-sweetened beverages (particularly those containing high-fructose corn syrup) also promote uric acid production.
- Dehydration, extreme temperatures, joint injury, stress, and poor sleep can further raise risk or trigger flares.

How Do Plant-Based Diets Impact Our Risk?

Plant-based diets can lower uric acid levels by reducing intake of animal purines and supporting kidney function. Whole plant foods are rich in fiber, polyphenols, and antioxidants, which may help to reduce inflammation and promote uric acid excretion. Compared to meat-heavy diets, plant-based patterns are associated with a lower risk of gout.

Do Plant-Based Diets Help with Treatment? Are Beans Bad for Gout?

Plant-based diets can help reduce both the frequency and severity of gout flares. Despite being modestly high in purines, plant foods like beans, lentils, and tofu do not increase gout risk. The body responds differently to plant-derived purines, likely due to their fiber content and accompanying anti-inflammatory compounds.

What Are the Best Dietary Patterns for Treating Gout?

For those managing gout, the ideal diet is low in animal purines and rich in anti-inflammatory, whole-plant foods. Animal-based purines, especially from red meat and certain fish, can increase uric acid production and the risk of painful flares. In contrast, plant-based proteins, including legumes, are associated with reduced risk.

Hydration is also essential. Drinking plenty of water helps the kidneys excrete uric acid more efficiently and may lower serum levels.

Key Dietary Tips Include:

- **Focus on plant proteins.** Include legumes, nuts, seeds, and soy foods, which are safe and beneficial for most people with gout.
- **Emphasize high-fiber, vitamin C-rich foods.** Enjoy plenty of fruits, vegetables, and whole grains to help reduce uric acid and inflammation.
- **Stay well hydrated.** Drink ample water throughout the day to support uric acid excretion through the kidneys.
- **Avoid purine-rich meats.** Limit or eliminate anchovies, sardines, herring, organ meats, and red meat, which raise uric acid levels.
- **Limit alcohol and sugar-sweetened beverages.** These include beer, liquor, and beverages sweetened with sugar or high-fructose corn syrup, which can increase gout risk.
- **Minimize ultra-processed and high-fat foods.** These may impair gut microbial diversity and reduce the body's ability to metabolize uric acid.

What Other Lifestyle Factors Are Important?

Weight management, physical activity, stress reduction, and sleep are all essential for preventing and managing gout. Excess body weight raises uric acid levels and increases the likelihood of flares, so achieving and maintaining a healthy weight can significantly reduce symptoms.

Regular, low-impact exercise, such as walking, swimming, or yoga, not only supports weight management but also improves circulation and reduces inflammation. Managing stress and getting adequate sleep help regulate hormonal and immune function, which may lower flare frequency. In more advanced cases, lifestyle strategies may need to be combined with medications for effective long-term control.

3 KEY TAKEAWAYS

1. Gout is driven by elevated uric acid levels, most often linked to animal-based foods, particularly organ meats and certain seafood, alcohol, and ultra-processed foods. While some plant-based foods also contain purines, they are less strongly linked to gout.

2. A high-fiber, plant-forward diet rich in vegetables, fruits, legumes, whole grains, nuts, and seeds can help manage and prevent gout by reducing inflammation and enhancing uric acid excretion.

3. Hydration, weight management, regular movement, and stress reduction are critical lifestyle tools that support joint health and reduce gout flare frequency and severity.

9. Hypertension

What Is Hypertension?

Hypertension, commonly called high blood pressure, is a condition in which the force of blood pushing against the artery walls is consistently too high. Over time, this extra pressure can damage arteries and organs, increasing the risk of heart disease, stroke, kidney failure, and dementia. In the United States, nearly half of all adults, and about 70 percent of those over age sixty-five, live with hypertension.

What Factors Increase the Risk of Hypertension?

While aging and genetics can raise hypertension risk, lifestyle is the biggest driver. The most common contributors include excess body weight, physical inactivity, smoking, high alcohol intake, chronic stress, inadequate sleep, and diets high in sodium, animal fat, and ultra-processed foods. Underlying conditions like kidney disease, diabetes, and hormonal imbalances can also play a role.

The good news? Many of these risk factors are modifiable. Healthy lifestyle habits can significantly lower blood pressure and prevent complications.

How Do Dietary Patterns Impact Risk?

Diets that emphasize whole-plant foods are consistently linked with lower blood pressure. These include the DASH (Dietary Approaches to Stop Hypertension), Mediterranean, and plant-based diets. In the Adventist Health Study-2, vegans had a 75 percent lower risk of hypertension compared with similar, health-conscious nonvegetarians while lacto-ovo vegetarians had a 55 percent lower risk.

Well-designed, plant-based diets are rich in vegetables, fruits, legumes, whole grains, nuts, and seeds, and naturally low in sodium and high in fiber, potassium, magnesium, and antioxidants. In contrast, Western-style diets, high in processed meats, refined grains, added sugars, and sodium, are closely tied to elevated blood pressure. Shifting to a minimally processed, low-sodium, plant-forward diet is one of the most powerful tools for prevention and treatment.

Where Does Most Sodium Come From?

Sodium lurks in more places than you might think. Here's where it typically comes from:

- Over 70 percent of sodium in the diet comes from processed and restaurant foods, especially bread and rolls, sandwiches, pizza, deli meats, cheese, soups, and salty snacks.
- 10 to 15 percent is added during cooking or at the table.
- 5 to 10 percent occurs naturally in whole foods like vegetables and seaweed.

Even foods that don't taste salty, such as bread and breakfast cereal, can be significant sodium sources.

Are Plant-Based Diets Effective for Treating Hypertension?

Absolutely, but their impact is determined by the quality of the plant-based diet. While healthful, whole-food plant-based diets decrease hypertension risk, plant-based diets that rely on processed foods are high in sodium and increase risk as much as Western-style diets.

The DASH diet, though not strictly vegetarian, was originally designed to capture the blood pressure–lowering benefits of a vegetarian diet while including small amounts of animal products to appeal to the general public. Its success highlights the power of plant-forward eating patterns.

What Dietary Strategies Help Lower Blood Pressure?

To support healthy blood pressure, focus on dietary choices that reduce inflammation, support vascular health, and moderate sodium. Simple daily habits can make a big difference:

- Base your meals on fiber-rich vegetables, fruits, legumes, whole grains, nuts, and seeds.
- Limit sodium intake to under 1,500 mg/day. The best way to do this is by avoiding ultra-processed foods, choosing no-, low-, or reduced-sodium versions of packaged items, and cooking your own food.

- Read labels carefully, especially on sauces, dressings, breads, veggie burgers, and canned vegetables and soups that often contain hidden sodium and choose products with lower levels.
- Canned beans often contain significant amounts of sodium, although no-salt-added varieties are widely available. Draining and rinsing reduces sodium by about 40 percent.
- Cut back on added sugars and saturated fats, especially from processed meats and tropical oils.
- Stay hydrated with water and avoid sugary drinks and excess caffeine.

If you're reducing or eliminating iodized table salt to lower sodium intake, it's important to ensure you're still getting enough iodine, which is essential for thyroid and cognitive function. Good alternatives include iodine supplements (including multivitamins with iodine) and appropriate amounts of sea vegetables (such as nori, wakame, or dulse). Be cautious with kelp and other seaweeds as their iodine content can be extremely concentrated and inconsistent, making it easy to exceed safe intake levels. (See page 168). Some seaweeds are also high in sodium (check labels).

What Other Lifestyle Changes Help Reduce Blood Pressure?

While diet is foundational, long-term blood pressure control depends on a combination of healthy lifestyle practices. These habits not only lower blood pressure but also improve heart function, reduce stress, and enhance overall well-being:

- **Move more.** Regular physical activity strengthens the heart, improves blood vessel function, and supports weight management.
- **Maintain a healthy weight.** If you are overweight or obese, losing just 5 to 10 percent of your body weight can significantly reduce blood pressure, improve insulin sensitivity, and lower cardiovascular risk.

- **Avoid tobacco and limit alcohol.** Both can elevate blood pressure and damage blood vessels. Reducing or eliminating these substances supports cardiovascular and overall health.
- **Manage stress effectively.** Techniques such as meditation, deep breathing, yoga, or time in nature can help lower blood pressure and improve emotional resilience.
- **Get quality sleep.** Aim for seven to nine hours of restorative sleep per night to support healthy blood pressure regulation and hormonal balance.

3 KEY TAKEAWAYS

1. A healthful plant-based diet, regular movement, stress management, and good sleep are powerful tools for preventing and treating high blood pressure.
2. DASH, Mediterranean, and whole-food, plant-based diets are effective in reducing blood pressure and improving overall heart health.
3. Western-style diets rich in salt, processed foods, and added sugars raise blood pressure. Cut back on ultra-processed foods, minimize restaurant meals, and aim to use less sodium.

10. Macular Degeneration and Cataracts

What Are Common Age-Related Eye Problems?

As we age, it's common to experience vision changes, such as difficulty reading fine print or seeing clearly in low light. Two of the most prevalent conditions are age-related macular degeneration (AMD) and cataracts.

AMD affects the macula, the central part of the retina responsible for sharp, central vision. This results in difficulty seeing objects directly in front of you. Cataracts occur when the lens of the eye becomes cloudy, leading to blurry vision, glare (or lens cloudiness), light sensitivity, and trouble seeing at night. These and other eye conditions affect millions of older adults, and as the population ages, their prevalence is expected to rise.

What Factors Increase the Risk of These Eye Conditions?

While aging is the biggest risk factor for vision problems, it's far from the only one. Fortunately, many other factors are within our control. Smoking, high blood pressure, excess weight, and diets high in unhealthy fats or low in carotenoids from orange-fleshed vegetables and fruits can increase the risk of macular degeneration.

Cataracts, on the other hand, are more strongly linked to diabetes, long-term steroid use, past eye surgeries, and excessive sun exposure without protection. The encouraging news? Small lifestyle changes can make a big difference. Wearing UV-protective sunglasses, staying smoke-free, and having regular eye exams can help protect your vision and detect issues early.

Do Dietary Patterns Impact Eye Disease Risk?

Yes—diet plays a critical role in preserving vision as we age. Nutrient-dense eating patterns reduce oxidative stress and chronic inflammation, both key drivers of age-related eye diseases. Whole-food, plant-based diets, rich in vegetables, fruits, legumes, whole grains, and healthy fats, provide a wide range of protective compounds that support long-term eye health:

- **Antioxidants,** including vitamin C, vitamin E, and provitamin A carotenoids (like beta-carotene), help neutralize free radicals that damage eye cells.

    - Vitamin C supports the health of blood vessels in the eye and may reduce cataract risk (page 153.)
    - Vitamin E helps protect retinal cells from oxidative damage (page 154.)
    - Beta-carotene and other provitamin A carotenoids function as antioxidants and are converted to vitamin A as needed.
- **Vitamin A** (retinol) is essential to support night vision and the health of the retina and cornea. While retinol is not an antioxidant, adequate vitamin A, whether from provitamin A carotenoids (from colorful plant foods like carrots, sweet potatoes, and dark leafy greens), supplements, or animal sources (such as eggs, and dairy), is critical for preventing night blindness and xerophthalmia (page 151.)
- **Macular carotenoids,** particularly lutein and zeaxanthin, are not converted to vitamin A but play a key role in eye protection.
    - These pigments accumulate in the macula, where they act like internal sunglasses, filtering harmful blue light, reducing oxidative stress, and supporting visual sharpness.
    - They are abundant in dark leafy greens (spinach, kale, collards, and bok choy), corn, and colorful vegetables like orange peppers, yams, sweet potatoes, and carrots.
- **Omega-3 fatty acids,** especially DHA, are structural components of the retina.
    - DHA helps preserve photoreceptor function and may reduce the risk of age-related macular degeneration (AMD) and dry eye disease.
    - ALA (from flax, chia, hemp, walnuts) provides modest conversion to DHA and EPA while algae-based supplements offer a direct plant-based DHA source.

Together, these nutrients help protect against macular degeneration, cataracts, and dry eye syndrome, and may also support optic nerve health and intraocular pressure regulation in glaucoma—preserving visual function well into later life.

Can Plant-Based Diets Help with Treatment?

While high-quality diets may not reverse conditions like AMD or cataracts, they can help slow progression, reduce inflammation, and support the health of the remaining eye tissue. Diets rich in whole plant foods have been associated with slower AMD progression and may also improve outcomes in other age-related eye diseases. Ensuring adequate intake of protective nutrients, such as lutein, zeaxanthin, other carotenoids, omega-3 fatty acids, and antioxidants, can make a meaningful difference in preserving vision over time.

What Other Lifestyle Factors Are Important for Eye Health?

Beyond diet, several lifestyle habits can make a meaningful difference in preserving vision and preventing disease:

- **Protect your eyes from UV rays.** Wear sunglasses with full-spectrum UV protection or a wide-brimmed hat when outdoors to reduce cumulative sun damage.
- **Stay physically active.** Regular movement supports healthy blood flow to the eyes, which helps deliver essential nutrients and oxygen to retinal tissues.
- **Don't smoke.** Smoking increases oxidative stress and inflammation, dramatically raising the risk of both AMD and cataracts.
- **Schedule regular eye exams.** Routine checkups help detect changes early and allow for timely treatment to slow progression and protect remaining vision.

3 KEY TAKEAWAYS

1. Age-related eye conditions like AMD and cataracts are common but not inevitable. Diet and lifestyle choices play a key role in their prevention and management.

2. Plant-based diets rich in antioxidants, carotenoids, and healthy fats help protect the eyes from oxidative stress and inflammation.

3. Sun protection, regular exercise, and avoiding smoking are critical to maintaining lifelong vision health.

11. Osteoporosis and Osteopenia

What Are Osteoporosis and Osteopenia?

Osteoporosis is a condition marked by porous, fragile bones that break more easily, often without a major fall or injury. Osteopenia is a less severe form of bone loss, in which bone density is lower than normal but not yet in the osteoporotic range. Think of osteopenia as an early warning sign: Bone loss has begun, but proactive steps can help preserve bone strength and prevent progression.

How Common Is Osteoporosis?

Osteoporosis is very common in older adults, especially women. In the United States, about one in four women over age sixty-five and roughly one in seventeen men in the same age group have osteoporosis. Even more concerning, around 54 million Americans have low bone density (osteopenia), increasing their risk for future fractures.

What Dietary Factors Increase the Risk of Osteoporosis?

Some of the common dietary habits that undermine bone health include:

- **Diets low in calcium and vitamin D.** These fail to provide the raw materials needed to build and maintain strong bones. Vitamin D also plays a critical role in helping the body absorb and retain calcium efficiently.
- **Inadequate intake of other bone-supportive nutrients.** Low intake of nutrients such as magnesium, potassium, vitamin K, and vitamin C can impair bone formation and increase inflammation, which may accelerate bone loss.
- **Inadequate protein intake.** Protein is essential for maintaining the mineralized structure of bone and supporting muscle strength. Insufficient intake can weaken both bone and muscle, increasing fracture risk. Adequate protein, from either plant or animal sources, supports bone density, particularly when calcium intake is sufficient. Plant-based protein sources such as legumes, soy foods, nuts, and seeds offer additional benefits, providing calcium, magnesium, potassium, fiber, and antioxidant compounds that support bone health.
- **Diets high in salt, soda, ultra-processed foods, and alcohol.** These dietary patterns may increase urinary calcium losses and displace more nutrient-dense foods, contributing to reduced bone strength over time.

Which Other Lifestyle Factors Increase Osteoporosis Risk?

Smoking, inactivity, excessive alcohol intake, and chronic diseases like diabetes or inflammatory conditions can all contribute to bone loss. A sedentary lifestyle leads to weaker bones while smoking can interfere with calcium absorption and reduce bone-forming cells.

Can Plant-Based Diets Help Prevent and Treat Osteoporosis?

Yes, when well-planned plant-based diets can support bone health and play a meaningful role in osteoporosis prevention and management. However, it is important to note that several studies have reported a higher risk of low bone mineral density and fractures among vegetarians, and particularly vegans, compared with omnivores, especially when key nutrients are not adequately supplied. The increased risk appears to be largely explained by modifiable factors, including lower intakes of calcium, protein, and vitamin D, as well as lower body weight. Bone is a dynamic, living tissue that is constantly being broken down and rebuilt. To maintain strength and structure, it requires weight-bearing exercise and a steady supply of nutrients, including calcium, magnesium, potassium, protein, and vitamins C, D, and K. Vitamin K, which is essential for both blood clotting and bone metabolism, exists in two main forms:

1. **Vitamin K1 (phylloquinone)** is found abundantly in leafy green vegetables such as kale, collards, spinach, turnip greens, beet greens, bok choy, and Swiss chard. It supports normal blood coagulation.
2. **Vitamin K2 (menaquinone)** is present in smaller amounts in plant-based diets, primarily through fermented foods like natto (a particularly rich source), tempeh, and sauerkraut. Trace amounts may also be produced by gut bacteria, though the extent of this contribution remains uncertain. Vitamin K2 plays a key role in bone mineralization.

To Optimize Bone Health on a Plant-Based Diet:

- **Boost Calcium.** Choose calcium-set tofu and fortified plant-based milks for calcium and vitamin D. Also include low-oxalate leafy greens like bok choy, broccoli, collards, kale, and turnip greens for well-absorbed calcium. If using calcium supplements, take just enough to meet the RDA, typically about 400 to 600 mg. Divide into two doses (200-300 mg per dose).

- **Prioritize Plant Protein.** Get adequate protein from beans, lentils, soy foods, and fortified plant-based milks to support bone structure and remodeling.
- **Supplement Smartly.** Consider supplements for vitamin D, vitamin B_{12}, and possibly vitamin K_2, especially for older adults or those at risk of deficiency.
- **Eat Sufficient Calories.** Inadequate calorie intake can lead to low body weight, which is associated with reduced bone density and increased fracture risk.

Emerging research suggests that plant-based diets may also support bone health by reducing inflammation, improving calcium retention, and promoting a healthy gut microbiome—all of which contribute to stronger bones.

What Other Lifestyle Factors Help Maintain or Build Strong Bones?

While diet is important, maintaining strong and healthy bones depends on a combination of healthy lifestyle practices. These habits also support mobility, independence, and overall well-being:

- **Move with Purpose.** Staying physically active is one of the most powerful ways to support bone health. Weight-bearing and resistance exercises, such as walking, dancing, hiking, stair climbing, strength training, and vigorous gardening, stimulate bone formation. While swimming is great for cardiovascular health, it doesn't offer the same bone-building benefits.
- **Ensure Adequate Vitamin D.** Whether from regular sunlight exposure or supplements, vitamin D is essential for calcium absorption and overall skeletal strength.

- **Limit Harmful Habits.** Avoid smoking and limit alcohol, as both can contribute to bone loss and increase the risk of fractures.
- **Prevent Falls.** Consider balance training, home safety modifications, and fall-prevention programs to help reduce fracture risk and maintain independence as you age. Fall prevention is just as important as building bone.

3 KEY TAKEAWAYS

1. Osteopenia and osteoporosis are common in older adults, especially in women who are thin.
2. A well-designed plant-based diet can help prevent and manage osteoporosis by supplying calcium, vitamin D, protein, and other key nutrients.
3. Regular weight-bearing activity, avoiding smoking, limiting alcohol, and preventing falls are all essential to lifelong bone strength.

12. Overweight and Obesity

How Are Overweight and Obesity Defined?

Overweight and obesity are typically measured using Body Mass Index (BMI), which compares your weight to your height. You can search for BMI Index and for waist to hip ratio online. A BMI between 25 and 29.9 is considered overweight while a BMI of 30 or higher falls into the obese category.

Simple measurements that can be done at home may be more reliable indicators of health risk than BMI. These include measuring the circumference of your waist or measuring your waist-to-hip ratio.

In the United States, over 73 percent of adults age twenty and older are either overweight or obese. About 31 percent are classified as overweight, and more than 40 percent meet the criteria for obesity. Among seniors, approximately 41 percent of those aged sixty-five to seventy-four and nearly 28 percent of those over seventy-five are classified as obese. The somewhat lower rates in the oldest adults may partly reflect age-related muscle loss, illness-related weight loss, survival bias, and limitations of BMI in older populations.

Does Aging Impact Weight Gain?

Yes, aging brings changes that make weight gain more likely. As we get older, our hormone levels change and metabolism naturally slows down, so we burn fewer calories at rest. Muscle mass also tends to decline with age, which further reduces calorie burning, especially if physical activity drops off. If eating habits stay the same while fewer calories are being burned, weight gain can sneak up on us.

How Do Plant-Based Diets Reduce the Risk of Weight Gain?

Plant-based diets can be a powerful ally in maintaining a healthy weight. Diets centered around vegetables, fruits, legumes, whole grains, nuts, and seeds are typically lower in calories and saturated fats than Standard American Diets. They're also high in fiber, which helps us feel full and satisfied, and support steady blood sugar levels.

What's more, these foods contain antioxidants and phytochemicals that reduce inflammation—a key factor in obesity-related conditions. Well-planned plant-based diets have been shown to support fat loss while preserving muscle, making them ideal for older adults who want to stay strong, mobile, and metabolically healthy.

What Are the Risks and Benefits of GLP-1 Medications?

GLP-1 receptor agonists (e.g., Ozempic, Wegovy, and Mounjaro) were originally developed to help manage type 2 diabetes, but they've gained popularity for weight loss. These medications work by mimicking glucagon-like peptide-1 (GLP-1), a natural gut hormone released after eating.

GLP-1 reduces appetite, slows gastric emptying, and enhances feelings of fullness, all of which can lead to reduced calorie intake and weight loss. Emerging research suggests they may also help preserve muscle during weight loss, which is an important benefit for older adults. But these drugs are not without downsides:

- **Cost.** Without insurance, monthly costs range from $900 to $1,350.
- **Side effects.** Common issues include nausea, vomiting, and diarrhea; more serious risks include pancreatitis, gallbladder problems, and kidney damage.
- **Temporary results.** Weight loss often plateaus, and weight regain is common once the medication is discontinued, as appetite typically returns.

While GLP-1 medications may offer important benefits, especially when combined with healthy lifestyle changes and appropriate medical supervision, they do not replace the long-term value of a nutrient-rich, plant-based diet, regular physical activity, and supportive behaviors.

What Other Lifestyle Factors Help Manage Body Weight?

Healthy weight management is about more than just food. Lifestyle habits play a major role, especially as you age:

- **Physical activity.** Boosts metabolism, helps preserve muscle, and burns calories. Strength training and aerobic exercise are especially helpful.
- **Sleep.** Impacts hormones that regulate hunger and fullness. Aiming for seven to eight hours of quality rest can support healthy weight.
- **Hydration.** Supports metabolism and may help reduce unnecessary snacking by controlling feelings of hunger.
- **Social connection.** Provides encouragement and accountability, whether it's a walking buddy, a fitness class, or simply a shared commitment to healthy living.

3 KEY TAKEAWAYS

1. Aging increases the risk of weight gain due to slower metabolism, reduced muscle mass, and lower activity levels, all of which make weight management more challenging.
2. GLP-1 medications support weight loss, but they are costly, carry risks, and weight regain is common once they are stopped.
3. A well-planned plant-based diet, regular physical activity, good sleep, hydration, and meaningful social connections offer safe, sustainable ways to maintain a healthy weight and preserve muscle as we age.

13. Respiratory Disorders

What Are the Most Common Respiratory Conditions in Older Adults?

As we grow older, it's normal to experience changes in breathing, but persistent shortness of breath, coughing, or wheezing may signal something more than aging. The most common respiratory conditions among seniors include chronic obstructive pulmonary disease (COPD), asthma, chronic bronchitis, and pneumonia.

COPD, which includes emphysema and chronic bronchitis, is especially prevalent, with over 10 percent of older adults in the United States being affected. The rate increases sharply with age, exceeding 25 percent among those eighty-five and older. COPD is frequently underdiagnosed, and many seniors live with the condition but do not have a formal diagnosis. Asthma, too, may persist or worsen with age and is often underdiagnosed in older adults because its symptoms can mimic other conditions.

Does Age Increase Respiratory Disease Risk?

Yes. Aging naturally brings changes that affect lung health. Lung tissue becomes less elastic, respiratory muscles weaken, and the immune system loses some of its strength, making it harder to fend off infections and recover from illness. Older adults may also have long-term exposure to air pollution, occupational hazards, or a past history of smoking.

But aging is only part of the equation. Diet, physical activity, and other lifestyle choices play a powerful role in preserving respiratory health, and a much bigger role than many realize.

Can Eating a Plant-Based Diet Play a Role in Respiratory Health?

Absolutely. Plant-based diets, rich in colorful fruits, vegetables, legumes, whole grains, nuts, and seeds, are naturally high in antioxidants and anti-inflammatory compounds that protect lung tissue. These nutrients help reduce oxidative stress and inflammation, two key drivers of chronic respiratory diseases.

Studies show that people who consume more fruits and vegetables tend to have better lung function and are less likely to develop conditions like COPD. Leafy greens, berries, citrus fruits, and cruciferous vegetables like broccoli are especially beneficial for lung health.

Can Diet Actually Reverse These Conditions?

While plant-based diets won't reverse structural damage caused by diseases like COPD, they can help manage symptoms, slow disease progression, and in some cases, improve overall lung function. This is especially true for those who are overweight. Excess weight can press on the lungs and diaphragm, making breathing more difficult.

Even modest weight loss, achieved through a fiber-rich, plant-based diet, can ease shortness of breath and reduce flare-ups. One study published in *The Lancet* found that individuals who adopted a plant-forward lifestyle, including diet, exercise, and smoking cessation, experienced measurable improvements in respiratory health.

Can Other Lifestyle Changes Make a Difference?

Yes. In addition to dietary strategies, several lifestyle modifications can significantly support respiratory health:

- **Engage in regular physical activity.** Gentle exercises such as walking, tai chi, or chair yoga can improve lung capacity and strengthen respiratory muscles. More vigorous exercise is suitable for many.
- **Avoid tobacco and second-hand smoke.** Smoking cessation and smoke-free environments are critical for lung preservation and disease prevention.
- **Minimize exposure to indoor air pollutants.** Reduce contact

with dust, mold, pet dander, and chemical irritants from household cleaners.

- **Prioritize adequate sleep and stress management.** Both support immune function and reduce inflammatory burden on the respiratory system.
- **Stay informed about vaccinations.** Vaccines such as those for influenza, COVID-19, pneumococcal disease, and RSV may help reduce the risk of respiratory infections, complications, and hospitalizations, particularly in older adults. Discuss with your healthcare provider what may be appropriate for you.

3 KEY TAKEAWAYS

1. Older adults are more susceptible to respiratory conditions like COPD and asthma, but lifestyle changes can help prevent or manage them.
2. A plant-based diet rich in, vegetables, fruits, legumes, and whole grains supports lung function by lowering inflammation, improving immune response, and helping with weight management.
3. Regular physical activity, avoiding smoke, maintaining a healthy weight, and staying up-to-date on vaccines all contribute to healthier lungs as we age.

14. Sarcopenia

What Is Sarcopenia, and How Common Is It?

Sarcopenia is the age-related loss of muscle mass, strength, and function. Unlike frailty, a broader condition that may include weakness, weight loss, fatigue, and reduced resilience, sarcopenia refers specifically to the decline in muscle tissue and physical strength. It can begin as early as age fifty and tends to accelerate after age sixty. This muscle loss is more than just a normal part of aging, it's a serious health issue that raises the risk of falls, disability, hospitalization, and loss of independence.

Sarcopenia can affect people of all body sizes, including those who are overweight or obese. When muscle loss occurs alongside excess body fat, it can trigger a condition known as sarcopenic obesity. This further impairs mobility and makes everyday activities, like climbing stairs or carrying groceries, more difficult. Estimates of how common sarcopenia is vary by age and how it's defined, but research suggests that between 5 percent and 13 percent of adults in their sixties and seventies, and up to 50 percent of those over eighty, may be affected.

How Does Aging Impact Our Risk?

As we grow older, several changes in the body contribute to muscle loss: Hormone levels decline, inflammation tends to rise, and we move less than we used to. In addition, many older adults lose muscle while gaining fat, especially around the abdomen. This shift not only affects strength and balance, but it also impacts metabolism, blood sugar control, and overall vitality.

How Do Plant-Based Diets Impact Our Risk?

A well-planned plant-based diet, built around fruits, vegetables, legumes, whole grains, nuts, and seeds, can help reduce the risk of sarcopenia and excess weight gain. These foods provide fiber, antioxidants, and anti-inflammatory compounds that support muscle and metabolic health.

Protein remains essential for maintaining muscle, and plant-based sources like beans, lentils, tofu, tempeh, edamame, quinoa, nuts, and seeds can supply what aging muscles need. Protein powders, for example, as part of smoothies can also be a convenient option. (See page 127.)

Research shows that older adults who follow healthful plant-based diets tend to have better body composition, stronger muscles, and less chronic inflammation compared to those who consume more animal-centered Western diets. It may surprise you to learn that plant protein is not only adequate but also protective, with higher intakes associated with a reduced risk of low muscle mass.

Can Plant-Based Diets Help Reverse This Condition?

While sarcopenia is challenging, it's not irreversible. Studies show that with the proper nutrition and sufficient physical activity, it's possible to slow or even partially reverse muscle loss. Plant-based diets that provide adequate protein, especially when combined with resistance training, can support muscle maintenance and growth in older adults.

Emerging evidence also shows that when total protein and calorie intake are sufficient, well-balanced vegan diets support muscle protein synthesis at levels comparable to omnivorous diets in older adults. The key is to eat a variety of protein-rich plant foods throughout the day to meet amino acid needs for muscle repair and maintenance.

What Other Lifestyle Factors Matter?

Exercise is vital, particularly strength training exercises like using resistance bands, lifting light weights, or doing bodyweight exercises such as squats, push-ups, planks, and lunges. Even simple routines done consistently can help maintain or rebuild muscle.

Getting enough sleep, managing stress, and avoiding smoking or excessive alcohol use are also vital for muscle and metabolic health. And staying socially connected matters, too! Older adults who remain socially engaged tend to move more and have better overall well-being.

3 KEY TAKEAWAYS:

1. Sarcopenia affects an estimated 5 percent to 13 percent of adults in their sixties and up to 50 percent of those over eighty, increasing the risk of falls, frailty, and loss of independence.

2. A plant-based diet rich in protein, fiber, and anti-inflammatory nutrients can help preserve muscle mass and support healthy aging.

3. Resistance exercise, good sleep, and staying socially active are essential strategies for preventing and managing sarcopenia.

15. Stroke

What Is a Stroke?

A stroke is a medical emergency that occurs when blood flow to part of the brain is interrupted, either by a blockage such as a blood clot (ischemic stroke) or by a burst blood vessel (hemorrhagic stroke). Without oxygen and nutrients, brain cells begin to die within minutes, which can result in lasting brain damage, disability, or even death.

Strokes can affect movement, speech, memory, and balance, depending on which part of the brain is impacted. They are especially important to watch for in older adults. Each year nearly 800,000 Americans have a stroke, and about three out of four cases occur in people over sixty-five. Estimates suggest that around 7 percent to 13 percent of older adults report having had a stroke during their lifetime.

What Raises Your Risk?

Several common health issues increase the risk of stroke, especially high blood pressure, high cholesterol, type 2 diabetes, and atrial fibrillation. Other contributors include smoking, obesity, physical inactivity, and poor dietary habits.

Age is another factor. Stroke risk doubles every ten years after age fifty-five. Family history, race, and previous heart problems also play a role. The good news is that many of these risk factors are modifiable, and up to 80 percent of strokes can be prevented through proactive lifestyle and medical management.

Do Plant-Based Diets Protect Against Stroke?

Plant-based diets built around vegetables, fruits, legumes, whole grains, nuts, and seeds are associated with a lower risk of stroke, particularly ischemic stroke. These foods are naturally low in saturated fat, cholesterol-free, and rich in fiber, antioxidants, potassium, and magnesium—nutrients that help regulate blood pressure, reduce inflammation, and support vascular health. Some studies, however, have reported a higher risk of hemorrhagic stroke among vegetarians and vegans, particularly when diets are not well planned and low in key nutrients such as vitamin B_{12}.

Can Plant-Based Eating Help After a Stroke?

Yes. After a stroke, adopting a well-balanced plant-based diet can help control underlying conditions like high blood pressure, cholesterol, and diabetes, which reduces the chance of having another stroke. These diets can also promote better recovery by supporting healthy weight, circulation, and brain function. Key strategies include:

- **Focusing on nutrient-dense plant foods** like leafy greens, berries, legumes, whole grains, nuts, and seeds to support vascular and brain health

- **Ensuring adequate protein intake** from sources such as tofu, tempeh, lentils, and fortified soy, pea, or hemp milks to aid in healing and muscle maintenance
- **Including reliable sources of vitamin B_{12},** either through fortified foods or supplements, to support nerve and cognitive function
- **Getting enough omega-3 fats,** especially DHA and EPA from algae-based supplements, to help reduce inflammation and protect the brain

A registered dietitian can help tailor a post-stroke eating plan that meets individual needs, especially when appetite, chewing, or swallowing have been affected.

What Other Lifestyle Choices Help Reduce Stroke Risk?

Your daily habits matter. Staying physically active, even a brisk walk for thirty minutes most days, helps protect your heart and brain. Not smoking, managing stress, getting good quality sleep, and taking medications as prescribed all work together to reduce stroke risk. Getting regular checkups to monitor blood pressure and cholesterol is key to prevention.

3 KEY TAKEAWAYS

1. Most strokes are preventable, and healthy lifestyle choices can dramatically lower your risk.
2. A plant-based diet supports heart and brain health, reducing the chance of both initial and repeat strokes.
3. Daily movement, stress management, and regular checkups are just as important as healthy eating for keeping your brain strong and your body resilient.

Summary

In this chapter, we've explored how specific dietary and lifestyle adjustments can help address many of the health conditions that become more common with age. While it's easy to assume that each chronic condition requires its own unique diet, the evidence tells a different story. A whole-food, plant-based diet, rich in vegetables, fruits, legumes, whole grains, nuts, and seeds, not only helps prevent many chronic diseases, but can also support their management and, in some cases, even contribute to reversal. That's because many of these conditions share underlying root causes, including:

- **Chronic inflammation:** a persistent, low-level activation of the immune system that can damage tissues and organs over time
- **Oxidative stress:** an imbalance between harmful free radicals and the body's ability to neutralize them, leading to cell and tissue damage
- **Dysbiosis:** an imbalance in the gut microbiome that can impair digestion, weaken immunity, and promote inflammation
- **Lipotoxicity:** the buildup of excess fat in organs and muscles where it doesn't belong, interfering with their normal function

All of these factors are heavily influenced by what we eat, and can be improved with a thoughtful, plant-forward approach.

KEY TAKEAWAYS

A well-planned, nutritionally adequate, whole-food, plant-rich diet, featuring a variety of colorful vegetables, fruits, legumes, whole grains, nuts, and seeds, offers broad protection and support for most chronic conditions that arise with aging.

Plant-based diets are a powerful complement to medical treatment. Let your healthcare provider know if you make dietary changes, as doing so may affect your medication needs and overall treatment plan.

Lifestyle habits matter! Regular physical activity, including both cardio and strength training, is essential for staying strong and independent. Other key healthy habits include not smoking, limiting or avoiding alcohol and other addictive substances, managing stress, getting restful sleep, and nurturing social connections. A healthy diet can make it easier to feel energized and motivated to be active and engaged!

From Healing to Nourishing

Understanding the role of plant-based eating in managing chronic conditions is only part of the story. The next step is learning how to meet your body's evolving needs with intention and balance. As we grow older, our nutrient requirements shift, even as our appetite or energy intake may decline. In the next chapter, we'll explore the individual nutrients delivered by a plant-based diet as support for strength, vitality, and well-being at every stage of aging.

CHAPTER 5

NUTRITION ESSENTIALS

This Chapter at a Glance

In this chapter, we explore how nutrient needs change with age, and how to meet those needs through thoughtful, plant-based choices. You'll learn how to maintain strength, energy, and resilience with nutrition strategies that are tailored to the later decades of life.

You will:

- Understand why nutrient density matters more than ever as energy needs decline with age.
- Learn how macronutrients, especially protein, fiber, and healthy fats, support strength, immunity, and metabolic health.
- Get practical guidance on meeting micronutrient needs, including vitamins B_{12}, D, and A, the minerals calcium, iron, iodine, zinc, and more.
- Gain tools to manage age-related challenges like reduced appetite, digestion issues, and medication-nutrient interactions.

Maria's Story: The Power of Precision

Maria took a thoughtful and well-informed approach to her transition to a plant-based lifestyle. From the outset, she began taking daily vitamin B_{12} and vitamin D supplements. Her meals reflected a well-planned routine: oatmeal with ground flaxseed in the morning, abundant salads at lunch, and a variety of creative bowls, salads, stews, casseroles, and ethnic dishes for dinner.

Despite her progress, Maria recently began to feel unusually fatigued, particularly in the late afternoon. Climbing stairs left her legs feeling heavy, and she noticed bruises appearing without apparent cause. At her most recent wellness check, her physician told her that her iron status was borderline and suggested adding a supplement. In addition, her doctor noted that her easy bruising and general fatigue could suggest marginal protein intake.

This feedback surprised Maria. Like many, she had embraced a common belief within some plant-based circles that if you eat enough calories, you'll naturally get enough protein. Maria began to realize that a successful plant-based diet, particularly in later life, is not simply about avoiding animal products. Rather, it requires a deliberate focus on ensuring that each bite delivers essential macro and micronutrients that her body needs to maintain function, resilience, and vitality.

Meeting Changing Plant-Based Dietary Needs with Confidence

Maria's experience highlights a pivotal truth: Thriving on a plant-based diet in later life demands an informed, proactive approach that accounts for shifting nutrient needs, metabolic adaptations, and age-related physiological changes. As we age, we experience a decline in lean body mass, reduced energy expenditure, changes in digestive efficiency, and evolving hormone and kidney function—all of which influence not just what we need to eat but also how we absorb and utilize nutrients.

To address these changes, we must rethink both what and how much we eat. Energy needs typically decline, making nutrient density increasingly important. This means that every bite matters. Foods rich in protein, micronutrients, healthy fats, fiber, and antioxidants become central to preserving muscle mass, immune function, and cognitive health.

In this chapter you'll learn how to strike the right calorie balance while avoiding undernutrition or unintentional weight loss. You'll learn how macronutrients, especially the quality, quantity, and timing of protein, contribute to maintaining strength and mobility while complex carbohydrates and anti-inflammatory fats support digestive and metabolic resilience. You'll also find evidence-based guidance on meeting micronutrient needs, particularly for nutrients like vitamin B12, vitamin D, calcium, iodine, magnesium, iron, and zinc, through strategic food choices, fortification, and supplementation when needed.

Finally, we offer practical tools for adapting plant-based eating to common age-related challenges such as reduced appetite, chewing or swallowing difficulties, medication-nutrient interactions, and financial limitations. With the right strategies, a plant-based diet in later life becomes not only feasible but a powerful, sustainable path to vitality and independence.

Let's begin by looking at how our energy needs change with age and why choosing nutrient-dense foods becomes increasingly important.

The Need for Fewer Calories

As we get older, our need for calories typically declines due to several physiological and lifestyle-related factors:

- **Reduced resting metabolic rate.** The amount of energy required to sustain basic functions such as breathing, circulation, and cellular maintenance tends to decrease with age.
- **Loss of lean body mass.** Muscle tissue, which is more metabolically active than fat, often diminishes over time.
- **Lower physical activity levels.** Although staying active brings considerable benefits, many older adults move less as they age.
- **Hormonal shifts.** Changes in thyroid function, sex hormones, and other regulatory systems can reduce energy needs.
- **Decreased appetite.** Many older adults experience a natural decline in hunger, which can affect food intake.

Yet, while total energy needs may fall, needs for most essential nutrients remain the same and, in some cases, even increase, such as for protein, vitamin D, and vitamin B_6. This means that nutrient density, or the amount of nutrition delivered per calorie, becomes increasingly important.

In other words, as our calorie "budget" shrinks, the quality of what we eat must improve. Individual energy needs vary based on gender, body weight and composition, age, and activity level. However, a common challenge in later life is striking the right balance between too many and too few calories.

Too Many Calories

Excess calorie intake, particularly from low-nutrient, highly processed foods based on refined carbohydrates and added fats, can lead to increased body fat, which is associated with chronic diseases such as type 2 diabetes, cardiovascular disease, and certain cancers. Regular physical activity and a healthy, whole-food, plant-based diet are key to achieving and maintaining a healthy body weight. (For more on this, see the Overweight and Obesity section in Chapter 4, page 105.)

Too Few Calories

Conversely, some older adults struggle to consume enough calories to meet their basic energy and nutrient needs. This may be due to:

- **Oral health issues,** such as poor dentition, chewing difficulty, or dysphagia (difficulty swallowing)
- **Gastrointestinal discomfort** when consuming bulky or high-fiber foods
- **Acid reflux or GERD,** which can reduce appetite and make eating uncomfortable
- **Psychosocial and financial factors,** including isolation, mobility challenges, depression, grief, or limited access to fresh, nutrient-rich foods
- **Appetite suppression** due to medications, chronic illness, or loss of taste due to zinc deficiency

In these situations, even normally healthful habits, such as beginning meals with a large salad, may unintentionally displace calorie-dense foods and lead to under-eating.

Nourishing, High-Energy Plant Foods

For older adults with reduced appetite or difficulty meeting energy needs, it's helpful to prioritize plant foods that are both calorie-dense and nutrient-rich. Examples include avocados, nuts, seeds (and their butters), dried fruits, whole grains, legumes, and tofu. For those with chewing or swallowing issues, smoothies and blended soups can help meet energy needs. Cooked, steamed, or sautéed vegetables, which are easier to chew and digest, can also feature prominently.

Rather than relying on two or three large meals daily, small, frequent meals and snacks can boost energy intakes. For snacks, you can include trail mix, oatmeal with seeds or walnuts and raisins, whole grain bread or pita with hummus, nut butter, or avocado, and Tasty Tofu cubes (page 299). For more on this topic, see the sections on Frailty and on Sarcopenia in Chapter 4 (pages 86 and 111).

Protein

Protein plays a vital role in keeping us strong, steady, and resilient as we age. It supports everything from muscle maintenance and immune defense to hormone production and wound healing. Even though our cells continue to renew themselves throughout life, the body becomes less efficient at building and maintaining muscle as we get older. That's why older adults actually need *more* protein per kilogram of healthy body weight, not less. And if you're managing a chronic condition, healing from illness or surgery, or experiencing frailty, your needs go even higher.

Ironically, many older adults end up unintentionally eating less protein. Appetite may decline, chewing may become difficult, and long-standing habits may lean more toward tea and toast than protein-rich meals. The good news is that a few small changes, such as adding tofu to a salad, choosing a protein-rich plant milk, or sprinkling a couple of tablespoons of hempseeds on your breakfast bowl, can make a big difference.

How Much Protein Is Needed?

The Recommended Dietary Allowance (RDA) for protein in North American adults of all ages is 0.8 grams of protein per kilogram (kg) of healthy body weight/day (g/kg/day). (Note that 1 kg = 2.2 pounds.) However, in Australia and many European countries, official recommendations are higher for older adults. Today, expert consensus is building that seniors need about 25 to 50 percent more protein than younger adults. The PROT-AGE Study Group recommends 1.0–1.2 g/kg/day for healthy older adults. They advise the high end of this range for those who are active.

To estimate your protein needs, start by determining your "healthy body weight." This is a weight that supports overall health, energy, and function. You can use an online tool like the Ideal Weight Calculator to get a general estimate: https://calculator.net/ideal-weight-calculator.html. Then, refer to the box below to calculate your personalized protein target.

Here's How to Calculate Your Recommended Daily Protein Intake

For a senior whose healthy weight is 61 kg (135 pounds), multiply 61 by 1 g to get 61 g of protein.

For an active senior whose healthy weight is 61 kg (135 pounds), multiply 61 by 1.2 to get 73.2 g of protein.

For you:

STEP 1. Divide your healthy weight* in pounds____lbs by 2.2 lbs to get your weight in kilograms =____kg.

STEP 2. Multiply your weight____kg by 1.0 or by 1.2 =____g to get your recommended protein intake for the day.

*A healthy body weight is one that promotes good overall health. This generally means a BMI of between 18. 5 and 24.9. You can calculate your BMI at http://www.calculator.net/bmi-calculator.html.

The reason we base protein recommendations on healthy body weight is that adipose (fat) tissue requires far less protein for maintenance than lean tissue. So, if you are overweight or obese, calculating protein needs based on your actual weight would overestimate your true requirement. Similarly, if you are underweight, it's more appropriate to base your needs on a healthy target weight rather than your actual weight, since the goal is to rebuild lean tissue.

If you have a chronic illness or inflammatory condition you may require more protein, around 1.2–1.5 g/kg/day, while those experiencing severe illness, injury, or malnutrition may need up to 2.0 g/kg/day. At these higher levels, it can be challenging to meet protein needs using whole-plant foods alone. In such cases, strategically using plant-based protein supplements, such as soy, pea, hemp, pumpkin, potato, or rice protein powders, can be a practical and clinically appropriate solution. (See page 127 for more on protein powders.)

Table 5.1 Recommended Protein Intakes in Grams per Kilogram of Healthy Body Weight

Population Group	Protein Recommendation
Healthy adults	0.8 g/kg/day*
Older adults, ≥65 years	1.0–1.2 g/kg/day
Older adults with chronic illness, ≥65 years	1.2–1.5 g/kg/day
Older adults with severe illness, injury, malnutrition, ≥65 years	Up to 2.0 g/kg/day

*0.8 g/kg/day is the RDA for this group. Many experts suggest that slightly higher intakes may better support optimal health.

Where Do I Get Protein on a Plant-Based Diet?

We can get all the protein we need by eating a variety of plant-based foods throughout the day, as shown in Your Plant-Powered Day (page 42). When we consume and digest any protein, it is broken down into its constituent amino acids, which are then absorbed and rebuilt into the proteins we need.

Many of us think of protein in relation to animal products such as meat, chicken, fish, dairy, and eggs. However, all the essential amino acids from which we build protein actually originate from plants, so it makes good sense that plants are reliable sources.

Table 5.2 A Few Examples of Plant-Based Protein Sources*

Food	Protein per Serving
Tempeh (1 cup, ~6 oz)	31 g
Seitan (3 oz)	21 g
Tofu (½ block, ~ 5 oz)	20 g
Cooked lentils (1 cup)	18 g
Chickpeas (1 cup cooked)	15 g
Hempseeds (3 tbsp)	10 g
Quinoa (1 cup cooked)	8 g
Almonds (¼ cup)	7 g
Oats (1 cup cooked)	6 g
Chia seeds (2 tbsp)	5 g

*Also check labels.

Should I Supplement with Protein Powder?

While most older adults can meet their protein needs through whole plant foods, some may benefit from including a plant-based protein powder, especially if appetite is reduced or needs are elevated due to illness or recovery. Powders made from soy, pea, hemp, pumpkin, rice, potato, or a blend of these are all suitable options. These can easily be added to smoothies, soups, or porridge for a protein boost.

When choosing a protein powder, look for products with minimal added ingredients (avoid unnecessary sweeteners, flavors, or fillers) and ensure they have been third-party tested for quality and purity. Reputable certification programs, such as NSF Certified for Sport, USP, or Informed Choice, help verify that products meet strict standards and contain contaminant levels (such as heavy metals or pesticides) that fall within established safety limits.

Check the labels on plant-based milks for protein content. Soy and pea-based milks, as well as certain protein-fortified milk blends, typically provide 7–10 grams of protein per cup, making them excellent choices for meeting daily protein needs. In contrast, oat and hemp milks offer a more modest 2–4 grams per cup, while almond, cashew, and rice milks tend to be lower in protein, with only 1–2 grams of protein per cup.

Research shows that higher protein intake (in line with the recommendations in this section) is associated with better physical performance, greater muscle mass, and lower mortality. With a bit of planning and moderate exercise, you can meet or exceed your protein needs and preserve your strength, mobility, and quality of life well into older age. Also, see the sections on Frailty and Underweight and Sarcopenia in Chapter 4 (pages 86 and 111).

What About Essential Amino Acids?

There's a long-standing myth that plant proteins are "incomplete" and must be carefully combined at each meal. In reality, all plant foods contain all twenty amino acids, including the nine essential amino acids that your body cannot produce on its own. As long as you're consuming enough total protein and enjoying a variety of plant foods throughout the day, your body can draw from its amino acid pool to build the proteins it needs. There is no need to pair foods like rice and beans at the same meal.

One essential amino acid that deserves special attention as we age is leucine. Leucine plays a key role in triggering muscle protein synthesis—the process your body uses to build and maintain muscle tissue. Older adults often experience anabolic resistance, meaning the body needs a higher leucine "signal" to stimulate muscle maintenance and growth.

That's why it's helpful to include at least one leucine-rich food at every meal. Excellent plant sources of leucine include soy products (e.g., tofu, tempeh, edamame, and soy milk), seitan, legumes, pumpkin seeds, hempseeds, peanuts, and many protein powders.

Choosing a mix of these foods throughout the day and aiming for 20–30 grams of protein per meal, helps ensure that you're getting not just enough protein overall but also the right amino acid profile to support muscle strength, recovery, and independence in later life.

Maria's Protein Peril

After reviewing her food records with a dietitian, Maria was surprised to learn that she was averaging only 42 grams of protein per day. At a healthy weight of 60 kilograms (132 pounds), her estimated needs are 60–72 grams daily (1.0–1.2 g/kg), meaning she was falling short by 20 grams or more.

Fortunately, with a few strategic tweaks, she bridged the gap. Her dietitian suggested replacing almond milk with fortified soy milk and adding baked tofu cubes and a protein-rich dressing to her lunch salad. In Table 5.3, you can see how quickly these small changes brought her protein intake from 42 to 75 grams, an increase of 33 grams!

Table 5.3 Maria's Dietary Adjustments to Reach Her Protein Goal

Meals	Maria's Original Diet	Protein Content	Dietary Changes	Protein Content
Breakfast	Oatmeal, 1 cup	6	Oatmeal, 1 cup	6
	Almond milk, 1 cup	1	**Soy milk, 1 cup**	**8**
	Blueberries, ½ cup	0.5	Blueberries, ½ cup	0.5
	Flaxseeds, 2 tsp	1	Flaxseeds, 2 tsp	1
			Hempseeds, 1tbsp	**3**
Lunch	Mixed green salad, 3 cups	3	Mixed green salad, 3 cups	3
	Fat-free dressing, 2–3 Tbsp	0	**Tahini-Balsamic Dressing, ¼ cup, (page 271)**	**4**
			Tofu cubes, 1/3 cup	**15**
	Wholegrain bread, 1 slice	3	Wholegrain bread, 1 slice	3
	Hummus, ¼ cup	3	Hummus, ¼ cup	3
	Tomato, 2 slices	0	Tomato, 2 slices	0
	Fresh orange, 1	1	Fresh orange, 1	1
Dinner	Sweet potato, 1 cup	2	Sweet potato, 1 cup	2
	Broccoli, 1 cup	4	Broccoli, 1 cup	4
	Black beans, ¾ cup	11	Black beans, ¾ cup	11
	Avocado, ½ small	2	Avocado, ½ small	2
	Creamy Chia Pudding (almond milk), ¾ cup	4	**Creamy Chia Pudding (soy milk), ¾ cup (page 314)**	**8**
	Strawberries, ½ cup	0.5	Strawberries, ½ cup	0.5
Total Protein		42		75

Note: Items added or changed are bolded. These small adjustments add 33 grams of protein.

Carbohydrates

Carbohydrates, often called carbs, have received a great deal of bad press, mainly because nearly half (42 percent) of the calories in a typical American diet come from refined carbohydrate sources such as white flour and added sugars. These ultra-processed foods have been stripped of key nutrients and are digested rapidly, leading to blood sugar spikes, weight gain, and an increased risk of chronic diseases.

But carbohydrates themselves are not the problem. In fact, they are the body's preferred energy source, especially for the brain. When blood glucose drops too low, we may feel tired, irritable, anxious, confused, or intensely hungry.

By contrast, carbohydrates from whole plant foods deliver energy in a way that is steady and sustained while supporting emotional and metabolic well-being. When we focus on quality, carbohydrates can be powerful allies in promoting resilience, vitality, and disease prevention.

Getting Carbohydrates Right: Focus on Carb Quality

Not all carbohydrates are created equal. What matters most is their source and nutritional content. High-quality carbohydrates are found naturally in whole-plant foods, including legumes, vegetables, whole grains, and fruits. These foods provide complex carbohydrates (starches) and naturally occurring sugars, packaged together with fiber, resistant starch, essential vitamins and minerals, and a broad spectrum of protective phytochemicals and antioxidants. This synergy slows digestion, moderates blood sugar response, and supports the growth of beneficial gut microbes.

In contrast, low-quality carbohydrates, such as refined grains, sugary beverages, and foods with added sugars, provide little to no fiber and few protective dietary components. They are rapidly absorbed, can destabilize blood glucose levels, and tend to feed gut microbes associated with inflammation and metabolic dysfunction.

Smart Swaps for Better Carbs

Enhancing carbohydrate quality isn't about restrictions; it's about making smarter, more purposeful choices. Try these practical substitutions to elevate nutrient density and metabolic benefit:

- Replace white rice with brown rice, quinoa, barley, or other intact whole grains.
- Swap white bread for sprouted or dense whole grain varieties.
- Choose whole grain or legume-based pasta instead of traditional white flour pasta.
- Use dried or fresh fruit to sweeten foods and recipes, instead of added sugars.
- Choose water, herbal tea or other unsweetened beverages rather than sugar-sweetened beverages.

Fiber

Fiber is a type of carbohydrate that we don't digest, but our gut bacteria do. It plays a central role in digestive function, immune support, and metabolic regulation while promoting regularity, blood sugar control, cardiovascular health, and a balanced gut microbiome.

Many older adults fall short of the recommended 14 grams per 1,000 calories, which translates to about 21 grams a day for women over fifty and 30 grams a day for men over fifty. In fact, most American adults consume less than 15 grams per day, or roughly half the recommended amount. Those following plant-based diets tend to fare much better, often coming closer to or even exceeding recommended fiber intakes. Table 5.4 provides a brief summary of the fiber content in common foods.

Table 5.4 Fiber Content of Common Foods (Approximate Values per Serving)

Food Category	Fiber per Serving	Examples
Vegetables	2–5 g per 1 cup (raw or cooked)	Broccoli (1 cup cooked): 5 g Carrots (1 cup raw): 3.5 g
Fruits	2–8 g per medium piece or 1 cup	Berries (1 cup): 5–8 g Apple, with skin (1): 4 g Banana (1): 3 g
Whole Grains	3–8 g per 1 cup cooked	Quinoa (1 cup cooked): 5 g Oatmeal (1 cup cooked): 4 g Brown rice (1 cup cooked): 3.5 g
Legumes (Beans, Lentils, Soy)	12–20 g per 1 cup cooked	Lentils (1 cup cooked): 16 g Black beans (1 cup cooked): 15 g Chickpeas (1 cup cooked): 12 g
Nuts & Seeds	2–5 g per 1 oz (3–4 tbsp)	Almonds: 4 g Pumpkin seeds: 2 g
Processed Plant Foods	2–10 g per slice/ item	Whole grain bread (1 slice): 2–3 g High-fiber cereal (1 cup): 5–10 g
Refined Grains	1 g or less per serving	White bread (1 slice): 1 g White rice (1 cup): 1 g
Animal Products	0 g	Meat, fish, eggs, dairy—all contain no fiber

Source: USDA FoodData Central. U.S. Department of Agriculture. https://fdc.nal.usda.gov.

Soluble Fiber Versus Insoluble Fiber and More

Dietary fiber is often categorized as either insoluble or soluble, based on its behavior in water. Almost all whole-plant foods contain both types, though in different proportions.

Insoluble fiber travels through the gastrointestinal tract, binding to carcinogens and other toxic substances, helping to eliminate them in the feces. This type of fiber absorbs and retains water, increasing stool volume, making it easier to pass, and promoting regularity. Bulky, softer stools reduce the risk of diverticulitis, in which pouches form in the colon. Some of the most notable sources include whole grains, vegetables (such as broccoli, carrots, corn), beans, lentils, and the skins of apples and pears.

Soluble fiber dissolves in water to form a gel-like substance in the gut. It is most concentrated in beans, vegetables (such as Brussels sprouts, broccoli, carrots, sweet potatoes, turnips), fruits (such as apples, apricots, avocadoes, figs, guavas, nectarines, pears), nuts and seeds (flaxseeds, sunflower seeds, hazelnuts), and grains (oats, barley). It slows digestion, helps balance blood sugar, improves insulin sensitivity, and can help manage or prevent type 2 diabetes. Viscous fibers such as beta-glucan in oats and barley can help lower LDL cholesterol. It's wise to drink plenty of water when consuming foods rich in soluble fiber. This helps the fiber form a gel, which aids digestion and prevents constipation.

Resistant starch isn't technically fiber, but it acts much like it. It resists digestion in the small intestine and is fermented in the colon, just like fiber. This fermentation process produces short-chain fatty acids (like butyrate), which support colon health, immune function, and insulin sensitivity. Present in whole grains, seeds, legumes, green bananas, and cooked and cooled starchy foods such as pasta, potatoes, and rice, resistant starches work with fiber to promote health.

Prebiotics are compounds that nourish beneficial gut bacteria, helping them thrive. Many soluble fibers and resistant starches have prebiotic effects. When gut bacteria ferment these substances, they produce compounds that protect the gut lining and support immune health. Prebiotics are found in a variety of foods, including asparagus, avocado, garlic, leeks, onions, oats, barley, flaxseeds, cocoa, apples, and underripe bananas.

Probiotics are live microorganisms found in fermented foods like tempeh, miso, sauerkraut, kimchi, and yogurts with live and active cultures. While they don't typically establish permanent residence in the gut, they can still offer important benefits. These live microbes interact with the gut lining and immune system, stimulating immune cells, enhancing gut barrier function, and helping maintain a healthy microbial balance.

In summary, carbohydrates from whole, unprocessed plant foods that are rich in soluble and insoluble fiber, resistant starch, prebiotics, and probiotics, are far more than a source of energy. They support a healthy gut microbiome, help regulate blood sugar and cholesterol, and play a critical role in cognitive function, including memory, mood, and mental clarity. A balanced plant-based diet built around whole-plant foods provides the full spectrum of these powerful, health-promoting compounds to support well-being as we age.

Aren't Beans Notorious Gas Producers?

Some people are hesitant to eat legumes because of their reputation as the "musical fruit." This is due to a type of fiber called oligosaccharides, which are fermented by gut bacteria, producing gas as a normal byproduct. When legumes are new to the diet, gas may be more noticeable at first, but this typically improves as the gut microbiome adapts. The good news is that this adjustment happens naturally over time. Here are some practical tips to help ease the transition:

1. **Start small and choose gentle options.**
   Begin with small portions of easier-to-digest legumes such as red lentils, split peas, or mung beans. Cook them well.
2. **Rinse canned beans thoroughly.**
   This helps remove some of the oligosaccharides found in the canning liquid.
3. **Soak and drain dried beans.**
   Presoak beans and discard the soaking water before cooking.
4. **Skim during cooking.**
   Remove any foam that rises to the surface.

5. **Cook until very soft.**
   Beans should be soft enough to mash easily against the roof of your mouth.
6. **Include lower-gas options.**
   Tofu (lower in fiber) and tempeh (fermented) tend to be easier to digest.
7. **Reduce swallowed air.**
   Eating quickly, gulping air, or poorly fitting dentures can increase intestinal gas.
8. **Eat mindfully.**
   Stop eating when comfortably full—about 80 percent.
9. **Use traditional digestive aids.**
   Many cultures use ingredients such as ginger, epazote, kombu, or hing (asafoetida) to improve legume digestion.

A FINAL NOTE: Passing gas twelve to twenty-five times per day is completely normal. For more on cooking beans, see page 229.

Fat: Friend or Foe?

Fat has often been portrayed as a dietary villain, but the truth is more nuanced. While some types of dietary fat are linked to conditions such as coronary artery disease, type 2 diabetes, stroke, and excess weight, fat itself is not inherently harmful. In fact, healthy fats are essential, supporting everything from brain function and hormone production to nutrient absorption, and cell membrane integrity, throughout life.

Rather than trying to minimize fat intake, choose the right types of fats from healthy sources. Just as with carbohydrates, there are fats that can be harmful and fats that are beneficial. The highest quality fats are found naturally in a variety of whole-plant foods. For example, 13 percent of the calories in lettuce come from fat, as do 4 percent in black beans and a remarkable 55 percent in hempseeds.

The goal isn't to eliminate fat but to be intentional in our food choices. We want to favor whole foods that deliver healthy fats, minimize those known to promote disease, and, in some cases, moderate overall intake depending on individual health goals.

What Types of Fats Should We Minimize?

Although animal products such as beef, cheese, and eggs are typically viewed as "protein foods," they could be regarded as "fat foods" since typically more than half their calories come from fat, and much of it is saturated fat.

Saturated Fat. Decades of research have established a strong association between saturated fat intake and elevated LDL cholesterol, a major contributor to atherosclerosis, coronary artery disease (CAD), and stroke. Saturated fat also raises levels of apolipoprotein B (ApoB), the structural protein found on all particles that deliver cholesterol into artery walls, including LDL, VLDL, and Lp(a). This means that on a lab test, ApoB provides a better measure than does LDL alone of the number of particles contributing to plaque formation. Many experts now consider it a stronger predictor of cardiovascular risk than LDL cholesterol.

Higher saturated fat consumption is also linked to increased risk of type 2 diabetes, likely due to its impact on insulin resistance and chronic inflammation. Limiting saturated fat is an effective strategy in reducing chronic disease risk, particularly in older adults. About 33 percent of the fat in poultry, 40 percent to 44 percent of the fat in red meat, and 60 percent of the fat in dairy products is saturated.

In contrast, most high-fat plant foods contain only 5 percent to 20 percent saturated fat. Notable exceptions include coconut oil and palm oil, which contain approximately 85 percent and 50 percent saturated fat, respectively, and are best avoided or used sparingly.

While everyone should aim to keep saturated fat intake in check, individuals seeking to prevent or treat coronary artery disease, stroke, and diabetes are advised to minimize saturated fat intake, especially from concentrated sources.

Cholesterol. Cholesterol is found in all animal products, with eggs and organ meats being especially concentrated sources. Although cholesterol is technically a fat-like substance called a sterol and does not provide calories, it is often grouped with dietary fats because it travels through the bloodstream alongside them. Excess cholesterol intake may increase the risk of cardiovascular disease in some individuals.

While cholesterol is essential for building cell membranes, producing hormones, and synthesizing vitamin D, we do not need to obtain it from food because nearly every cell in the body can produce cholesterol, with the liver serving as the primary site of production. We are, in essence, cholesterol-making machines, and like other animals, our bodies easily produce all the cholesterol we need.

Trans Fats. Trans fats exist in two forms: those industrially produced through the partial hydrogenation of vegetable oils, and those naturally occurring in small amounts in the milk and meat of ruminant animals like cows, sheep, and goats.

Industrial trans fats, once widely used in margarine, baked goods, and processed snacks, were created to improve shelf life and texture. However, they raise LDL cholesterol, lower HDL, and significantly increase cardiovascular disease risk. Because of these well-documented harms, partially hydrogenated oils have been banned in the United States, Canada, Brazil, and other countries, and restricted in many parts of Europe.

Natural trans fats are produced in the stomachs of ruminant animals during digestion and enter the food supply via dairy and meat. While structurally different, emerging evidence suggests these too may contribute to inflammation and heart disease, particularly in vulnerable individuals. Although industrial trans fat exposure has decreased dramatically, minimizing all sources of trans fat remains a prudent strategy for reducing chronic disease risk.

How Much Fat Is Healthy?

The Dietary Reference Intakes (DRIs) for the United States and Canada recommend getting 20 percent to 35 percent of total calories from fat, with saturated fat as low as possible. The World Health Organization recommends 15 percent to 30 percent of calories from fat, with saturated fat under 10 percent. For individuals aiming to reverse or manage heart disease or type 2 diabetes, intakes at the lower end of these ranges (15 percent to 20 percent) are often recommended, with some experts suggesting even lower (10 percent to 15 percent).

Unsaturated Fats. For health, our best fat sources are the unsaturated fats in seeds, nuts, grains, legumes (including soy), and other plant foods (in smaller amounts). When unsaturated fats replace saturated fats, trans fats, and refined sugars in the diet, levels of total cholesterol, LDL cholesterol, and ApoB tend to decrease.

Omega-3 Fatty Acids. Especially important allies are the omega-3 fatty acids. ALA is an essential omega-3 fat that must be obtained from food. The richest plant sources are flaxseeds, chia seeds, hempseeds, and walnuts, with amounts featured in the food guide (page 45). Although the body can convert ALA into the long-chain omega-3 fatty acids EPA and DHA, this process is inefficient. DHA and EPA are important building blocks for the brain, nervous system, and cell membranes.

An emerging field of research shows that consuming direct sources of DHA may slow cognitive decline, lower the risk of Alzheimer's disease, and support mental and retinal health. EPA also plays a critical role, particularly in mood regulation; several studies have found that

EPA-rich supplements may reduce symptoms of depression, especially in older adults or those with low baseline omega-3 status.

While some people obtain DHA and EPA from fish, it is interesting to note that fish don't produce these fatty acids themselves—they accumulate them by eating microalgae, which is the original source. On plant-based diets, we can obtain DHA and EPA from microalgae-based supplements.

There are currently no official RDAs for DHA and EPA, but we suggest a daily microalgae-based supplement of 500 to 1,500 mg DHA/EPA, though this can vary with the individual's omega-3 status. Strive for an Omega-3 Index of at least 6 percent and preferably 8 percent or more. You can check if your blood is at an optimal level through Omega-3 Index tests from local lab tests or www.omegaquant.com.

In summary, to support heart, brain, and metabolic health, especially as we age, moderate intakes of healthy fats are beneficial. Here are some simple tips to help fine-tune your intake:

- Minimize saturated fats from animal products and tropical oils.
- Prioritize whole-food plants for health-supportive fats that come with fiber, antioxidants, and micronutrients.
- Limit concentrated fats and oils, especially from processed foods.
- Include reliable sources of omega-3 fatty acids daily, such as flaxseeds, chia seeds, hempseeds, walnuts, and microalgae-based DHA/EPA supplements.

Vitamins

The word *vitamin* comes from the Latin word *vita,* meaning life—a fitting name for compounds that are essential to our survival. The "amin" part of the word reflects an early twentieth century belief that these substances were amines (nitrogen-containing compounds).

Although we now know that not all vitamins contain nitrogen, the name stuck. Nutrition is, after all, a relatively young science that continues to evolve.

These essential compounds support a vast and growing list of functions throughout the body. They power immune defense, bone maintenance, energy metabolism, vision, blood formation, and more. Yet as we age, we may become more vulnerable to vitamin insufficiency or deficiency, not just because of what we eat, but also due to reduced absorption, medication interactions, reduced sun exposure, and physiological changes such as diminished gastric acid secretion and kidney function. In plant-based diets, two vitamins deserve special attention: vitamin B_{12}, which must be supplemented, and vitamin D, which is harder to obtain from food and very often requires supplementation, especially in older adults.

As you read about the vitamins and minerals that follow, you'll see how wise it is to base one's food choices around the food guide on page 43!

Vitamin B_{12}

Vitamin B_{12} is a complex, water-soluble vitamin. It is the largest and most structurally intricate of all vitamins. First isolated in 1948, its discovery led to a Nobel Prize in 1964. While often associated with animal products, it's important to understand that neither animals nor plants produce B_{12}.

This vitamin is synthesized exclusively by certain microorganisms. Animals acquire it through gut bacteria, by consuming food or soil that is contaminated with bacteria, or through B_{12} supplementation in their feed. So, when we obtain B_{12} from meat, eggs, or dairy, we're actually getting second-hand bacteria-derived B_{12}.

For those consuming exclusively plant-based diets, the only reliable sources of vitamin B_{12} are supplements and fortified foods such as plant milks, nutritional yeasts, meat analogs, and breakfast cereals. Check the label to ensure vitamin B_{12} has been added, as content can vary significantly by brand and product and is likely to be much lower than amounts that we recommend.

It's also important to note that certain fermented foods and seaweeds may contain inactive B_{12} analogs that do not support human metabolism and may interfere with the absorption of active forms. For this reason, supplementation remains the safest and most consistent way to ensure adequate intake.

Vitamin B_{12} is essential for converting food into energy, for building red blood cells, and for maintaining the myelin sheaths (protective insulation) around nerve fibers, ensuring that nerve impulses can be transmitted properly. Deficiency can lead to a range of symptoms, including:

- Fatigue, weakness, or lightheadedness
- Tingling or numbness in the hands and feet
- Poor balance, memory problems, or vision changes
- Digestive issues and, in some cases, depression or mood disturbances.

B_{12} absorption becomes less efficient with age, including among those who regularly consume animal products. The process requires adequate stomach acid and digestive enzymes to cleave B_{12} from the protein to which it's bound in animal products. It then must bind with a compound called intrinsic factor, secreted by the stomach, to be absorbed in the small intestine.

However, an estimated 10 percent to 30 percent of older adults (on any diet) produce insufficient gastric acid (a condition known as *atrophic gastritis*), which impairs the release of protein-bound B_{12}. Because of these age-related challenges, the Institute of Medicine recommends that all adults over age fifty obtain vitamin B_{12} from fortified foods or supplements, which contain B_{12} in its free (crystalline) form—unbound to protein and therefore absorbable without the need for gastric acid.

Additionally, a subset of seniors do not produce enough intrinsic factor, leading to insufficient absorption. For individuals with intrinsic factor deficiency, monthly B_{12} injections are an effective therapeutic option.

Getting Enough B_{12} from Supplements

For adults aged sixty-five and older, a daily vitamin B_{12} supplement providing 500 to 1,000 micrograms is recommended. Cyanocobalamin is the most stable form, although methylcobalamin and other forms may also be used. Supplementation helps offset age-related declines in B_{12} absorption.

For younger adults, 1,000 mcg taken two to three times per week may be sufficient as long as status is periodically monitored. The RDA for adults is only 2.4 mcg, based on getting tiny amounts throughout the day, but only about 1 percent or less of a high-dose supplement is absorbed. This is why much larger doses are needed to meet physiological needs, particularly in later life.

Several laboratory markers can be used to assess B_{12} status:

- **Serum B_{12}** is the most commonly ordered test, though there are limits on its usefulness.
- **Methylmalonic acid (MMA)** and **homocysteine** both rise early in B_{12} deficiency.
- **Holotranscobalamin II (holo-TCII)** reflects the biologically active fraction of B_{12} and is a sensitive marker for early deficiency.
- **Complete Blood Count (CBC)** may reveal macrocytic anemia in more advanced stages of deficiency.

B_1–B_6 and Folate: The Spark Plugs of Your Body

When it comes to keeping our energy up, our brain sharp, and our heart and bones strong, few nutrients work harder than these B vitamins. This team of water-soluble nutrients, especially thiamin (B_1), riboflavin (B_2), niacin (B_3), pyridoxine (B_6), and folate, plays key roles in everything from energy metabolism to nerve function, red blood cell production, and DNA maintenance.

As we get older, our need for some B vitamins increases while our ability to absorb them may decline. Appetite changes, medications, and certain health conditions can also affect intake and absorption. Let's take a closer look at each of these nutrients.

Thiamin (B_1), Riboflavin (B_2), and Niacin (B_3)

Thiamin (B_1), riboflavin (B_2), and niacin (B_3) are essential for converting carbohydrates, proteins, and fats into energy, fueling every cell in the body. They also contribute to healthy nerve function, support skin vitality, and help maintain strong bones and a resilient cardiovascular system.

Deficiencies in one or more of these B vitamins can lead to fatigue, mood or memory changes, and visible changes in skin or circulatory function. Recommended intakes for these vitamins do not increase with age, but ensuring adequate intake remains critical throughout the lifespan.

The RDAs for adults nineteen years and older are:

- Thiamin—1.1 mg/day (women), 1.2 mg/day (men)
- Riboflavin—1.1 mg/day (women), 1.3 mg/day (men)
- Niacin—14 mg/day (women), 16 mg/day (men)

Top plant-based sources include legumes (such as beans, peas, lentils, and soyfoods), whole and enriched grains, seeds, nuts, and nutritional yeast.

Vitamin B_6 (Pyridoxine)

Vitamin B_6 is a multitasking nutrient involved in over a hundred enzymatic reactions. It plays a critical role in the production of neurotransmitters that support brain function, facilitates the metabolism of protein and fat, supports immune system function, and helps regulate homocysteine levels (a compound associated with cardiovascular risk).

As we age, the body's requirement for B_6 increases due to changes in absorption, metabolism, and physiological demand. In fact, vitamin B6 is one of the few nutrients with a higher RDA for older adults. While adults under fifty-one require 1.3 mg/day, the RDA for those ages fifty-one and older is:

- 1.5 mg/day for women
- 1.7 mg/day for men

Low B_6 status in older adults may result from reduced appetite, limited dietary variety, or the use of medications that interfere with absorption or metabolism. Excellent plant-based sources include bananas, potatoes, sweet potatoes, squash, spinach, bell peppers, okra, peas, lentils, peanut butter, avocados, and seeds.

Folate

The word *folate* comes from *folium*, the Latin word for leaf, and leafy greens are indeed one of its richest sources. Folate is essential for red blood cell production, and this vitamin helps build and repair DNA, protecting it from changes that may lead to cancer. It supports thinking, memory, and mental health, and plays a vital role in cardiovascular health by helping to process and eliminate homocysteine. The RDA for all adults ages nineteen and older, including seniors, is 400 mcg of dietary folate equivalents (DFE) per day. While folate from food is highly beneficial, large doses of synthetic folic acid (the form used in most supplements, fortified foods, and nutritional yeast) can mask a vitamin B12 deficiency, which is a concern for older adults. Folic acid is also in enriched flour and fortified breakfast cereals, though in smaller amounts.

Some research also suggests that excessive folic acid intake (above 1,000 mcg/day) may be linked to an increased risk of certain cancers, though the evidence is not yet conclusive. For these reasons, it may be prudent to obtain folate primarily from food, unless your healthcare provider advises otherwise.

Folate is abundant in greens, beans, and oranges. Cooking can reduce folate levels, so it's smart to emphasize raw or lightly cooked greens. Other good sources are almonds, asparagus, avocados, beets, cashews, kelp, kiwi fruit, lentils, quinoa, soy, spinach, and sunflower seeds.

Choline

Choline is often grouped with B vitamins because of its similar functions in the body, but it is not officially classified as one. Although our bodies can produce some choline, this internal synthesis is typically not enough to meet our full needs, so choline is considered an *essential nutrient* that must also come from food.

It plays many important roles, including supporting liver function, maintaining healthy cell membranes, and producing acetylcholine, a neurotransmitter involved in memory and muscle control. Choline also works alongside folate and vitamin B_{12} in regulating homocysteine levels, an action that supports cardiovascular and brain health. Emerging research suggests that choline may be especially important for preserving cognitive function as we age.

Unlike most B vitamins, there is no RDA for choline. Instead, the Adequate Intake (AI) has been established to guide intake:

- 425 mg/day for women
- 550 mg/day for men

Because choline is found more abundantly in animal products, individuals following a plant-based diet, particularly older adults, may need to be more intentional about including choline-rich plant foods, such as soyfoods (tofu, tempeh, soy milk), quinoa, broccoli, Brussels sprouts, pinto beans, and peanuts.

It may be beneficial to discuss choline intake with a healthcare provider, especially if there are memory concerns, dietary restrictions, or metabolic factors. In some cases, a choline supplement may be appropriate. While meeting daily needs is important, excessive intake of choline from high-dose supplements may lead to side effects, including low blood pressure, sweating, gastrointestinal upset, or a fishy body odor. Food-first strategies are generally safest and most effective for supporting long-term health.

Vitamin D

Vitamin D deserves special attention, not just for those on plant-based diets, but for all older adults. This essential nutrient plays a critical role in bone health, muscle function, immune defense, and possibly even healthy aging.

One of vitamin D's most important jobs is to help the body absorb and retain calcium efficiently. Without enough vitamin D, we absorb only 10 percent to 15 percent of the calcium from our food. With adequate vitamin D, that figure can rise to 30 percent to 40 percent, significantly improving the body's ability to keep calcium in the bones and prevent losses through the urine. In this way, vitamin D helps maintain strong bones and teeth while reducing the risk of fractures. It also helps regulate calcium and phosphate levels in the blood, supporting muscle contraction and preventing cramps or spasms.

Beyond bone health, vitamin D supports the immune system, may help regulate blood sugar, and may even contribute to healthy aging by helping preserve telomere length, a marker of cellular longevity. Low vitamin D levels have been linked to osteoporosis, infections, some cancers, and other chronic conditions. While research continues to evolve, one thing is clear: Maintaining healthy vitamin D status becomes increasingly vital as we age.

Our bodies can produce vitamin D when our skin is exposed to sunlight containing ultraviolet B (UVB) rays. However, this process depends on several conditions and is more complex than many realize. For example, UVB radiation does not penetrate glass, meaning that sunlight exposure through windows doesn't contribute to vitamin D synthesis. In addition, several factors can significantly limit the skin's ability to produce adequate vitamin D, including:

- Living at higher latitudes, where winter sunlight is too weak to trigger synthesis
- Air pollution or cloud cover that blocks UVB radiation
- Limited time spent outdoors, or consistent use of sunscreen or protective clothing
- Having darker skin, which reduces vitamin D synthesis due to higher melanin content
- Aging, which naturally lowers the skin's production capacity

Other factors may interfere with the body's ability to convert or absorb vitamin D, including:

- Declining kidney function, which reduces conversion of vitamin D to its active form

- Use of certain medications that impair vitamin D absorption or metabolism

As a result, many older adults do not generate sufficient vitamin D from sunlight alone, particularly in colder climates and during seasons with limited sun exposure. Population data suggest that 25 percent to 75 percent of seniors may have suboptimal vitamin D status, with a higher risk in men, individuals with obesity (BMI >30), and those who do not take vitamin D supplements.

While the sun is our most potent natural source of vitamin D, a few foods can also provide modest amounts. In omnivorous diets, vitamin D is primarily found in fatty fish (such as salmon, sardines, and mackerel), egg yolks, and fortified dairy products. In plant-based diets, the primary dietary sources are fortified foods, including vitamin D-fortified plant milks, breakfast cereals, orange juice, or margarine (amounts vary, check labels).

Mushrooms exposed to ultraviolet (UV) light can also be rich sources of vitamin D_2, a plant-derived form of the vitamin. You can boost the vitamin D content of store-bought mushrooms by placing them gills-up in direct sunlight before cooking or storing in the refrigerator (see page 151). However, unfortified plant foods do not naturally provide vitamin D, so for those on a plant-based diet, especially seniors with limited sun exposure, supplementation remains the most consistent and reliable source.

The North American Recommended Dietary Allowance Is:

- 600 IU (15 mcg) for adults ages fifty one to seventy
- 800 IU (20 mcg) for adults older than seventy

These values assume some sun exposure, which many older adults do not consistently receive. For this reason, we recommend a daily supplement of 2,000 IU (50 mcg) of vitamin D for most seniors, particularly those who receive limited sun exposure, have darker skin, or live in northern latitudes. This level is safe, well-tolerated, and sufficient to help most people maintain optimal vitamin D levels year-round.

However, individual needs can vary based on absorption, health conditions, body weight, and medications. To fine-tune your intake, ask your healthcare provider to check your serum vitamin D [25(OH) D] and adjust your dose to stay in the optimal range (typically 30–50 ng/mL or 75–125 nmol/L).

Vitamin D is available in two forms: vitamin D2 (ergocalciferol) and vitamin D_3 (cholecalciferol). Vitamin D_2 is always plant-based and vegan, typically derived from irradiated fungi or yeast. Historically, vitamin D_3 was available only from animal-derived sources, such as fish liver oil or lanolin extracted from sheep's wool. However, a lichen-derived form of vitamin D_3 is now widely available in supplement form, offering a vegan alternative that is biologically equivalent to conventional D_2 in raising serum 25(OH)D levels.

The Tolerable Upper Intake Level (UL) for vitamin D is 4,000 IU (100 mcg) per day for adults. Intakes above this level should be medically supervised. Excessive doses, particularly those exceeding 10,000 IU (250 mcg) daily, can lead to hypercalcemia, resulting in calcium deposits in soft tissues and potential damage to the heart, kidneys, and other organs.

Please note that Vitamin D supplements may interact with certain medications, including statins, corticosteroids, thiazide diuretics, and orlistat, so it's important to review your intake with a healthcare provider. For more detailed information, consult the NIH Office of Dietary Supplements: https://ods.od.nih.gov/factsheets/VitaminD -HealthProfessional.

Smart Strategies for Ensuring Adequate Vitamin D

Getting enough vitamin D on a plant-based diet, especially as we age, takes some planning, but it's entirely achievable with the right strategies:

- **Take a reliable supplement:** A daily dose of 2,000 IU (50 mcg) of vitamin D_2 or D_3 is appropriate for most seniors. Some individuals may need more or less depending on their vitamin D status, sun exposure, or medication use. Choose a lichen-derived D_3 supplement if you're looking for a vegan option.
- **Choose fortified foods:** If you use plant-based milk, ready-to-eat breakfast cereal, orange juice, or margarine, check the label and select an option that is vitamin D-fortified (though amounts are low).
- **Make the most of mushrooms:** UV-exposed mushrooms naturally contain vitamin D2. Boost levels further by placing fresh mushrooms gills-up in direct sunlight for fifteen to sixty minutes, (ideally midday), before cooking.
- **Test your levels:** If you're unsure whether you're getting enough, ask your healthcare provider to check your blood vitamin D [25(OH)D] level and tailor your intake accordingly.

Vitamin A

You may remember hearing in grade school that carrots help you see in the dark, and there's truth to that! Vitamin A is essential for vision, particularly night vision, and for maintaining the health of the eyes, skin, and mucous membranes. It also plays important roles in immune function, cellular integrity, and protection against infections, certain cancers, and cardiovascular disease. Vitamin A comes in two main forms:

- Preformed vitamin A (retinol and retinyl esters) is found only in animal-derived foods, such as liver, eggs, and dairy.
- Provitamin A carotenoids are plant-based compounds (most notably beta-carotene) that the body can convert into active vitamin A.

Carotenoids are naturally occurring pigments responsible for the vibrant orange, yellow, red, and dark green hues in many vegetables and fruits. Some carotenoids, like lutein and zeaxanthin, are not converted into vitamin A but still play critical roles in eye health, especially in protecting the retina and helping reduce the risk of cataracts and age-related macular degeneration.

Carotenoids also act as potent antioxidants, supporting healthy aging by protecting cells from oxidative damage. Carotenoid-rich foods include apricots, broccoli, cantaloupe, carrots, leafy greens, mangos, nectarines, papaya, peppers, persimmon, plantains, prunes, pumpkin, purple cabbage, seaweeds, squash, sweet potatoes, turnips, tomatoes, and yams. Including a wide variety ensures a broad spectrum of protective phytochemicals.

The RDA for adults ages nineteen and older is:

- 700 mcg Retinol Activity Equivalents (RAE) for women
- 900 mcg RAE for men

RAE accounts for the differences in bioavailability and activity between preformed vitamin A and provitamin A carotenoids. You can meet your daily needs with two-thirds of a baked sweet potato or yam, or a combination such as half a cup of carrots plus a quarter cup of cooked spinach.

Although the RDA doesn't increase with age, vitamin A status can be a concern for some seniors due to reduced absorption or intake of carotenoid-rich foods, chronic health conditions or medications affecting digestion or metabolism, and limited appetite or restrictive diets.

In general, it is safer to obtain vitamin A from these plant foods rather than from vitamin A supplements. Excess intake of preformed vitamin A (from supplements or liver) can pose risks for older adults. High levels may increase the risk of hip fractures, interfere with vitamin D metabolism, and be toxic to the liver.

Vitamin C

Vitamin C plays a vital, wide-ranging role in maintaining strength, resilience, and repair, and is particularly important as we age. It's essential for the synthesis of collagen, the structural protein in blood vessels, bones, skin, tendons, and ligaments. When intake is insufficient, wound healing slows, tissues weaken, and immune function declines.

This water-soluble vitamin is also a potent antioxidant, helping protect cells from oxidative damage and regenerating other antioxidants, such as vitamin E. In addition to bolstering immune defense, vitamin C supports the synthesis of key compounds, including thyroid hormone, carnitine (which transports fat into cells for energy), and norepinephrine, a neurotransmitter essential for brain function and mood regulation. Vitamin C also enhances the absorption of iron from plant foods. Eating a vitamin C–rich food, such as red bell pepper, kiwi, or citrus, with an iron-rich plant food can significantly improve iron uptake.

The RDA for vitamin C is:

- 75 mg/day for women
- 90 mg/day for men

These values apply to all adults ages nineteen and older, including older adults. However, some researchers and clinical nutrition experts suggest that higher intakes of 100–200 mg/day may offer additional benefits for seniors, including improved immune resilience, reduced inflammation, and compensation for age-related declines in absorption efficiency. While not yet reflected in official guidelines, these targets are considered safe and potentially advantageous for healthy aging.

The richest sources of vitamin C include fruits such as blackberries, cantaloupe, citrus, kiwi, guava, mango, papaya, pineapple, raspberries, and strawberries, as well as vegetables like broccoli, Brussels sprouts, cabbage, cauliflower, daikon radish, green peas, leafy greens, onions, red bell peppers, sweet potatoes, and tomatoes. Because vitamin C is sensitive to heat, light, and air, it's ideal to enjoy some fruits and vegetables raw or lightly cooked to preserve their vitamin C content.

Vitamin E

Vitamin E is a powerful antioxidant that helps protect our cells from damage caused by free radicals. It supports immune function, helps maintain healthy skin and eyes, and may reduce the risk of blood clots by supporting normal blood vessel function. It is fat-soluble, meaning it is absorbed along with dietary fat. If our intake of healthy fats is too low, especially from whole-plant foods, we may not get enough. Fortunately, many nutrient-rich plant foods provide vitamin E, particularly nuts, seeds, avocados, and leafy green vegetables. The RDA for all adults ages nineteen and older, including seniors, is 15 mg (22.4 IU) of alpha-tocopherol per day. Most people can meet their needs through food. Very high doses from supplements may increase the risk of bleeding, especially for individuals taking blood thinners or anticoagulant medications. For this reason, routine high-dose vitamin E supplementation is not recommended unless medically advised.

Vitamin K

Vitamin K is a relative newcomer in the world of nutrition, officially recognized as an essential nutrient in 1974. The *K* comes from the German word *Koagulation,* reflecting one of its most important functions: helping blood clot properly in response to injury. Without enough vitamin K, clotting may be delayed or impaired, increasing bleeding risk.

Vitamin K also plays a critical role in regulating calcium in the bloodstream and supporting bone health, particularly important as we age. There are two main forms: vitamin K_1 (phylloquinone), abundant in leafy greens and essential for blood coagulation, and vitamin K_2 (menaquinone), which plays a role in bone metabolism and is found in some fermented foods and produced in small amounts by gut bacteria and by conversion from vitamin K_1. (For more details, see page 103 in Chapter 4.)

The RDA for all adults, including seniors, is:

- 90 mcg per day for women
- 120 mcg per day for men

Leafy greens are vitamin K superstars! Just 1 cup of raw spinach or 1½ cups of kale provides around 145 mcg. Other excellent sources include avocado, broccoli, Brussels sprouts, cabbage, cauliflower, grapes, green peas, green tea, kiwi fruit, lentils, nori, pumpkin, and soy foods.

Although our gut bacteria can produce small amounts of vitamin K, this source can be disrupted by antibiotics. Eating a varied plant-based diet, especially one rich in leafy greens, is the best way to ensure consistent intake. Because vitamin K can interfere with blood-thinning medications like warfarin (Coumadin), those taking such drugs are often advised to maintain a consistent intake of vitamin K-rich foods and work with their healthcare provider to adjust medication dosing as needed.

In summary, well-designed plant-based diets typically provide more folate, higher levels of vitamins C, E, and K than omnivorous diets, and tend to supply adequate amounts of most other vitamins. Special attention must be paid to vitamins B_{12} and D, as these are not consistently available from plant foods and are more likely to fall short without fortified foods or supplements.

Minerals

We've all seen the messages from the food industry linking calcium to dairy and iron to meat, but those aren't the only paths to strong bones or healthy blood. With a bit of care, plant-based diets will provide all the essential minerals needed for strength and lifelong health. What matters is knowing where to find these minerals and how to help your body absorb them. Here's your guide to a mineral-rich diet, powered by plants.

A unique feature of minerals is that their absorption is highly variable, depending on a range of factors, including how foods are prepared, how they're combined, and your body's physiological state. Here are a few key examples:

- **Food preparation.** Techniques like soaking, sprouting, fermenting, and cooking can increase the bioavailability of calcium, iron, zinc, copper, magnesium, and manganese from beans, grains, seeds, and other mineral-rich foods.
- **Timing.** For certain minerals, splitting intake can improve absorption and reduce gastrointestinal discomfort. For example, calcium is best absorbed in doses of 200–300 mg at a time, so if you supplement, it's more effective to take divided doses with meals rather than all at once. Similarly, minerals like magnesium

and iron may also be better tolerated and absorbed when taken in smaller, spaced doses, depending on individual needs and gastrointestinal tolerance.

- **Combinations.** The presence of certain nutrients can enhance or inhibit mineral absorption. For example, pairing iron-rich foods with vitamin C–rich produce (like citrus, bell peppers, berries, or tomatoes) boosts iron absorption. Similarly, consuming calcium and magnesium together in moderate amounts may support synergistic intake. In contrast, excessive calcium or zinc taken at the same time may interfere with iron uptake.
- **Your body's condition.** Physiological state influences mineral absorption efficiency. When your body is deficient or under increased demand for a particular mineral, such as iron, zinc, or magnesium, it often adapts by increasing absorption. Conversely, absorption may decline when stores are adequate. Age, inflammation, digestive health, and chronic disease can all impact this regulatory balance.
- **Age or digestion.** As we age, lower stomach acid production can reduce the absorption of key minerals, including calcium, iron, and zinc.

With so many delicious and nutrient-packed plant foods to choose from, it's easier than you might think to get all the minerals you need—without the empty calories. Your body deserves more than just fuel—it deserves nutrition that works for you. The food guide (see pages 42–46) was designed with this in mind—highlighting mineral-rich choices that support bone health, blood function, metabolism, and more. Let it be your road map to building a well-balanced, plant-powered day.

Calcium

Our bones are living tissues that are constantly rebuilt and remodeled throughout life. Calcium is critical in this process, essential not only for maintaining strong bones and teeth but also for proper muscle contraction, nerve signaling, blood clotting, and blood pressure regulation.

Alongside vitamin D (which helps us absorb calcium), this mineral plays a central role in reducing the risk of osteoporosis and fractures as we age. It also helps maintain the jawbone, keeping teeth anchored and reducing tooth loss. Of course, regular brushing, flossing, and dental checkups are essential too.

Bone loss accelerates after menopause, making calcium especially important for postmenopausal women. Men over age seventy also face an increased risk of age-related bone loss.

Calcium needs shift across the lifespan, with higher requirements later in life due to changes in bone remodeling, absorption efficiency, and hormonal regulation. Here are the current RDAs for adults:

- Women ages nineteen to fifty: 1,000 mg/day
- Women older than fifty: 1,200 mg/day
- Men aged ages nineteen to seventy: 1,000 mg/day
- Men older than seventy: 1,200 mg/day

Almost half of North American adults fail to meet these targets. So plan ahead! Reliable plant-based calcium sources include fortified plant milks, low-oxalate dark leafy greens (such as bok choy, broccoli, collard greens, kale, and napa cabbage), calcium-set tofu (check labels), almonds, chia seeds, sesame seeds (especially unhulled), tahini, and fortified orange juice. See Table 3.1 on page 43 for further information.

In contrast, high-oxalate greens, including spinach, Swiss chard, beet greens, and rhubarb, contain calcium, but it is poorly absorbed because oxalates bind to it and limit its bioavailability. These foods should not be relied on as meaningful sources of calcium. Individuals prone to oxalate kidney stones may also need to limit their intake of these vegetables.

National guidelines recommend meeting calcium needs through food first, using supplements only as needed. For many older adults, a practical strategy is to consume at least two servings of calcium-fortified foods daily and, if necessary, take a calcium supplement of 400–600 mg to fill the gap. Because the body absorbs calcium best in smaller amounts, it's ideal to divide supplemental doses, for example taking 200–300 mg with breakfast and another 200–300 mg with lunch or dinner.

While the UK recommends a lower intake of 700 mg/day for adults over sixty-five, we recommend aiming for the North American RDAs of 1,200 mg/day for women over fifty and men over seventy, as these higher targets better reflect current evidence on bone preservation in aging. Avoid exceeding 2,000 mg/day of total calcium intake from food and supplements combined. High intakes, particularly from supplements, may increase the risk of kidney stones and, in some cases, vascular calcification.

Iron

Iron is a central component of hemoglobin, the protein in our red blood cells that transports oxygen from the lungs to our tissues, and myoglobin, which stores oxygen in muscles. Iron also supports the immune system, helps produce hormones and neurotransmitters, and contributes to our overall energy and vitality.

As we age, iron needs change, especially for women. For men, the recommended intake remains steady at 8 mg/day throughout adulthood. But for women, the RDA increases to 18 mg due to menstruation during the childbearing years, then drops significantly to 8 mg at age fifty-one, reflecting the average age of menopause and the end of menstrual blood losses. This shift can make meeting iron needs easier for older women, but thoughtful food choices remain essential.

Iron-deficiency anemia is not uncommon among older adults and can cause fatigue, weakness, reduced immunity, and even cognitive changes. It is reassuring to know that rates of anemia are similar in vegans and non-vegans. While iron from plants is absorbed at a slightly lower rate than from meat, plant-based diets often provide more total iron overall.

Hemoglobin levels, a measure of working iron, tend to be similar between dietary groups. However, serum ferritin, which reflects iron stores, is typically lower in vegans. It is worth noting that ferritin levels at the lower end of the normal range and energy levels are fine, as high serum ferritin is linked to elevated risk of chronic disease. Overall, it's important to regularly include iron-rich foods and combine them with strategies that support absorption.

Legumes (such as beans, lentils, and soy foods) and seeds (such as pumpkin, hemp, and chia) are among the best plant sources of iron. Including these with each meal can help meet your needs. Other helpful sources include whole grains, nuts, dried fruit, and many vegetables. Eating these foods alongside sources of vitamin C, such as citrus fruits, strawberries, tomatoes, bell peppers, and broccoli, can significantly boost absorption.

The menus on page 51 each provide well over our needed 8 mg/day. We get about 2 mg of iron from any of these:

- ¼ cup of seeds (poppy, pumpkin, sesame, sunflower), cashews, or pine nuts
- 2 tablespoons of hempseeds or 3 tablespoons of chia seeds
- ½ cup of cooked beans or tofu
- 2 cups of soy milk
- ¾ cup of cooked quinoa
- 1 baked potato
- ⅓ cup of dried currants
- 1 ounce of dark chocolate

It Is Not Hard to Get Enough Iron When We Consume a Variety of Whole-Plant Foods!

Should your doctor determine that you have anemia or low iron stores, you may need to supplement your iron intake. However, taking high dosages of iron supplements can cause gastrointestinal distress: upset stomach, nausea, constipation, vomiting, and diarrhea, and some forms, such as ferrous bisglycinate, are more easily tolerated than others. Ask your healthcare provider to recommend a form of iron that will work for you.

Maria's Experience: Building Back Iron Stores

When Maria's blood work showed her iron stores were low, her doctor recommended a low-dose iron supplement. But Maria also changed the way she ate, again. With guidance from a dietitian, she began to build meals around iron-rich plant foods. She added lentils to her soups, black or kidney beans to her tacos, and pumpkin seeds to her morning oatmeal. To her delight, she discovered that even a few squares of dark chocolate could make a contribution!

In addition, she added vitamin C–rich foods like oranges and grapefruit to her breakfast and bell peppers to her lunch salads and to the stir-frys she made for dinner to boost iron absorption. Maria also made a small but important change to her routine: She started enjoying her tea between meals rather than with them, since tea contains tannins that can reduce iron absorption. After a few consistent months of these simple strategies, her iron levels improved, and so did her energy.

Zinc

If your sense of smell or taste has faded, a shortage of zinc could be to blame. This essential mineral is a component of gustin, a protein in saliva that supports taste bud function, and it helps maintain our olfactory receptors, which detect odors. Zinc also plays a critical role in immune defense, DNA synthesis, protein production, cell division, gastrointestinal health, and wound healing, functions that become even more important with age.

Zinc deficiency can lead to increased infections, slower wound healing, hair loss, changes in appetite, and reduced senses of taste and smell. It may also increase susceptibility to toxin-producing bacteria and viruses by compromising the integrity of the intestinal lining, allowing harmful microbes to enter the bloodstream more easily.

The RDA for adults, including seniors, is:

- 8 mg/day for women
- 11 mg/day for men

Older adults may be at greater risk for zinc deficiency due to several factors:

- Reduced absorption of zinc in the gut
- Lower dietary intake due to appetite changes, limited variety, or chewing difficulties
- Health conditions, such as diabetes, chronic kidney disease, or gastrointestinal disorders, may increase zinc losses or needs

Because of these challenges, some older adults may benefit from slightly higher zinc intake within a safe, moderate range, guided by a healthcare provider. The most effective strategy is to include a variety of zinc-rich plant foods in your daily diet. Choosing a multivitamin that contains zinc can also help boost intake without exceeding safe levels.

The best plant-based sources of zinc are like the ones that provide iron: legumes, whole grains, nuts, and seeds. You'll get about 1 mg of zinc from each of the following:

- ½ cup cooked beans (such as black beans, kidney beans, lentils, or soybeans)
- ½ cup cooked chickpeas, peas, tofu, or tempeh
- ½ cup cooked whole grains (like oatmeal, quinoa, or spelt)
- 2 slices of whole wheat bread
- 2 tablespoons almond butter, cashews, chia seeds, pine nuts, pumpkin seeds, or sesame seeds (or tahini)
- ¼ cup almonds, Brazil nuts, peanuts, pecans, sunflower seeds, or walnuts

Adding one or two of these to each meal or snack can help you meet your daily needs. Vegetables such as avocado and mushrooms also contribute smaller amounts. Using food preparation techniques like soaking beans and grains, sprouting lentils, fermenting soy, or choosing leavened breads can enhance zinc absorption.

Taking too much zinc (above the upper limit of 40 mg/day) can cause side effects such as nausea, cramps, and headaches, and may interfere with copper absorption, potentially leading to deficiency. For this reason, it's best to aim for steady intake from food and avoid high-dose supplements unless medically advised.

Magnesium

Magnesium works hand in hand with calcium and vitamin D to support bone strength, which becomes increasingly important as we age. Magnesium also helps regulate muscle contraction, nerve function, and heart rhythm while playing a key role in hundreds of enzymatic reactions for energy production, protein synthesis, blood pressure, and blood sugar control.

The RDA for adults, including seniors, is:

- 320 mg/day for women
- 420 mg/day for men

Older adults following plant-based diets often enjoy higher magnesium intakes than nonvegetarians—sometimes even exceeding the RDA—thanks to their naturally nutrient-dense food choices. Still, some older adults may fall short, especially if they have a reduced appetite, impaired absorption, or are taking medications such as diuretics, proton pump inhibitors, antacids, or laxatives, all of which can deplete magnesium. A deficiency can lead to muscle cramps or weakness, fatigue, tremors, or irregular heartbeat.

Magnesium is the central mineral in chlorophyll, the pigment that gives plants their vibrant green color. So, every time you eat a leafy green, you're getting a boost of magnesium! Other excellent sources include legumes, cashews, seeds, whole grains, and even dark chocolate (made from magnesium-rich cacao or cocoa beans). The recipes in Menus 1 to 3 (see Table 3.3, page 51) each provide more than 420 mg/day of magnesium.

A small supplemental dose of magnesium may help with leg cramps or occasional constipation. However, excess magnesium from supplements (above 350 mg/day) can cause diarrhea, nausea, or abdominal cramping. People with impaired kidney function should only take magnesium supplements under medical supervision, since their bodies may not be able to excrete excess amounts effectively.

For most of us, though, the best approach is simple: Focus on magnesium-rich whole foods every day! Your bones, heart, and muscles will thank you.

Potassium

When we think of potassium, bananas often come to mind, and while they do provide a reasonable amount, many other whole-plant foods offer even more. Vegetables, legumes, and potatoes are especially rich in this essential mineral. Potassium plays a vital role in regulating fluid levels, relaxing blood vessels, and counterbalancing the effects of sodium on blood pressure.

It supports healthy nerve signaling, muscle contraction, kidney function, and a steady heart rhythm. In addition, potassium helps protect bones by reducing calcium loss. A potassium-rich diet can lower the risk of high blood pressure, stroke, and heart disease, which are pressing concerns as we age.

The AI for potassium is:

- 2,600 mg/day for women
- 3,400 mg/day for men

Note that potassium does not have an RDA. Instead, the AI represents an amount that is assumed to support nutritional adequacy in healthy people.

Unfortunately, most older adults don't meet these targets, regardless of dietary pattern. However, those following Your Plant-Powered Day (see page 42), which includes at least eight servings of fruits and vegetables daily, along with legumes and whole grains, tend to get much closer to ideal intakes.

Here's how much potassium you can get from some everyday whole foods:

- 900 mg from a medium baked potato
- 400–500 mg from a banana, half an avocado, ⅓ cup of pistachios or pumpkin seeds, or ½ cup of cooked spinach, sweet potato, acorn squash, yam, lentils, or beans (such as white, aduki, black turtle, or soy)

Potassium needs and tolerance can vary depending on health status. For example, diuretics, often prescribed for high blood pressure or heart failure, can increase potassium losses, which means you may need more from your diet to compensate. On the other hand, individuals with chronic kidney disease or those taking medications such as ACE inhibitors, Angiotensin II Receptor Blockers (ARBs), or potassium-sparing diuretics, may need to monitor potassium intake to avoid elevated blood levels. While potassium from whole-plant foods is generally less problematic than previously thought, potassium supplements and additives can pose a higher risk and should only be used under medical supervision. Excess potassium can lead to abnormal heart rhythms or other serious complications, particularly when kidney function is impaired.

While salt substitutes made with potassium chloride can help lower sodium intake, they aren't right for everyone. Most healthy adults can use them in moderation. However, for individuals with kidney disease or those taking potassium-affecting medications, these products can pose serious health risks. If your kidneys can't excrete excess potassium efficiently, using salt substitutes could lead to dangerous potassium buildup. Always consult your healthcare provider before using them.

Sodium

Salt was once hard to come by in many parts of the world. It was so valuable that the word *salary* comes from the Latin *salarium*, as Roman soldiers used part of their wages to buy it. The phrase "salt of the earth" reflects its historic worth. Today, salt is no longer scarce, and for many, it's consumed in excess.

Sodium, the main component of salt, plays essential roles in the body. It helps regulate fluid balance, supports nerve impulses and muscle function, and contributes to the production of digestive secretions. A small amount of sodium is naturally found in celery, leafy greens, carrots, eggplant, sweet potatoes, and sea vegetables.

In developed countries, natural sources account for roughly 12 percent of total sodium intake. Another 6 percent comes from salt added during cooking, and 5 percent from salt added at the table. An estimated 77 percent comes from salt added to a great many foods during commercial processing.

Diets high in sodium can raise blood pressure, increasing the risk of stroke, heart disease, and kidney damage. Hypertension forces the heart to work harder and can damage arteries and vital organs, including the brain and eyes.

While the body needs only about 500 mg/day of sodium to function, most people consume far more. The Chronic Disease Risk Reduction (CDRR) intake level recommends limiting sodium to no more than 2,300 mg/day to lower the risk of hypertension, cardiovascular disease, and kidney damage.

Many experts, and some clinical guidelines, suggest even more conservative targets: 1,500 mg/day for most adults, and 1,200 mg/day for those over seventy, to better support heart and kidney health. Despite these recommendations, sodium intake remains high.

For American adults, the *average* is 3,400 mg/day, so clearly, it's even higher for some!

Seniors tend to do slightly better but still exceed optimal levels: Women over seventy *average* 1,950 mg/day, and men about 2,440 mg/day. For reference, just ½ teaspoon of salt contains roughly 1,150 mg of sodium—nearly half the CDRR limit—and also supplies the daily recommended intake of iodine (as discussed in the next section). The good news? Small, consistent changes can significantly reduce sodium intake, without sacrificing flavor or enjoyment.

Use These Strategies to Reduce Sodium Intake

1. **Read labels on packaged and processed foods, condiments, and snack products.** Select those with less sodium. Table 5.5 provides a guide to salt and sodium on food labels.

2. **Make more meals at home.** Limit or avoid added salt. Use herbs, spices, and salt-free seasonings along with lemon juice and exotic vinegars for flavoring.
3. **Request low-sodium options at restaurants.** You can also ask for sauces or dressings on the side.

Table 5.5 Terms and Their Meanings Related to Salt and Sodium

Salt/Sodium-Free	Less than 5 mg of sodium per serving
Very Low Sodium	35 mg of sodium or less per serving
Low Sodium	140 mg of sodium or less per serving
Reduced Sodium	At least 25% less sodium than the regular product
Light in Sodium/ Lightly Salted	At least 50% less sodium than the regular product
No-Salt-Added/ Unsalted	No salt is added during processing

When we sweat heavily, during hot weather, gardening, or exercise, sodium is lost through perspiration, and we may need a little extra in our diet. Sodium deficiency is uncommon but can occur, especially in older adults with certain medical conditions or those taking medications that affect sodium balance such as diuretics (often called water pills) like hydrochlorothiazide or furosemide, as well as some antidepressants, including sertraline and fluoxetine. Symptoms may include headache, nausea, muscle cramps, fatigue, and disorientation.

Iodine

Iodine is essential for thyroid hormone production, which regulates metabolism, supports immune function, and influences nearly every organ system in the body. Without sufficient iodine, the thyroid cannot function properly, which may lead to hypothyroidism, a condition linked to fatigue, weight gain, cold intolerance, constipation, depression, and reduced cognitive performance. In more severe or prolonged cases, iodine deficiency can result in goiter (a swelling in the neck) and, in rare cases, may increase the risk of thyroid nodules or cancer.

Although iodine deficiency is most commonly associated with an underactive thyroid, long-standing deficiency can sometimes lead to changes in the thyroid that increase the risk of hyperthyroidism, especially when iodine intake rises suddenly. In addition, autoimmune thyroid disorders—another common cause of hyperthyroidism—are generally not caused by iodine deficiency but may be influenced by both low and excessive iodine intake in susceptible individuals.

Iodine is present in iodized salt—a public health measure adopted just over a century ago to eliminate deficiency—but it is not typically added to specialty salts (see below). It is also found in foods such as eggs, poultry, fish, and meat, largely because iodine is added to animal feed. In dairy products, iodine content is due mainly to the use of iodine-containing disinfectants in dairy processing. The iodine content of plant foods varies by region, depending on soil levels. As a result, seniors following plant-based diets, as well as those who do not use iodized salt, may have relatively low dietary intakes that make them susceptible to both overt hypothyroidism and subtle thyroid dysfunction.

The RDA is 150 mcg/day for adults, including seniors. You can meet your daily iodine needs (150 mcg) with any one of the following:

- ½ teaspoon of iodized salt. This provides approximately 150 mcg of iodine along with about 1,150 mg of sodium. (Be sure to check the label—only iodized salt is a reliable source of iodine.)
- ½ teaspoon of arame or dulse granules. These sea vegetables naturally contain iodine, but levels may vary.
- 1½ sheets of nori. Nori is a mild-tasting, edible seaweed commonly used in sushi. It offers a moderate and relatively consistent source of iodine.
- A tiny amount of kelp powder. Use with caution, as kelp is extremely rich in iodine. Just 1/16 to ⅛ teaspoon may exceed

the daily requirement. Choose kelp products with standardized iodine content and follow dosage guidelines carefully to avoid excess.

- An iodine-containing multivitamin or supplement. Look for products that provide 150 mcg of iodine from potassium iodide or potassium iodate, the most reliable and consistent supplemental forms.

Many specialty salts, including Himalayan pink salt, kosher salt, and sea salt, are not iodized. Neither are soy sauce, tamari, Bragg's Liquid Aminos, or miso. Most of the salt used in processed foods is also non-iodized, despite contributing to the bulk of sodium in the modern diet. In the United States, iodizing table salt is voluntary, so not all brands contain iodine. In Canada, however, all table salt is iodized. Always check the label to be sure.

While ensuring adequate iodine intake is essential, excessive iodine intake can also be harmful. The upper intake level for adults is 1,100 mcg/day. Excessive iodine can disrupt thyroid function, particularly in individuals with existing thyroid conditions. If you're unsure about your iodine intake or have thyroid disease, speak with your healthcare provider before using seaweed or iodine supplements regularly.

Copper, Manganese, Selenium, and Chromium

These trace minerals are needed in small amounts but play essential roles in immune function, metabolism, and overall health. Most plant-based eaters meet their needs through a varied diet, though selenium may require a bit more attention.

- **Copper** is usually abundant in plant-based diets. The RDA is 900 mcg/day, and you can easily meet this through nuts, seeds, legumes, whole grains, and avocados.

- **Manganese** is found in all plant food groups. The RDA is 1.8 mcg/day for women and 2.3 mg for men. Deficiencies are rare when eating a variety of whole foods.
- **Selenium** is a trace mineral that supports immune function, thyroid hormone metabolism, and antioxidant activity. While deficiency is rare in North America, it can occur in individuals with low intake or malabsorption issues. The RDA for adults is 55 mcg/day, and the Tolerable Upper Intake Level is 400 mcg/day. Because selenium levels in foods depend heavily on soil content, they vary widely by region. Brazil nuts are exceptionally rich sources, with a single nut typically exceeding the adult RDA. While one Brazil nut daily can help meet selenium needs, regularly eating more than one may lead to excessive intake. Other good sources include sunflower seeds, brown rice, legumes, oatmeal, mushrooms, and tofu. A multivitamin containing selenium can also help.
- **Chromium** supports blood sugar control and is found in broccoli, potatoes and apples (especially the skins), whole grains, fruits, and other vegetables. While there is no RDA for chromium, the AI for those over fifty is 20 mcg/day for women and 30 mcg/day for men.

Supplements: Closing Nutritional Gaps

Supplements can help round out even the most well-planned diet, especially as we age. Certain nutrients deserve special attention in older adults following fully or mostly plant-based diets. Table 5.6 summarizes the official recommended dietary allowances (RDAs) for selected nutrients, along with practical guidance on supplements based on current evidence. Table 5.7 lists additional vitamins and minerals that are generally less likely to require supplementation but still play important roles in healthy aging.

Table 5.6 RDAs and Notes on Supplements for Older Adults

Nutrient	RDA (daily)	Notes on Intakes and Supplements
Protein	0.8 g protein/kg of healthy body weight	Many experts now advise 1–1.2 g protein/kg of healthy body weight per day, and more for those with certain health conditions (page 126). Protein powders may help (page 127).
Omega-3 fatty acids, ALA, DHA + EPA	About 2 g alpha-linolenic acid (ALA) per day (Table 3.1, page 43)	A microalgae-based supplement of 500–1500 mg of combined DHA/EPA daily is suggested. (Table 3.1, page 43).
Vitamin D3	600 IU (15 mcg) per day for men and for women ages 51–70, 800 IU (20 mcg) for women over 70*	2,000 IU (50 mcg) per day is suggested; however, dose should be based on serum 25(OH)D levels. Use vegan (lichen-derived) D3 (page 150).
Vitamin B_{12}	2.4 mcg/day**	1,000 mcg 2–3 times a week for those under 65 500–1,000 mcg/day for 65+
Calcium	1000 mcg/day for men ages 51–70 years 1,200 mg/day for older men and for women over age 50	Supplement if food intake is insufficient. Use small, divided doses such as 200–300 mg calcium, twice a day). Do not exceed 2000 mg/day calcium.
Iron *(if needed)*	8 mg/day	Supplement only if iron status is low. Monitor ferritin and hemoglobin.
Zinc	8 mg/day (women 11 mg/day (men)	Up to 15–20 mg if needed; do not exceed 40 mg/day.
Iodine	150 mg/day	A supplement is necessary if avoiding iodized salt, unless controlled amounts of seaweed are regularly included (page 46). Avoid excess from kelp.

* RDA may be too low; research has not been updated and there is extremely wide variation in needs.

**RDA may be far too low. Due to absorption issues in many individuals over age fifty, experts advise supplements as indicated or a combination of supplements and fortified foods.

If your diet is varied and based on Your Plant-Powered Day (page 42), you're likely well nourished and do not need a daily multivitamin-mineral supplement, but for added peace of mind, taking one once or twice a week can provide extra assurance without being excessive. In choosing such a supplement, Table 5.7 shows the recommended intakes for seniors for a number of minerals and vitamins that are not covered in Table 5.6 (page 172).

Table 5.7 Recommended Intakes for Select Vitamins and Minerals Not in Table 5.6*

Nutrient	Recommended Intake per Day (RDA or AI)
Vitamin A	700 mcg (women), 900 mcg (men)
Vitamin C	75 mg (women), 90 mg (men)
Vitamin E	15 mg
Vitamin K	90 mg (women), 120 mg (men)
Thiamin (B1)	1.1 mg (women), 1.2 mg (men)
Riboflavin (B2)	1.1 mg (women), 1.3 mg (men)
Niacin (B3)	14 mg (women), 16 mg (men)
Vitamin B6	1.5 mg (women), 1.7 mg (men)
Folate	400 mcg
Choline	425 mg (women), 550 mg (men)
Magnesium	320 mg (women), 420 mg (men)
Potassium	2,600 mg (2.6 g, women), 3,400 mg (3.4 g, men)
Selenium	55 mcg for women and men
Sodium	1,500 mg (1.5 g), also see page 166.

*There are additional vitamins and minerals beyond those in Tables 5.6 and 5.7; however, those are typically not an issue.

KEY TAKEAWAYS:

Aging Changes Our Nutrient Needs. As we get older, we typically require fewer calories, but our need for key nutrients changes. Our requirement for protein increases, and needs for essential vitamins and minerals stay the same, or increase. This makes nutrient density more important than ever!

A Varied Plant-Based Diet Can Meet Most Essential Nutrient Needs. As with any dietary choice, plant-based diets need to be planned, but they can provide nearly all the nutrients your body needs. In some cases certain fortified foods or supplements can bridge the nutritional gap.

Quality and Variety Matters. Focus on whole-plant foods as your primary sources of protein, carbohydrates, and healthy fats for long-term health.

Go for Variety! For color, for fun, and for a wealth of protective nutrients and phytochemicals.

Plant-Powered, Confident, and Connected

Eating well is one thing, but doing it with ease and confidence in social settings is another. Whether you're dining out, attending family gatherings, or fielding questions from curious friends, the next chapter offers practical tips and encouragement to help you stay true to your plant-based eating plan and your values without missing out on the joy of shared meals and connection.

CHAPTER 6

NAVIGATING PLANT-BASED LIVING IN SOCIAL SETTINGS

Chapter at a Glance

Will going plant-based strain your social life? Maybe, but it may also deepen it. Changing how you eat can shift how you relate to others, especially when food has been central to shared experiences. But plant-based living doesn't have to mean sacrificing connection. It can open the door to greater authenticity, creativity, and even new friendships.

In this chapter, we explore the social side of plant-based living, including how to:

- Navigate meals with family, friends, and guests who eat differently.
- Enlist support from doctors, dietitians, and other healthcare providers.
- Manage meals at hospitals and care facilities.

Maria's Story: Maintaining Social Ties Through Food Choices

Maria lives independently in the same cozy neighborhood where she raised her family. Her circle of friends, many of whom she's known for decades, meets monthly for dinner. These gatherings range from birthday celebrations to spontaneous potlucks, meals at restaurants, and dinners in one another's homes.

Since changing her diet to manage her hypertension and prediabetes, Maria has encountered new challenges during these get-togethers.

At first, she worried that her food choices might make others uncomfortable or disrupt long-standing traditions. But rather than withdraw, Maria approached the situation with warmth and grace. She decided to host one of the monthly dinners and prepared a beautiful Mediterranean-inspired spread: Tofu Cacciatore (page 309), fresh Italian bread, a gorgeous salad, and Tahini-Balsamic Dressing (page 271). For dessert, she served fresh grapes, Nutty Date Cookies (page 328), and dark chocolate. Her friends raved about the meal for weeks.

Over time, Maria's vibrant dishes became something her friends looked forward to. When dining out, she learned to call ahead or browse menus in advance, often suggesting restaurants with vegan options. At friends' homes, she often brought something to share, ensuring she had something satisfying to enjoy while sparking curiosity, not discomfort.

Maria didn't preach—she led with kindness, hospitality, and delicious food. Her gentle, consistent approach became a quiet inspiration. Friends noticed that she was losing weight and feeling more energetic. Some asked for recipes and even began incorporating more plant-based meals into their own lives.

Maria's story shows that you don't have to choose between your health and your relationships. With intention, confidence, and generosity, you can nourish both.

Plant-Based Eating and Connecting

Food is more than fuel—it's tradition, comfort, memory, and connection. As we age, its emotional and social significance often deepens. Choosing a plant-based lifestyle can be deeply empowering, with clear benefits for longevity, heart health, cognitive function, and energy. Yet the social and logistical hurdles, especially for older adults, can feel daunting, particularly when others are doing the cooking or when gatherings center around animal-based meals.

This chapter addresses those challenges and offers realistic, compassionate strategies to help you stay true to your values while continuing to build meaningful relationships. Living plant-based is an act of intention and courage but also one of joy, creativity, and shared purpose.

With thoughtful planning, honest communication, and great food, you can nourish your health and your relationships at the same time. Because in the end, what we bring to the table isn't just food—it's love, memories, and a vision of the future we hope to share.

How Do I Navigate Living with Family Members Who Are Not on Board?

Adopting a plant-based lifestyle is often deeply personal, motivated by health, ethics, or environmental concerns. But when you live with a spouse or share time with adult children or grandchildren who don't share your values, tensions can arise. Here are some thoughtful ways to coexist while staying true to your path:

- **Start with respect and empathy.** Change can be perceived as threatening to others, especially when it appears to challenge long-standing traditions or imply judgment. Approach the conversation with kindness, acknowledging that everyone is on their own journey. You might say, "This is something I'm doing for my health and well-being. I don't expect you to change your diet, just to support me as I explore what feels right for me."

- **Model; don't mandate.** Rather than persuading with arguments, let your actions and outcomes speak for themselves. As loved ones notice improvements in your energy, mood, or lab results, curiosity may grow. Prepare delicious, satisfying plant-based meals and invite others to taste, without pressure or expectation. Quiet consistency is often more impactful than debate.
- **Share kitchen space creatively.** If you share cooking responsibilities or have a small kitchen, consider a flexible system. Cook plant-based staples like rice, beans, or salads that everyone can enjoy. When both plant- and animal-based dishes are prepared, allow each person to customize their plate. Batch cooking, labeling, and using designated cutting boards can keep things organized and respectful.
- **Set gentle boundaries around shared meals.** It's okay to ask for small accommodations. For example, you might request one plant-based meal each week or ask that animal products be prepared separately. Framing these requests as health-related or values-based often increases understanding and cooperation.
- **Lean on outside support.** If support at home is limited, find community elsewhere. Join local plant-based groups, online forums, or connect with friends who share your values. Even a weekly call, walk, or shared recipe can boost your motivation and remind you that you're not alone.

How Can I Maintain Friendships and Traditions While Eating Differently?

Attending social events while following a plant-based lifestyle can feel challenging, especially as a guest. But with a little planning and a positive mindset, you can stay true to your values while enjoying the company and spirit of the occasion.

Here are some simple strategies to help you feel confident and comfortable:

- **Communicate ahead of time.** Let your host know in advance that you eat a plant-based diet and offer to bring a dish. If the main course is meat-centered, like barbecued chicken, consider bringing a flavorful plant-based alternative to throw on the grill for yourself, such as marinated tofu (page 299), veggie kabobs, or a veggie burger (whether store bought or homemade, such as the Best Black Bean Burgers [page 292]).
- **Bring something special.** Choose a dish that's festive, flavorful, and satisfying—something everyone will want to taste. A vibrant Rainbow Quinoa Salad (page 267), Marvelous Mushroom Ragout (page 307), Easy Chocolate Pudding (page 312) or a store-bought dairy-free ice cream can help spark curiosity and conversation. Think of it as an opportunity to delight and share, not simply to replace.
- **Eat a little something before arriving.** If you're unsure of the food offerings, eat a small meal or nourishing snack beforehand so you're not caught off guard.
- **Focus on connection, not confrontation.** Keep the spotlight on the gathering, not the menu. If asked about your dietary choices, speak from personal experience and health goals rather than trying to convert others. A friendly tone and nonjudgmental approach go a long way.
- **Respectfully decline, but don't isolate.** If a dish isn't suitable, simply say "no, thank you" with appreciation. There's no need to justify or explain. Your presence matters more than what's on your plate.

How Do I Entertain Non-Plant-Based Guests with Confidence?

Hosting a meal as a plant-based eater offers a unique opportunity to showcase how vibrant, satisfying, and delicious plant-based cuisine can be, without making your guests feel like they're missing out. With a bit of creativity and attention to flavor and presentation, you can impress even the most skeptical palates.

Here are some strategies to make your gatherings inclusive, nourishing, and memorable for everyone at the table:

- **Check in with your guests.** Ask ahead if anyone has food allergies, dietary restrictions, or strong dislikes. This simple gesture builds trust and ensures everyone feels welcome and cared for.
- **Focus on familiar flavors.** Here are a few guest-friendly, flavor-packed ideas:
  - **Tacos for All** (page 295): Offer seasoned black or pinto beans, shredded lettuce or cabbage, guacamole, salsa, lime wedges, and plant-based toppings.
  - **Easy Peasy Chili** (page 297): Serve with Double Corn Muffins (page 322) and toppings such as avocado, cilantro, and lime.
  - **Italian Comfort Night:** Serve Red Lentil Pasta Sauce (page 305) on pasta, topped with a cashew-based cheese alongside your favorite salad.
  - **The Multicolored Bowl** (page 304): Set out quinoa or rice, roasted vegetables, beans or tofu, a zesty sauce, and toppings like avocado, toasted nuts, or fresh herbs. Creamy sauces such as Perfect Peanut Sauce (page 273) appeal to everyone, regardless of dietary preferences.
- **Include a memorable dessert.** Finish the evening with something homemade and indulgent, like an Apple Pear Crisp (page 317) with Cashew Pear Cream (page 319), Easy Chocolate Pudding (page 312), or strawberries dipped in melted dark chocolate.

How Can I Dine Out Without Compromising My Values?

Eating out can be one of life's great pleasures, and with a little planning, it doesn't have to compromise your plant-based lifestyle. While restaurant offerings continue to improve, not all places are well-versed in plant-forward dining. These strategies can help you enjoy the experience while staying aligned with your values:

Strategies for Eating Out

- **Research in advance.** Use apps like *HappyCow* to find restaurants in your area that are entirely vegan or offer a variety of dietary options.
- **Browse the menu online.** Look for clearly labeled plant-based choices or customizable dishes that can easily be adapted.
- **Call ahead.** If in doubt, call the restaurant and ask whether they can accommodate a plant-based meal.
- **Request simple swaps.** Most kitchens are happy to adjust a dish, like using olive oil instead of butter, omitting cheese, or adding extra veggies or beans.
- **Be gracious but assertive.** Ask for what you need with a warm, respectful tone. Expressing appreciation often leads to extra effort from the staff.
- **Embrace global cuisines.** Many ethnic restaurants naturally feature plant-based staples—think Indian (dal, chana masala), Thai (vegetable tofu curries), Ethiopian (injera with lentils), and Mediterranean (hummus, falafel, tabbouleh).
- **Bring a little plant protein.** Sometimes, the best you will do is a baked potato or pasta and veggies, and protein falls short. To round out the meal, consider discreetly bringing baked marinated tofu cubes (page 299), roasted chickpeas, a small container of hummus, or a few nuts/seeds.

- **Eat a light meal or snack before you head out.** If you anticipate limited options, having something nourishing ahead of time, such as a smoothie or a handful of nuts and a piece of fruit, can help you enjoy the outing without feeling deprived or overly hungry.

How Can I Better Foster Inclusivity and Connection Around Food?

Food has the power to unite, heal, and build bridges, especially when shared with humility, creativity, and heart. Plant-based living doesn't have to mean eating separately or feeling set apart. In fact, many people are open, and even excited, to try new dishes, especially when they're shared with warmth and intention.

Tips for Strengthening Connection Through Food:

- **Host plant-based meals and invite participation.** Whether it's a casual dinner or a holiday celebration, inviting others to contribute dishes encourages inclusivity and sparks curiosity.
- **Share culturally meaningful recipes.** Re-create familiar family or cultural favorites with plant-based ingredients and invite conversations around their significance.
- **Bring plant-based options to gatherings.** Offering delicious, crowd-pleasing dishes at potlucks or work events lets others experience how satisfying and joyful plant-based eating can be.
- **Celebrate small moments.** If someone tries your dish or asks a question about your choices, acknowledge it with gratitude. Small acts of openness can lead to significant shifts over time.
- **Find common ground.** Focus on what unites people around the table—flavor, comfort, tradition, nourishment, and the joy of sharing good food.

What if My Doctor or Healthcare Provider Isn't on Board?

Choosing a plant-based lifestyle is a powerful step toward better health, but what if your healthcare provider isn't fully supportive or seems unsure about it?

Fortunately, plant-based eating is now increasingly recognized in clinical settings for its role in preventing and managing chronic diseases such as type 2 diabetes, cardiovascular disease, hypertension, and obesity. Providers with specialty training in lifestyle medicine are becoming more common.

Still, not all healthcare professionals have training in nutrition, and even fewer are well-versed in plant-based nutrition or lifestyle medicine. In some cases, they may express concern, not because the approach is unsafe, but because they are not yet familiar with the scientific evidence.

If this happens, try taking a team approach. Bring your questions, share your goals, and invite your provider into the conversation. You might say: "I've decided to follow a plant-based lifestyle to support my health. Could we talk about which lab tests might help ensure I'm meeting my nutritional needs?" By keeping the conversation open and respectful, you build trust—and turn your healthcare visits into a true partnership.

One powerful way to foster a supportive dialogue with your provider is to bring along credible, peer-reviewed resources that reflect the science behind your dietary choices. Consider printing or sharing:

- Melina V, Craig W, Levin S. Academy of Nutrition and Dietetics Position Paper on Vegetarian Diets. *J Acad Nutr Diet.* 2016;116(12):1970–1980.
- The Safe and Effective Use of Plant-Based Diets with Guidelines for Health Professionals. Craig WJ, Mangels AR, Fresán U., et al. *Nutrients.* 2021: 19;13(11):4144.

- Landry MJ, Ward CP. Health Benefits of a Plant-Based Dietary Pattern and Implementation in Healthcare and Clinical Practice. *Am J Lifestyle Med.* 2024;18(5):657–665.
- **American College of Lifestyle Medicine Guidelines**
  The American College of Lifestyle Medicine (ACLM) provides comprehensive resources. Their official website provides access to clinical practice guidelines, position statements, and educational materials for both healthcare professionals and patients. You can explore these resources directly at https://lifestylemedicine.org.

In some cases, your healthcare provider may advocate for a very different dietary approach—such as low-carbohydrate or animal-based patterns like keto or paleo. If this difference in perspective becomes a barrier to open communication or shared decision-making, you may find it helpful to seek out a provider who is knowledgeable about—and supportive of—plant-based nutrition. The goal is to work with someone who respects your choices and helps you monitor your health in a way that aligns with your values.

Are There Resources for Finding Plant-Based Physicians, Dietitians, or Coaches?

If you're seeking a provider who understands or supports your plant-based journey, these directories can help:

- **Plantrician Providers—Find Plant-Based Docs and Providers**
  https://plantrician.org/places/
  Their Find a Doc directory connects patients with healthcare professionals who are trained in or supportive of plant-based approaches to disease prevention and treatment.

- **Find a Plant-Based Dietitian**
  Look for dietitians via www.healthprofs.com, https://www.pcrm.org/findadietitian, or https://www.eatright.org/find-a-nutrition-expert, and filter by location and "vegetarian/vegan nutrition," or contact the authors:
  brendadavis@telus.net (brendadavisrd.com) or
  vesanto.melina@gmail.com (nutrispeak.com)
- **Plant-Based Telehealth**
  www.plantbasedtelehealth.com
  Connects patients with plant-based physicians across the United States via telemedicine.
- **Physicians Committee for Responsible Medicine (PCRM)**
  www.pcrm.org
  Offers educational materials and a directory of plant-based–aligned clinicians. Visit https://www.pcrm.org/findadoctor.
- **American College of Lifestyle Medicine (ACLM)**
  www.lifestylemedicine.org
  Has a directory of lifestyle medicine clinicians who are trained and board-certified, see www.lifestylemedpros.org/home.

Plant-Based Coaches: Another Layer of Support

In addition to healthcare providers and dietitians, many older adults find it helpful to work with plant-based health coaches—professionals trained to offer guidance, accountability, and encouragement throughout lifestyle transitions. Coaches trained through reputable programs, such as the Food Revolution Network, the American College of Lifestyle Medicine (ACLM) Certified Health Coach Program, or the Wellcoaches School of Coaching, often have a solid foundation in evidence-based nutrition, behavior change, and motivational strategies. While they don't diagnose or treat medical conditions, coaches can be valuable allies in setting goals, navigating social situations, and building sustainable habits for long-term success on a plant-based path.

How Can I Advocate for Plant-Based Meals in Hospitals, Retirement Communities, or Assisted Living?

It is paradoxical that many hospitals and healthcare institutions, places dedicated to healing, continue to serve meals based on dietary patterns that contribute to chronic diseases such as heart disease, type 2 diabetes, and certain cancers. In many facilities, standard menus still reflect the traditional Western diet, high in saturated fat (from fatty animal products), sodium, and ultra-processed foods.

Fortunately, this is beginning to change. A growing number of hospitals now offer plant-based options, though availability remains inconsistent. Patients and caregivers can play a pivotal role in accelerating this shift. By asking for plant-based meals, even when they are not explicitly listed, we not only advocate for our own health but also help normalize and encourage the inclusion of more health-promoting choices for all patients.

Over time, consistent advocacy from patients, families, and healthcare professionals is helping transform hospital menus to feature, or even prioritize, plant-based offerings. Some forward-thinking institutions are even integrating nutrition education into patient care, reinforcing the concept that *food is medicine.*

This Food Is Medicine approach, now championed by programs such as the American Heart Association's *Health Care by Food* initiative, emphasizes the power of whole, minimally processed foods in the prevention, treatment, and even reversal of chronic disease. Research shows that improved nutrition in healthcare settings can reduce complications, promote recovery, and decrease hospital readmissions.

For many older adults living in retirement communities, assisted living facilities, or long-term care homes, food service is centralized. In these settings, meals often default to conventional menus lacking adequate plant-based options. It's not uncommon to receive a plate of vegetables, rice, and potatoes, without a meaningful source of protein, such as tofu, beans, or veggie patties. Residents deserve better. Whether you're an individual advocating for yourself or a family member advocating for a loved one, you can be a catalyst for positive change.

Here are some simple strategies for success:

- **Build relationships with staff.** Request a meeting with both the culinary director and registered dietitian to explain your dietary preferences. Share information to help staff improve plant-based offerings (a sample 7-Day Meal Plan for staff is provided on page 190).
- **Frame requests around inclusivity and wellness.** Position plant-based options not only as a personal preference but also as part of a growing movement toward healthful eating.
- **Offer education and resources.** Share credible literature and recipes or invite a plant-based dietitian to speak to the culinary team.
- **Suggest simple plant-based additions.** Plant-based milk and veggie patties are a great place to start. Advocate for easy-to-prepare items such as lentil soup, black bean chili, chickpea salad, or tofu stir-fry. These meals require no specialty products but significantly boost nutrient adequacy.
- **Recruit allies.** Find other residents with similar preferences and voice concerns as a group.

To support these efforts, what follows is a practical guide for culinary directors, dietitians, administrators, and support staff in residential care environments. This resource outlines best practices for meeting the nutritional needs of plant-based residents while honoring their values and preferences.

It is designed to encourage inclusive, evidence-based food service that promotes well-being, cultural respect, and resident satisfaction. If you are a resident, family member, or caregiver, consider sharing this guide with your facility's food service team or dietitian. Doing so can open the door to collaborative conversations, raise awareness, and help foster a more supportive dining environment for yourself and others who follow plant-based diets.

Creating Plant-Based Dietary Change: A Practical Guide for Staff in Residential Care Facilities

Plant-based dietary patterns are increasingly common among older adults in residential care, driven by health, cultural, religious, ethical, and environmental motivations. Honoring these preferences is a cornerstone of person-centered care, supporting autonomy, dignity, and overall quality of life. This guide provides essential information for culinary teams, administrators, and support staff to ensure that plant-based residents are seen, supported, and nutritionally nourished.

Why Supporting Plant-Based and Plant-Forward Residents Matters

Healthcare facilities have a professional and ethical responsibility to support residents' dietary preferences, including those who choose plant-based diets. Doing so affirms residents' autonomy and values, promotes equitable care, and aligns with the principles of person-centered service delivery.

Moreover, when properly supported, plant-based diets can play a critical role in managing chronic conditions, improving quality of life, and even reducing the need for healthcare. Well-planned plant-based diets are endorsed by reputable organizations, including the American Heart Association and the Academy of Nutrition and Dietetics.

Supporting plant-based residents is about more than dietary preference; it is about providing care that reflects the whole person. In addition, plant-based diets can offer important benefits for residents, caregivers, and communities:

- **Health:** Reduce risk of heart disease, hypertension, type 2 diabetes, certain cancers, and cognitive decline, as outlined in Chapter 4.
- **Environment:** Help reduce our carbon footprint and support sustainability goals through lower greenhouse gas emissions and resource use.
- **Ethics:** Promote compassionate living and animal welfare.
- **Inclusion:** Support diverse cultural, religious, and spiritual dietary practices.

Nutritional Adequacy: A Professional and Moral Imperative

Older adults face increased risks of nutritional deficiencies due to physiological changes, chronic illness, and medication use. As with any diet, plant-based diets must be carefully planned to prevent specific nutrient shortfalls. Facilities are ethically and legally responsible for ensuring that menus meet residents' needs based on the Dietary Reference Intakes (DRIs), under the oversight of a registered dietitian. Table 5.6 on page 172 provides a list of nutrients that deserve special attention in the diets of seniors and provides practical suggestions for ensuring nutritional adequacy.

Menu Planning

Developing well-balanced plant-based meals in care settings requires thoughtful inclusion of protein-rich legumes, soy products, whole grains, vegetables, and fortified foods. At every meal, facilities should aim to offer at least one nutritionally adequate plant-based option that supports resident health and respects their dietary preferences. In addition to whole foods, consider incorporating fortified plant-based milks, as well as yogurts, cheeses, and meat substitutes to ensure nutritional completeness and variety.

Below is a sample seven-day plant-based menu plan that can serve as a flexible framework for meal planning and adaptation. Keep in mind that many vegetarian and plant-based alternatives to meat, dairy, and eggs are now widely available, making it easy to modify existing menus without starting from scratch. Be sure to include a fortified plant-based milk, such as soy milk or another calcium- and vitamin D–fortified option, as part of daily meals.

Sample 7-Day Meal Plan for Plant-Based Residents

Day	Breakfast	Lunch	Dinner
1	Oatmeal with berries, chia or hempseeds, fortified soy milk	Lentil vegetable soup, whole grain bread with hummus and tomatoes, apple slices	Tofu vegetable stir-fry with brown rice, plant-based brownies
2	Whole grain toast with almond butter, banana, plant-based yogurt parfait	Chickpea salad sandwich, vegetable crudites with dip, fresh orange sections	Pasta with red lentil marinara, mixed greens with vinaigrette, plant-based ice cream with blueberry sauce
3	Green smoothie bowl with berries, seeds, and granola as toppings.	Old-fashioned pea soup, fresh bread, carrot slaw with vegan mayo, grapes	Black bean chili with cornbread, apple crisp
4	Overnight oats with prunes, hempseeds, fortified soy milk, blueberries	Tofu and vegetable kebabs, couscous, green salad	Black bean tacos with shredded lettuce, grated carrots, peppers, salsa, and guacamole, fruit salad with pear cream

5	Chia pudding with fortified soy milk, mango or raspberries, toast	Refried bean and vegetable wrap, plant-based yogurt with mango	Vegetable curry with lentils over quinoa or rice, carrot cake
6	Pancakes (made with fortified soy milk), maple syrup, sliced strawberries	Greek salad, whole wheat pita, hummus, fruit salad	Old-fashioned bean stew with root vegetables, cabbage, and green beans, oatmeal cookies
7	Scrambled tofu with veggies, sweet potato hash browns, cantaloupe slices	White bean and tomato soup, whole grain crackers, nut cheese, pear	Veggie burgers on a wholegrain bun, coleslaw, chocolate pudding

5 Best Practices for Facility Staff

1. Engage with residents and families to identify dietary preferences and needs. Incorporate their feedback. Remember that inclusive food service honors the dignity, values, and health of each resident.
2. Provide education and training for culinary and support staff.
3. Consult regularly with a registered dietitian trained in plant-based nutrition to ensure variety and nutritional adequacy.
4. Provide education and host taste testing sessions for residents (regardless of dietary preferences). With exposure to plant-based options, residents may incorporate more whole-plant foods that will help with the prevention and treatment of chronic diseases.
5. Take steps to balance menus and boost flavor:
   - Offer at least one balanced plant-based meal option per service.
   - Avoid vegetable-starch combinations alone—include plant protein choices with each meal.
   - Use herbs, spices, and umami flavors (e.g., nutritional yeast, tamari) to build flavor.

KEY TAKEAWAYS

Be prepared. Portable snacks, communication in advance, and a gracious presence go a long way in social settings.

Kind communication builds bridges. Whether dining with family or friends, focus on connection and gratitude, not confrontation.

Share delicious food. Plant-based meals that are rich in flavor, texture, and tradition spark curiosity, open minds, and make others more receptive to plant-forward meals.

Stay nourished. Prioritize protein, B_{12}, omega-3s, calcium, and vitamin D—especially when relying on others for food prep.

Be your own advocate. In care or communal settings, advocating for balanced plant-based meals can improve both individual health and food culture for others.

Lead with joy. Food is not only fuel—it's a celebration of life and relationships. Use your plant-based lifestyle to invite curiosity, not judgment.

With Grace and Purpose

Choosing a plant-based lifestyle is about more than what's on your plate, it's about how you live, connect, and show up in the world. In this chapter, we explored the joys and challenges of navigating a social world that doesn't always align with our values. Whether it's dining with friends, sharing meals with family, or advocating for yourself in healthcare settings, these moments call for grace, confidence, and compassion—for others and for yourself.

In the next chapter, we widen the lens even further, exploring the other pillars of lifestyle medicine that support healthy aging, including physical activity, sleep, stress management, social connection, and avoidance of addictive substances. You have the power to build a life that feels truly fulfilling.

CHAPTER 7

OTHER IMPORTANT PILLARS OF HEALTH

Chapter at a Glance

In this chapter, we explore five essential lifestyle pillars that work alongside plant-based eating to promote health, vitality, and resilience in later life: physical activity, restorative sleep, stress management, social connection, and the avoidance of risky substances. Each pillar is grounded in the science of lifestyle medicine and plays a key role in extending not just lifespan but health span—the years we spend feeling strong, independent, and well.

With helpful tips, evidence-based strategies, and inspiration from Maria's ongoing journey, this chapter will support you so that you can build a balanced, purposeful life, one step at a time.

Maria's Story: Building a Life in Balance

Several months into her plant-based journey, Maria began gently layering in other health-supporting habits. Most mornings, she laces up her walking shoes for a forty-five-minute stroll around the neighborhood or local park. Twice a week, she attends a gentle yoga class, discovering both strength and peace in the slow, focused movements.

Sleep still has its ups and downs, especially when she's worried about her aging mother or managing the joyful chaos of grandchildren. But she now skips late-night TV in favor of a good book and a calming cup of herbal tea.

Yoga has become more than a class; it's a lifeline. It helps Maria manage stress and stay grounded as she navigates caregiving, grief, and growing older. She also prioritizes long-standing friendships: sharing meals, going for walks, and laughing over cards or board games. While she occasionally enjoys a glass of wine, she drinks mindfully and is grateful that substance use has never been a concern.

Maria's routines aren't perfect, and she's learned that they don't need to be. Like many older adults, she's found that steady, intentional steps, taken with self-compassion, can lead to deep, lasting change. Her evolving lifestyle now supports not just her body but her sense of purpose, peace, and connection.

Beyond Your Diet: Expanding the Foundations of Health

Maria's evolving routine reflects a powerful shift that extends far beyond what's on her plate. As she's discovered, eating well lays the foundation, but it's the daily patterns of movement, rest, connection, and care that build a truly resilient lifestyle.

These habits—staying active, sleeping well, managing stress, fostering meaningful relationships, and avoiding harmful substances—work in synergy with plant-based eating to support well-being on every level. They influence everything from our energy and mood to our immune function and independence. And while it may seem like a lot at first, each pillar offers practical, achievable ways to feel better, stay engaged, and thrive through every season of life.

Physical Activity

Do you ever feel like it's harder to stay active than it used to be? You're not alone. Many older adults face challenges staying active due to aches, energy changes, or simply not knowing where to start. The encouraging news? Even gentle movement can have a profound impact on how we age.

Physical activity is one of the most powerful predictors of healthy aging. Regular movement helps maintain a healthy weight, preserve muscle mass and bone strength, support blood sugar control, and enhance memory and mood. It also reduces the risk of chronic conditions such as heart disease, type 2 diabetes, and some cancers, while helping preserve mobility, balance, independence, and overall quality of life.

However, staying active can become more challenging with age, due to joint discomfort, muscle loss (sarcopenia), fear of falling, illness, or simply a lack of safe spaces. Chronic health conditions that require more medical visits, or caregiving duties may also disrupt usual routines. Fortunately, even small amounts of movement, adapted to your circumstances, can go a long way in supporting strength, confidence, and long-term vitality.

How Much Exercise Is Enough?

You don't need to train for a marathon to enjoy the benefits of physical activity. Leading health organizations like the World Health Organization and the Centers for Disease Control and Prevention (CDC) recommend:

- 150 minutes per week of moderate activity (such as brisk walking), or
- 75 minutes per week of more vigorous activity (like dancing, swimming, or hiking)

Add strength-building activities twice a week to help maintain muscle and bone strength. This might include bodyweight movements (like sit-to-stand or wall push-ups), and using free weights, resistance bands, or machines.

And don't forget balance and flexibility exercises such as yoga, tai chi, or stretching, which support stability, prevent falls, and improve daily function. Aim for some movement every day, even if it's just a few minutes.

Remember, the best movement is the one you'll keep doing. Start where you are and build from there!

Practical Tips:

- **Make it enjoyable.** Choose activities that are fun! Walk with a friend, join a senior fitness class at your local community center, play pickleball, dance to your favorite music, or spend time in the garden.
- **Try a group class.** Whether it's cardio, strength, or flexibility, group fitness classes are open to all ages and abilities. Many communities offer sessions designed for older adults, and these are a great way to stay motivated and socially connected.
- **Track your steps.** Use a pedometer or smartphone app to aim for 6,000–10,000 steps per day, or whatever target feels sustainable for you.
- **Build real-life strength.** Add functional movements like standing from a chair without using your hands, climbing stairs,

or carrying groceries to maintain everyday independence.

- **Be kind to your joints.** Swimming, walking poles, or stationary cycling offer gentle, low-impact options that still build stamina and strength.
- **Break it up.** Short sessions—just ten to fifteen minutes—done throughout the day can be just as effective as one longer workout.
- **Adapt as needed.** If you have limited mobility, try chair yoga, gentle stretching, or resistance-band exercises from a seated position. These activities are safe, simple, and surprisingly effective.

Supplement Guidelines

Note: Always check with your healthcare provider before starting any new supplement. Some may interact with medications or health conditions.

Strong Evidence (worth considering):

- **Creatine Monohydrate**–Supplementation with 3–5 g/day has been shown to enhance muscle strength, lean mass, and functional performance in older adults, particularly when combined with resistance training. Though this is not an essential nutrient, and our body can produce about 1 g/day, plant-based eaters consume little or no dietary creatine, so their baseline stores are often lower than those of omnivores. Some individuals may opt for a lower maintenance dose (e.g., 1–2 g/day) to maintain muscle creatine levels within the typical range observed in individuals following a mixed diet, even if they are not doing structured strength training.
- **Protein Supplements (Plant-Based)**–Supplementing with 20–30 g of high-quality plant-based protein, such as soy, pea, or blended protein powders, can help support muscle maintenance and prevent sarcopenia when daily protein intake

is otherwise low. While some evidence supports consuming protein after resistance training, meeting total daily needs by consuming some protein at each meal is more important than timing.

Limited Evidence (use only if advised by your healthcare provider):

- **Beta-Alanine–May** enhance endurance and delay fatigue, but more research is needed in older populations.

For individuals experiencing joint discomfort that limits physical activity, certain supplements may offer modest support when combined with exercise, weight management, and physical therapy.

- **Curcumin (from turmeric)**–Evidence suggests that curcumin can help reduce joint pain and stiffness when used for more than twelve weeks, particularly in individuals with osteoarthritis, due to its anti-inflammatory, antioxidant, and digestive properties. Absorption varies widely between products, and formulations that enhance bioavailability are typically required for clinical effect.
- **Palmitoylethanolamide (PEA)**–A naturally occurring fatty acid compound that may help reduce pain and inflammation by modulating the body's endocannabinoid system. Emerging research suggests potential benefits for chronic pain conditions, including joint discomfort for some individuals, but more high-quality studies in older adults are needed.
- **Glucosamine Sulfate**–Commonly used for joint health, particularly in osteoarthritis. Some individuals report modest improvements in pain and function although results across studies are inconsistent.

Insufficient Evidence (not recommended):

- **Testosterone Boosters**–Over-the-counter products claiming to boost testosterone are often ineffective and potentially risky.

Restorative Sleep

Do you sometimes wake up feeling unrefreshed, even after what seemed like a full night's sleep? Or find yourself lying awake with "monkey mind" in the middle of the night? Sleep challenges are common in later life, and while the nature of our sleep may change with age, the need for restorative rest does not. The good news is that small changes can lead to meaningful improvements.

Restorative sleep is essential for memory consolidation, immune support, reducing inflammation, metabolic balance, and emotional resilience. On the other hand, chronic sleep deprivation is associated with increased inflammation, impaired cognitive function, and a greater risk of cardiovascular and neurodegenerative diseases. A good night's sleep is one of the best things you can do for your body and your mood.

How Much Sleep Do We Need?

As we age, getting quality sleep may become more difficult, but it remains just as important as it was in our younger years. According to the National Sleep Foundation, adults over sixty-five need seven to eight hours of sleep per night to feel rested and maintain optimal health.

Unfortunately, many factors can interfere with restful sleep—frequent nighttime urination, sleep apnea, medications, pain, chronic conditions, stress, poor sleep habits, or a partner who snores. Sleep disorders like insomnia or sleep apnea are also more common in older adults.

There are several ways to improve the sleep we get every night. Surprisingly, what we do during the day can influence our sleep. Developing a strong circadian rhythm to set the body's internal twenty-four-hour clock, and working to improve sleep hygiene (the set of simple habits that support high-quality rest) can set us up to sleep well through the night. However, if these practices don't resolve your sleep challenges, talk to your doctor about a referral to a sleep specialist.

Sleep Hygiene Hacks

Cultivate healthy habits that support sound sleep.

- Establish a consistent wake-up time, and keep regular bedtimes.
- Get morning sunlight, and spend time in nature. Ideally, getting exposure to ten to twenty minutes of natural sunlight within the first hour of waking will boost alertness and suppress melatonin (the sleep hormone).
- Limit use of screens before bed. In addition, dimming indoor lights can encourage natural sleepiness.
- Be physically active, especially in the morning or early afternoon. Avoid strenuous exercise within ninety minutes of bedtime.
- Avoid smoking and minimize alcohol intake.
- Minimize caffeine, especially in the afternoon or evening.
- Stop eating after dinner, and if possible, finish dinner at least two to three hours before bedtime.
- If you need to snack before bed, choose one that provides both complex carbohydrates and tryptophan-rich plant foods (such as oatmeal with pumpkin seeds and soy milk or whole grain toast with hummus), which may boost the body's production of sleep-regulating hormones.

Make sleep a priority.

- Maintain a regular sleep schedule, even on weekends. This means going to bed and waking up at about the same time every day.
- Don't overdo naps, as they can throw off your sleep at night. If you do nap, you may find it helpful to keep it brief (twenty to thirty minutes) and not too late in the day.

Create a nightly sleep routine.

- Unplug from electronics at least sixty minutes before going to bed. Electronics emit blue light, which can have an alerting effect and affect sleep.
- About a half hour before bed, wind down with music, gentle relaxation exercises, meditation, or reading.
- Dim your lights to facilitate the production of melatonin, our sleep hormone.
- Establish a consistent bedtime routine, such as brushing your teeth, taking a hot bath, and reading a book.
- Listen to an audiobook before or even as you fall asleep. Just as in childhood, listening to a book prepares you for sleep. Audiobooks are available for free on libbyapp.com or whatever app your local library uses; choose light reading rather than thrillers so that the story won't keep you awake.

Optimize your sleeping environment.

- Invest in a comfortable mattress, pillow, and bedding.
- Set a cool, comfortable temperature for sleep.
- Block out light using heavy curtains or an eye mask.
- Drown out noise with earplugs or a white noise machine.

Supplement Guidelines

Note: Always check with your healthcare provider before starting any new supplement. Some may interact with medications or health conditions.

Limited Evidence (use only if advised by your healthcare provider):

- **Melatonin**–May help older adults who have trouble falling asleep, particularly those with naturally lower melatonin levels. Research shows benefits are modest but meaningful for improving sleep onset and adjusting sleep schedules, such as when traveling or shifting bedtime routines. Typical doses for older adults range from 1–3 mg. Take thirty to sixty minutes before bedtime.

- **Magnesium**–Can support relaxation and improve overall sleep quality and may help manage mild insomnia symptoms. Evidence suggests it may be especially helpful when combined with a calming bedtime routine. Typical doses range from 100–200 mg/day. Take in the evening, one to two hours before bed.
- **Valerian Root**–May reduce the time it takes to fall asleep and improve perceived sleep quality, though results are mixed. It is generally used for mild insomnia rather than severe sleep disorders. Effects may build over several days of regular use. Take thirty minutes to two hours before bedtime.

Insufficient Evidence (not recommended):

- **CBD Products**–Current studies do not offer consistent evidence of benefit for sleep. Product quality varies widely.

Stress Management

Do worries about your health, your loved ones, or the future feel heavier than they used to? Life brings many challenges, especially as we age, but learning how to manage stress can build resilience and bring lasting relief.

Chronic stress contributes to inflammation, weakens immune function, raises blood pressure, and accelerates cellular aging. It's also linked to depression and cognitive decline in older adults. But not all stress is bad. Some forms, like the excitement of learning something new, engaging in meaningful work, or rising to a challenge, can actually boost resilience, sharpen thinking, and increase vitality. The goal isn't to eliminate all stress but to reduce the kind that wears us down.

We can learn to respond to life's pressures in healthier, more balanced ways.

Ways to Manage Stress and Rediscover Purpose

We can't always control what happens, but we can learn to influence how we respond. There are things we can do to help us stay calm, focused, and emotionally balanced. Many older adults find that mindfulness practices, such as meditation, prayer, deep breathing, or gentle movement like yoga and tai chi, are especially effective. Even just five to ten minutes a day of intentional relaxation can help lower stress hormones and promote a sense of calm. The key is finding what works for you and making it part of your routine.

Life may have changed in ways that have altered your sense of purpose, whether through shifts in work, relationships, or family roles. Taking time to rediscover or clarify what brings meaning can reduce stress and enhance enjoyment. You might consider volunteering in areas that feel deeply meaningful, or exploring new interests such as art, music, or gardening. Reconnecting with friends or family, across generations, can also be deeply rewarding. You might find fulfillment in reflecting on and sharing your life story. You could focus on your physical well-being, perhaps even becoming the fittest senior you know. Here are a few practical tips:

- **Start your morning with mindfulness.** Take five to ten minutes for slow, deep breathing, guided meditation, or progressive muscle relaxation.
- **Set healthy boundaries.** Practice saying no to activities that are not aligned with your interests. You don't have to meet every demand.
- **Keep your to-do list realistic.** Focus on what matters most to you.

- **Know when to reach out.** Some stressors, like grief, are beyond your control. Talking to a trusted friend, therapist, counselor, or support group can help.
- **Try journaling.** Writing down what you're grateful for or reflecting on your day can ease stress and promote peace of mind.
- **Find community.** Meditation groups, walking clubs, and gentle yoga classes can offer both relaxation and connection.
- **Embrace simple joys.** Walk in nature, garden, paint, knit, play music, or go bird-watching. Creative and outdoor activities can soothe the mind and restore perspective.

Supplement Guidelines

Note: Always consult your healthcare provider before starting new supplements, especially if you take medication or manage chronic conditions.

Strong Evidence (worth considering):

- **B-Complex Vitamins**–Supplementation with a full B-complex may help reduce stress and support mood in adults, including seniors. Key B-vitamins in this mix include **B_{12}** (supports nerve function and energy, often low in older adults), **B_6** (helps make neurotransmitters that regulate mood), and **folate** (supports serotonin and dopamine production).

Limited Evidence (use only if advised by your healthcare provider):

- **Ashwagandha**–An adaptogenic herb that may modestly reduce stress and cortisol levels in the short term (up to 12 weeks). Typical doses range from 250–600 mg/day. While some studies suggest potential benefits, data in older adults are limited, and rare cases of liver injury have been reported.
- **Omega-3 Fatty Acids**–May support mood regulation and stress resilience; doses of 1–2 g/day of DHA and EPA are commonly suggested.

Insufficient Evidence (not recommended):

- **Kava and GABA Supplements**–Potential safety concerns and limited evidence make these less advisable for stress management in seniors.

Social Connection

Have you ever felt lonely, even in a room full of people? Or maybe you've lost touch with someone who once brought joy to your life. Staying socially connected takes effort, but it's one of the most powerful ways to protect your health and happiness.

While many of us are aware of the risks associated with smoking, poor diet, obesity, and inactivity, fewer realize that loneliness and social isolation carry comparable health risks. In fact, strong social relationships are among the most consistent predictors of longevity and quality of life. A systematic review and meta-analysis of ninety studies found that social isolation was associated with a 32 percent increase in overall mortality, a 34 percent increase in cardiovascular mortality, and a 24 percent increase in cancer mortality.

Investing time and energy in relationships isn't just emotionally fulfilling; it can be lifesaving. Regular, meaningful connections foster emotional resilience, reduce stress, enhance immune function, and provide a sense of belonging and purpose.

Social well-being is often overlooked, but it plays a vital role in protecting both mind and body as we age. That said, maintaining and building social ties can become more challenging in later life. Friends may pass away or relocate, especially in our eighties, nineties, and beyond. Although those relationships can never be replaced, it is essential to nurture existing connections and actively seek out new ones.

Practical Tips

- **Get involved in your community.** Join groups that align with your interests, such as art or exercise classes, book clubs, gardening groups, or lifelong learning programs.
- **Volunteer your time.** Contributing to a cause not only supports others but also fosters a strong sense of purpose and belonging.
- **Keep in touch regularly.** Schedule weekly phone or video calls with friends and family. If technology is a barrier, ask someone to help you get set up.
- **Nurture spiritual connections.** Participation in a faith-based or spiritual community can offer deep emotional support and meaningful connection.
- **Wear your hearing aids.** Untreated hearing loss is a common, and often overlooked, cause of social withdrawal. Using hearing aids can help you stay connected and confident in conversations.
- **Address mobility or other barriers.** If issues like transportation, mobility, or incontinence are keeping you isolated, talk to your healthcare provider or support network about practical solutions.
- **Plan regular social time.** Organize game nights, shared meals, or simple outings with others to keep connection part of your routine.
- **Make the first move.** Say hello to a neighbor, invite someone for a walk, or share a cup of tea. Small gestures can lead to meaningful friendship.
- **Consider a companion animal.** Whether you live alone or with a partner, pets can provide companionship, emotional comfort, and a sense of routine. They may also encourage daily movement, like regular walks, and can even spark social interactions in your community.

Check Out Cohousing

This way of creating community arose from a Danish concept of a modern village that that fosters connection, sustainability, and neighborhoods where everyone can thrive—together. Some are only for seniors, some for all ages, and examples exist in more than half the states and provinces.

See https://www.cohousing.org/find-cohousing/finding-cohousing/ and https://cohousing.ca/communities/.

Co-author Vesanto Melina lives in one and has visited twenty-four cohousing communities.

Supplement Guidelines

Note: Always consult your healthcare provider before starting new supplements, especially if you take medication or manage chronic conditions.

Limited Evidence (use only if advised by your healthcare provider):

- **Omega-3 Fatty Acids**–May support mood regulation and emotional resilience, which can help foster social engagement. Typical doses range from 1–2 g/day of combined DHA and EPA.
- **Vitamin D**–Low vitamin D levels have been linked to depressive symptoms in older adults. Maintaining adequate levels may support mood and social motivation.
- **B-Vitamins (especially B6, folate, and B_{12})**–Important for neurological function and mood regulation. Deficiencies can affect cognition and mood, potentially impacting social engagement.

Insufficient Evidence (not recommended):

- **Over-the-counter "mood enhancers" or "social anxiety remedies"**–These products often lack evidence, and some may have safety concerns or interact with medications.

Avoidance of Addictive Substances

Have you ever wondered if you, or someone close to you, might be struggling with substance use? What starts as a way to cope with pain, grief, loneliness, or a life transition may take root quietly and grow into a dependency that's hard to shake, even when there is a strong motivation to quit.

Understanding the risks and recognizing the signs are important steps toward regaining control. Warning signs of substance misuse can include changes in sleep or appetite, memory lapses, mood swings, social withdrawal, and an increase in falls or injuries. In older adults, these symptoms are sometimes mistaken for normal aging or overlooked altogether.

But misuse, whether of alcohol, tobacco, prescription medications, such as sleeping pills and painkillers, (see section added below for other substances not covered) raises the risk of nearly every major cause of premature death. Fortunately, recovery is possible at any age. With compassionate support and evidence-based strategies, many people find they can regain control, improve their health, and experience renewed purpose and connection.

How Much Is Too Much: What's a Healthy Relationship with Alcohol?

As we age, our bodies become more sensitive to addictive substances. The liver and kidneys may process alcohol more slowly, and medications can interact more strongly with even small amounts of alcohol or sedatives such as benzodiazepines (e.g., lorazepam and diazepam), as well as sleep medications like zolpidem.

Based on new evidence, the World Health Organization (WHO) states that there is no safe amount of alcohol and advises against drinking. Alcohol consumption, even in moderation, is associated with increased risks of cancer and cardiovascular disease. According to experts, any reduction in alcohol consumption is beneficial for health.

In the United States, the National Institute on Alcohol Abuse and Alcoholism (NIAAA) recommends no more than one standard drink per day for older adults. Many may benefit from drinking less, or not at all, especially if they take medications that interact with alcohol or have health conditions like diabetes, heart disease, or liver disease.

Canada's 2023 Guidance on Alcohol and Health, from the Canadian Centre on Substance Use and Addiction (CCSA), states that for general health, less alcohol is better. They provide the following guidelines:

- **Zero drinks/week:** Not drinking has benefits, such as better health and sleep.
- **Two standard drinks or less per week:** Likely to avoid alcohol-related consequences.
- **Three to six drinks per week:** Increased risk of several types of cancer, including breast and colon cancer.
- **Seven or more drinks per week:** Increased risk of heart disease or stroke.

The Canadian Coalition for Seniors' Mental Health (CCSMH) advises older adults to consume no more than five drinks per week, with several alcohol-free days.

If You Smoke, Quit

When it comes to tobacco, there's no safe level of use. The good news is that quitting brings health benefits at any age, often starting within days. Support from a healthcare provider, counseling, nicotine replacement therapy, or group programs can greatly improve success. Replacing smoking-related habits with meaningful routines, like gardening, walking, staying active, or engaging in creative hobbies, can also help sustain long-term change.

Overuse of Prescription Medications and Other Substances

In addition to alcohol and tobacco, the overuse or long-term reliance on certain prescription medications is an important and often overlooked concern in older adults. Medications commonly used to manage pain, sleep, or anxiety, such as opioid pain relievers, benzodiazepines, and sleep aids, can lead to dependence, especially when used regularly over time or at higher doses than prescribed.

For example, opioid medications such as oxycodone and hydrocodone may be effective for short-term pain relief but carry risks of tolerance, dependence, and increased sensitivity to pain with prolonged use. Similarly, sedative medications, including benzodiazepines and sleep medications such as zolpidem, are associated with increased risks of falls, confusion, memory problems, and daytime drowsiness in older adults.

Even over-the-counter medications can pose risks when used frequently. Sedating antihistamines (often found in sleep aids) and certain pain relievers may contribute to drowsiness, dizziness, or interactions with other medications.

Regular review of all medications, including prescriptions, over-the-counter products, and supplements, is essential for healthy aging. Working with your healthcare provider or pharmacist to reassess ongoing need, adjust dosages, or explore safer alternatives can help minimize risk.

Practical Tips

Build Awareness and Intention

- **Practice mindful awareness.** Take time to notice when, why, and how much you drink. If you choose to consume alcohol, do so consciously, remembering that less is better for your health.
- **Reflect on your habits.** Consider how alcohol or sedatives fit into your routine and whether they align with your physical and emotional goals.

Find Support That Works

- **Choose evidence-based help.** Explore programs like Alcoholics Anonymous, Nicotine Anonymous, nicotine replacement therapy, cognitive behavioral therapy (CBT), or group counseling.
- **Stay accountable.** Share your goals with a trusted friend, loved one, or support group to stay motivated and connected.

Create Healthier Routines

- **Build positive rituals.** Swap alcohol for herbal teas, sparkling water, or other enjoyable nonalcoholic alternatives.
- **Celebrate small wins.** Acknowledge your progress along the way. Every step forward matters.
- **Review medications regularly.** Work with your healthcare provider to assess any risks of alcohol interactions or overuse of prescription medicines such as opioid pain relievers (e.g., oxycodone), antianxiety medications like lorazepam, and sleep aids such as zolpidem, as well as over-the-counter products with sedating effects.

Supplement Guidelines

Note: Always consult your healthcare provider before starting new supplements, especially if you take medication or manage chronic conditions.

Strong Evidence (worth considering):

- **Vitamin B_1 (Thiamine)**–Routinely used in clinical settings to prevent Wernicke's encephalopathy, which is a serious neurological condition caused by thiamine deficiency that can lead to confusion, memory problems, and poor coordination. If untreated, it can cause permanent brain damage. It is most common in individuals with chronic alcohol use, as alcohol interferes with thiamine absorption and utilization.

Limited Evidence (use only if advised by your healthcare provider):

- **Vitamin C and E**–May alleviate withdrawal symptoms in substance use disorders, though more research is needed.

Evidence Lacking (not recommended):

- **Herbal Detox Supplements**–Many lack scientific validation and may pose health risks; professional medical guidance is essential for substance cessation.

Final Thoughts

By integrating these five lifestyle pillars alongside a nourishing plant-based diet, older adults can meaningfully enhance the quality of their later years. These changes aren't about perfection or restriction; they're about reclaiming energy, purpose, and vitality for the years that matter most.

KEY TAKEAWAYS

Small, consistent changes can make a big difference in energy, mood, and overall well-being.

Move with intention. Regular physical activity helps preserve strength, flexibility, and independence.

Make rest a ritual. Prioritizing restorative sleep supports memory, immune health, and emotional resilience.

Manage stress mindfully. Gentle practices like deep breathing, stretching, or meditation can help you stay grounded and calm. Build on interests that give your life purpose.

Cultivate connection. Strong social bonds nourish emotional health, reduce isolation, and even extend lifespan.

Choose wisely. Limit or avoid tobacco, alcohol, and other risky substances to protect your body's healing capacity.

Be supplement smart. Some supplements can help, but others may be unnecessary or even harmful. Always check with your healthcare provider.

Each pillar reinforces the others. Start where you are. Choose one area to focus on this week, just like Maria, and take one mindful, manageable step at a time.

Your Next Step: Cooking with Purpose

As we've seen, a healthy, purposeful lifestyle is built on more than just food, but food remains a central pillar. What we choose to eat, and how we prepare it, can powerfully influence every other area of well-being, from energy and immunity to sleep, strength, and social connection. That's why your kitchen matters.

In the next chapter, we'll show you how to make plant-based eating and cooking work for you. Whether you're a seasoned cook or just getting started, you'll discover that cooking isn't just a chore; it's a superpower for healthy aging, joyful living, and plant-forward vitality.

CHAPTER 8

PLANT-BASED COOKING IS YOUR SUPERPOWER!

Chapter at a Glance

This chapter invites you to rediscover the kitchen as a place of nourishment, confidence, and joy. Whether you're a lifelong cook or just getting started, you'll find the guidance and practical tools to make plant-based meals a rewarding part of your daily life.

You'll learn how to:

- Set up a senior-friendly kitchen with tools that support safety and success.
- Build a well-stocked pantry for simple, satisfying meals.
- Master techniques and time-saving strategies that reduce effort, maximize nourishment, and make your time in the kitchen a pleasure.

Maria: Learning to Cook with Confidence

When Maria first began exploring a plant-based lifestyle, the idea of cooking without meat or dairy felt unfamiliar, and a little intimidating. She'd always prepared meals for her family but not plant-based entrées. Now, some of her go-to recipes no longer fit her new lifestyle and values and she wasn't sure what ingredients belonged in her new pantry, let alone how to season lentils or bake tofu.

So, she started small, taking it one meal at a time. At first, she leaned on simple swaps, like adding beans to her soups or pouring nondairy milk over her morning oats. Slowly, her confidence grew. She found a handful of core recipes she loved and learned to batch cook grains and prep vegetables ahead of time. A once-foreign pantry began to feel like home, with jars of dry black beans, fragrant spices, and whole grains lining the shelves.

Before long, Maria began to have more energy and fewer aches in her joints. Her digestion improved. But perhaps most important of all, she rediscovered something unexpected: joy in the kitchen. Now, when her grandkids come over for dinner, Maria sees it as a chance to show them how fun and flavorful plant-based eating can be.

On their last visit, the children built their own bowls and learned how to make peanut sauce from scratch, laughing and taste testing as they went. She's taught her walking group how to cook her famous Tofu Cacciatore. Every Wednesday evening, she joins a plant-based cooking class at her community center, and it's the highlight of her week.

For Maria, meals are no longer just about nutrition or managing health conditions. They're about creativity, connection, and care. Cooking has become more than a daily task—it's now a source of pleasure, purpose, and empowerment. And she's just getting started.

Welcome to Your Plant-Based Culinary Adventure!

Making a shift to plant-based cooking might feel like learning a new language, but the encouraging news is that it's simpler than you think, and the benefits are deeply rewarding. Whether you've been cooking for decades or you're just beginning to explore the kitchen, you'll find the information and support you need here.

Plant-based cooking is not about fads or restrictions; it's a return to wholesome, time-honored simplicity. It's about preparing meals with ingredients your parents or grandparents would recognize, such as garden vegetables, hearty whole grains, nourishing legumes, fresh fruits, and wholesome nuts and seeds. These aren't just ingredients; they're the foundation of meals that nourish your body, sustain your energy, and leave you feeling well fed.

When you cook with intention and care, you're doing more than making meals—you're activating a superpower that supports your health, your independence, and your joy in daily living.

Getting Comfortable in Your Kitchen

Start with what you know. Any kitchen experience you have is valuable. Take it one step at a time—you'll build confidence with each meal.

Top 5 to Get You Started

If you're just getting started, begin with:

- A good knife
- A cutting board
- One pot and one pan
- A set of mixing bowls
- Measuring cups and spoons

Kitchen Starter Cheat Sheet: Your Plant-Powered Kitchen

Start Here (Essentials)	Add Next (Helpful)	Optional Extras (Nice to Have)
Chef's knife + paring knife	Steamer basket	Air fryer
Cutting board	Citrus juicer	Food processor
Mixing bowls	Grater	Immersion blender
Measuring cups/spoons	Salad spinner	Instant Pot/pressure cooker
1–2 pots with lids	Baking dish	Slow cooker
Frying pan	Cookie sheet	Spray oil bottle
Wooden spoon + spatula	Loaf pan/muffin tin	Knife sharpener
Colander	Parchment paper/ silicone mat	Rasp-style zester
Can opener		
Blender		
Storage containers		

You don't need everything at once. Many delicious, nourishing meals can be made with just the essentials. Add tools gradually as your confidence and interest grow. Arrange the kitchen so that your most-used tools are within easy reach. When everything has its place and is easily accessible, cooking becomes a pleasure rather than a chore.

Building Your Plant-Based Pantry

Think of stocking your fridge and pantry like a painter's palette. You want a rich variety of colors and textures to create beautiful, nourishing meals. Transitioning doesn't have to be overwhelming. Start with what you have, take it one step at a time, and build a pantry that inspires you.

Step-by-Step Pantry Transformation

Step 1: Take Inventory. Start by going through your current pantry and fridge. Set aside the foods that align with your new plant-based approach. You might be surprised by how many suitable items you already have! Refer to the shopping list on page 240 for inspiration. You don't need everything on that list, but it can help you identify gaps and fill them.

Step 2: Make Space. Donate unopened items that no longer fit your eating style to a family member, friend, neighbor, or local food bank. This not only creates space, but it also marks the beginning of your new adventure.

Step 3: Organize with Care. Invest in or find a few simple storage tools: glass jars with tight-fitting lids for storing grains, beans, nuts, and seeds, and microwave-safe glass bowls for leftovers. Clear labeling makes it easy to find what you need. Use paper and tape for a simple solution or try a handheld label maker. Label the sides of jars for pantry shelves, and label the lids for items stored in drawers or the freezer. When your pantry is organized, food prep becomes faster and more enjoyable.

Step 4: Stock Up Thoughtfully. Rather than buying everything at once, begin with the ingredients you need for recipes you're excited to make. As you discover new favorites, your pantry will grow naturally, supporting the meals you most enjoy.

How to Stock Your Plant-Based Pantry

It's good to have a small notepad or whiteboard nearby to track staples you're running low on. This reduces last-minute store trips.

Whole Grains: Energy Boosters

Start with several familiar grains. Oats make a comforting breakfast (see pages 250–252); quinoa cooks very quickly and is rich in protein;

barley is perfect in soups and pilafs; and brown rice pairs beautifully with stir-fries, beans, and curries. As you become more adventurous, you might experiment with ancient grains like amaranth, farro, sorghum, Kamut, or spelt. These grains are fun additions to breakfast bowls, salads, and stews.

Pantry Tip: Cook a batch of grains ahead of time and store them in the refrigerator or freezer to save valuable meal prep time!

Legumes: Protein Powerhouses

Beans, lentils, and tofu are nutritional superstars. Start with versatile staples like black beans, chickpeas, and lentils. They are easy to cook and adapt well to a variety of dishes. You might stock both canned and dried legumes: Canned varieties offer unbeatable convenience and are great for quick meals while dried beans are economical, shelf-stable, and ideal when you have time to cook in bulk. Nutritionally, they deliver comparable amounts of protein, fiber, and key minerals.

Tofu is an especially senior-friendly food. It checks all the boxes: nutrient-rich, easy to chew and digest, and quick to prepare. It's also wonderfully versatile! Try it blended into smoothies or scrambles for breakfast; added to soups, sandwiches, or salads for lunch; or baked, grilled, or stir-fried for dinner. Legume-based pastas, made from black beans, chickpeas, edamame, or lentils, are another great option, offering about three times the protein of their grain-based counterparts.

Keep shelled edamame in your freezer, and, if you like, a few plant-based meat alternatives. While veggie burgers and sausages can add variety and familiarity to meals, they're often higher in sodium and more processed, so compare labels and choose wisely.

Pantry Tip: Purchase canned beans without added salt. If using regular canned beans, rinse first to cut sodium by nearly half.

Nuts and Seeds:

As nutrition powerhouses, nuts and seeds add richness, texture, and satisfaction to meals. Just a small daily amount provides essential fats, plant-based protein, fiber, and a broad range of important micronutrients. Every nut and seed contributes a distinct set of nutrients and benefits. For example, hempseeds are rich in protein; chia seeds, sesame tahini, and almonds are high in calcium; Brazil nuts are loaded with selenium; pumpkin seeds provide protein, iron, and zinc; and all provide vitamin E.

Cashews are good sources of zinc and work like magic for creamy sauces, cheeses, and other dairy replacements. Walnuts, flax, chia, and hempseeds are all excellent sources of plant-based omega-3 fatty acids. To preserve their valuable fats, store shelled seeds and nuts in the refrigerator or freezer. Just an ounce or two a day helps to support heart and brain health.

Pantry Tip: Keep a jar of mixed omega-3-rich seeds, such as chia, hemp, and ground flax, in the refrigerator or freezer for quick additions to cereals, smoothies, or baked goods.

Vegetables: Powerful Phytochemical Protection

Buy fresh produce as needed and in season, choosing organic and local when possible (see page 227). Aim to purchase only what you'll use within a week, except for long-lasting vegetables like winter squash and root vegetables, which keep well in a cool, dry place. A fun goal when selecting vegetables is to include something from every color of the rainbow. Each hue brings different nutrients and phytochemicals.

You'll find a wide variety of delicious, nutrient-rich vegetables in every color group. Here are just a few to explore:

- **Green:** Leafy greens such as kale, spinach, lettuces, collard greens, Swiss chard, parsley, bok choy, and napa cabbage (include daily), asparagus, broccoli, broccolini, Brussels sprouts, cabbage, celery, cucumbers, green beans, green onions, green peppers, peas, sprouts, and zucchini.

- **Yellow-orange:** Carrots, corn, golden beets, orange or yellow peppers, squash, sweet potatoes, yams
- **Pink-red:** Beets, radishes, red chard, red leaf lettuce, red onions, red peppers, red potatoes, tomatoes
- **Purple-blue:** Eggplant, red or purple cabbage, purple cauliflower, purple asparagus, purple carrots, purple potatoes
- **White-beige:** Cauliflower, daikon, garlic, kohlrabi, onions, potatoes

Pantry Tip: For convenience, keep frozen vegetables, such as peas and corn, on hand. Frozen greens, stir-fry mixes, broccoli, and riced cauliflower are great time-savers and often just as nutritious as their fresh counterparts. Canned vegetables can be handy, but some are high in sodium, so check the labels.

Fruits: Antioxidant Allies

Choose a wide range of fruits throughout the year: citrus (oranges, grapefruit, lemons, limes), berries, melons, and in-season local options like apples, grapes, peaches, pears, and plums. Dried fruits, such as apricots, cherries, dates (medjool or the more common deglet noor), figs, mangos, peaches, pears, prunes, and raisins, serve as ideal sweeteners and treats. Keep fruits on hand to top oatmeal, to enhance salads, as a base for desserts, or to enjoy as a refreshing snack. They provide fiber, hydration, and potent antioxidants to help protect your health.

Pantry Tip: When fruits like banana, mango, or pineapple become very ripe, peel, cut, and freeze them. Berries can be frozen as-is—no peeling or chopping required. For best results, spread fruit pieces in a single layer on a baking sheet and freeze until firm, then transfer to airtight containers or freezer bags. This prevents clumping and makes it easier to use only what you need. Label with the date and use within six to twelve months for best quality. These frozen fruits are perfect for smoothies and fruit-based "ice creams."

Fortified Plant-Based NonDairy Products

Plant-based milks, cheeses, yogurts, and other dairy alternatives are widely available in supermarkets. Choose milk that is unsweetened and fortified (enriched) with calcium, vitamin D, and vitamin B_{12}. Soy, pea, and some blended milks stand out for their protein content (check labels to find options with at least 6 g protein per cup).

Plant-based yogurts can be very healthy, especially if they contain active live cultures. As with milks, look for options that are fortified with calcium, vitamin D, and vitamin B_{12}, and prioritize those that have no added sugars and are low in saturated fat. Vegan cheeses vary wildly in their nutritional value, with some being predominantly oils and starches (less nutritious), while others, especially those made from cultured nuts or seeds, offer greater nutritional value. Be mindful of added sugars in nondairy yogurts and frozen desserts as they generally contain just as much sugar as their dairy counterparts.

Pantry Tip: Unopened, shelf-stable plant milks can be kept on hand for times when you run out of fresh. Once opened, refrigerate and use within seven to ten days.

Herbs and Spices: Flavor Boosters

Herbs and spices elevate simple meals into something extraordinary. Stock your pantry with basics like garlic (whole, minced, powdered), oregano and basil (fresh or dried), cumin, and cinnamon. Seasoning blends, including salt-free options, can be delicious and convenient. Fresh herbs like parsley, dill, and cilantro add bright, fresh flavors. Freeze herbs for instant flavor additions.

Pantry Tip: Purchase jars of pre-minced garlic and ginger for instant use. Plant-based bouillon pastes and stock or broth cubes or powders add depth to soups and sauces.

Salt, Oil, and Sugar: Flavor Boosters to Limit

Some whole-food, plant-based enthusiasts avoid added salt, oil, or sugar for health reasons while others use them thoughtfully. In many culinary traditions, even small amounts of these ingredients play an important role in enhancing flavor, texture, and authenticity, particularly in cultural dishes where their use carries deep-rooted significance. A drizzle of oil, a pinch of salt, or a touch of sweetness can go a long way in making a dish feel satisfying and familiar. As a general guideline, it's best to use as little salt, oil, or sweetener as possible, without compromising flavor. Get in the habit of checking food labels for added sugar, saturated fat, and sodium (look at the amounts per serving).

In the recipes you'll find in this book, we limit added oil and keep salt moderate or optional. Over time, you will find that your taste buds adjust to healthier foods, and often within a few weeks you will become more sensitive to natural flavors. Recipes can be adapted to suit your preferences or health needs. Listen to your body and consult your healthcare provider as needed.

Minimize Added Sugar, Fat, and Salt

Instead of refined sugar, try:

- Fresh or dried fruits
- A drizzle of maple syrup, date syrup, or molasses
- Vanilla and cinnamon to enhance natural sweetness

Cooking Oils/Fat

Instead of cooking oil, try:

- Water or vegetable broth for sautéing
- Steaming or roasting without added fat

- Cashews, nut butters, tahini, or mashed avocado for creamy dressings or sauces
- Oil spray, for tiny amounts, when needed

Salt

Instead of adding extra salt, try:

- Fresh lemon or lime juice to brighten dishes
- Herbs, spices, and salt-free seasoning blends
- Nutritional yeast for a savory, cheese-like flavor

Plant-Based Cooking Wisdom: Six Keys to Cooking Success

1. **Read First, Cook Second.** Always read the entire recipe before you begin. This prevents surprises, helps you plan your steps, and ensures that you have all the necessary ingredients on hand.
2. **Prepare Before You Cook.** Chop, measure, and organize your ingredients before you start cooking. Professional chefs refer to this as "mise en place," a simple practice that makes cooking smoother, easier, and more enjoyable.
3. **Measure with Care.** Accurate measuring, especially in baking, often makes the difference between success and disappointment.
4. **Choose Quality Ingredients.** Fresh, seasonal ingredients make everything taste better. When possible, choose organic and local produce for optimal flavor and nutrition.
5. **Start Simple with Substitutions.** Follow a recipe exactly as written the first time. Once you're familiar with the method and flavor profile, you may wish to adapt it to suit your own preferences or dietary needs.
6. **Create a Comfortable Workspace.** Organize your counter so that you have everything within reach. Good lighting and a clean workspace make cooking more enjoyable.

Time-Saving Strategies

Meal prep doesn't have to be time-consuming. With a few smart strategies, you can enjoy home-cooked meals without spending hours in the kitchen.

- **Plan a Weekly Prep Session:** Set aside one or two afternoons or evenings each week to prepare basics that will simplify weekday meals. Listen to music, a podcast, or invite a friend to join you in your kitchen, or even join a cooking club online.
- **Presoak Ahead:** Soaking beans and grains overnight can significantly reduce cooking time the next day and improve digestibility.
- **Batch Cooking Is Your Secret Weapon:** Cook a large pot of beans and another of grains. When making soups, stews, or casseroles that you love, freeze the extras in labeled containers for later.
- **Premake a Salad Base:** Wash and chop a large container of hearty greens (like romaine, kale, or spinach). You can also add other crisp, sturdy vegetables that hold up well over several days, such as shredded carrots, chopped broccoli or cauliflower, and sliced celery. Just before serving, add delicate items like tomatoes, cucumbers, or avocado. A ready-to-go salad base makes it easy to build nourishing meals in minutes and have salad every day.
- **Mix a Dressing or Sauce:** Prepare a jar of your favorite salad dressing to keep in the fridge for a week or more (See pages 270–272). You may also wish to prepare a favorite such as the Peanut Sauce on page 273 to create tasty bowls in short order.
- **Wash and Prep Sturdy Veggies:** Chop carrots, cabbage, or celery and store them in airtight containers. This keeps them crisp and ready for meals or snacks.

- **Roast a Rainbow Tray:** Roast a big tray of vegetables such as sweet potatoes, carrots, zucchini, potatoes, cauliflower, broccoli, or yams. Store them in the fridge, reheat, and mix into bowls, wraps, or soups.

Quick Meal Ideas with Prepped Ingredients:

- **Breakfast:** A hearty bowl of precooked grains topped with nuts, seeds, fresh, stewed or dried fruit, and plant-based milk or yogurt (page 235).
- **Lunch:** A quick salad with prepped greens, cooked beans, grains, seeds, and a drizzle of homemade dressing (pages 270–272).
- **Dinner:** A warm grain bowl with marinated tofu (page 299), steamed or roasted vegetables, and a flavorful sauce (page 273).

A few hours of prep can lead to days of ease—and energy to enjoy the things you love.

Cooking Beans: Easier Than You Think

Looking for something that's kind to your wallet and good for your health? Legumes are your best friends in the kitchen! They're nutritious, full of fiber, and easy to cook in big batches, so you can "cook once and eat smart all week." Pick a day each week, simmer a pot of beans or lentils, and whip up a recipe or two from this book. You'll thank yourself later when you have ready-to-go meals waiting in the fridge or freezer.

Legume Prep for All Cooking Methods

Even after commercial cleaning, uncooked legumes may contain tiny pebbles or bits of field debris. Here's how to prepare them properly:

1. **Sort and Rinse:** Remove visible debris or damaged beans, as necessary.

2. **Soak:** Place legumes in a large bowl or pot and cover with water to several inches above the beans (they will expand as they soak). Let them soak for at least six hours or overnight.
   Why soak? Even when using an Instant Pot or pressure cooker, soaking beans reduces cooking time, improves texture, enhances digestibility, and minimizes gas-producing compounds called oligosaccharides—a type of carbohydrate that can be difficult to digest and may cause bloating or flatulence. While soaking isn't essential for small, quicker cooking legumes like lentils, mung beans, and split peas, it improves their digestibility as well. For legumes that are not soaked, rinse before cooking.
3. **Drain and Rinse:** After soaking, discard the soaking water and rinse the legumes well. This further reduces compounds that may cause digestive discomfort.
4. **Cook:** Each type of bean has a different cooking time, which may vary depending on your cooking device. Refer to your Instant Pot, pressure cooker, or slow cooker manual for specific times and water-to-bean ratios. Stovetop guidance is below.

Cooking Legumes on a Stovetop

1. Add presoaked, rinsed legumes to a large pot with the amount of water indicated in Table 8.1.
2. Bring to a boil, then reduce heat, cover, and simmer gently.
3. Skim off any foam that rises to the top, as this contains indigestible oligosaccharides.
4. Add more water as needed to avoid drying out.
5. Beans are done (and are most digestible) when you can soften them on the roof of your mouth with your tongue or by pressing lightly with a fork.

Table 8.1 Cooking Legumes

Legume	Presoak, Yes, No, or Optional?	Ratio Legumes: Water Cups	Cooking Time, Minutes*	Approximate Yield from 1 Cup Legumes, Cups
Beans bigger than lentils and mung beans (e.g., black, kidney, navy, pinto, white)	Yes	1:4	45–90 Check for tenderness	2½–3
Lentils: split red	Optional	1:3	15–20 Fastest cooking legumes	2¼
Lentils: brown, green, or gray	Optional	1:2 for firm lentils used in loaves or patties 1:3 or 1:4 for soupier textures or stews (depending on thickness desired)	45 Faster cooking than larger legumes	2¼ or more
Peas, split, green or yellow, or mung beans	Optional	1:3	30–45 Faster cooking than larger legumes	2¼
Soybeans	Yes	1:4	180–240	2½–3

*Cooking time can vary considerably. Larger beans and older beans that have been stored for a longer period can take longer to cook. Check them toward the end of the estimated cooking time.

Freezing Cooked Legumes and Soups

Cooked legumes freeze well, on their own or in soups or stews. Invest in freezer-safe containers such as wide-mouthed mason jars, leak-proof glass containers, or labeled freezer bags.

- Once cooked, wait for your legumes and soup to cool before freezing.
- Leave at least 1 inch of headspace in jars to allow for expansion.
- Freeze in 1 or 2 serving portions for convenience.
- Label clearly with the name and date.
- Use within six months for optimal texture and flavor.

Canned Legumes for Convenience

Pressed for time? Canned beans and lentils are a nutritious, convenient option. They retain their protein, fiber, and minerals during canning. To reduce sodium, rinse them well or select "no salt added" or "low-sodium" varieties.

Cooking Grains

Whole grains are nutritious, satisfying, and versatile. Processed grains can be cooked according to package directions. Unprocessed whole grains are perfect for batch cooking. Use them throughout the week at breakfast and in soups, salads, bowls, and sides. For added flavor, use vegetable broth in place of water. For cooking oats, see recipe section, pages 251–252.

Whole Grain Prep for All Cooking Methods

1. **Rinse.** Rinse grains to remove any soil and drain before cooking.
2. **Optional Soak.** Soak grains overnight to reduce cooking time and improve digestibility. This is especially helpful for large,

chewy grains like wheat, spelt, Kamut berries, farro, and hulled barley.

Cooking Whole Grains with a Slow Cooker, Pressure Cooker, or Instant Pot

1. Follow the instructions that accompany your device for cooking whole grains.

Stovetop Method

1. Place rinsed grains in a pot with a lid and add the amount of water indicated in Table 8.2.
2. Bring to a boil; lower heat, cover, and simmer for the time indicated. Add water if needed. These times and yields are approximate.

Table 8.2 Cooking Grains

Grain	Ratio Grain: Water, Cups	Cooking Time, Minutes*	Approximate Yield from 1 Cup Grain, Cups	Notes
Barley, whole grain or scotch	1:3	60	3½	
Buckwheat groats or kasha	1:2	20	3	
Kamut berries	1:3	70–80	3	Presoaking for 8–10 hours reduces cooking time to 60 minutes
Millet	1:2	18–20; then let stand 10 minutes after cooking Quick cooking	3½	Serve warm

Grain	Ratio Grain: Water, Cups	Cooking Time, Minutes*	Approximate Yield from 1 Cup Grain, Cups	Notes
Quinoa	1:2	15; then let stand 15 minutes after cooking Quickest cooking of all whole grains	3	Most quinoa has been thoroughly pre-washed, but it can also be rinsed in a mesh strainer to remove a soapy or bitter tasting coating called saponin
Rice, brown*	1:6*	40–60, then drain*	3½	Cooking time can vary with the variety of rice so check after 40 minutes
Spelt berries	1:3	45–60	2½	
Wheat berries	1:3	45–60	3	
Wild rice	1:3	40–45; then let stand 10 minutes after cooking	3½–4	

*To reduce arsenic that is present in some rice, use 6 or more cups of water instead of the usual 2 cups of water per cup of rice, and drain after cooking. For added benefit, soak rice for 8–12 hours, drain, and rinse before cooking. This reduces both cooking time and arsenic levels.

After Cooking: Fluff and Release

Once your grains are cooked, remove the pot from the heat and let the grains rest, covered, for five to ten minutes. This helps the moisture redistribute evenly and makes it easier to fluff the grains with a fork, giving you a lighter, more separated texture. If any grains have stuck to the bottom of the pot, simply turn off the heat, add water, and cover the pan for a few minutes. This will help loosen the grains naturally, making serving and cleanup easier.

Storing Cooked Grains

To prevent cooked grains, especially rice, millet, and quinoa, from becoming overly soft or clumpy:

- **Option 1: Spread on a tray**
  After cooking, spread grains on a baking sheet or tray to allow steam and excess moisture to evaporate. Let them cool completely before transferring to an airtight container, which helps preserve their structure and fluffiness.
- **Option 2: Rinse and drain**
  For sticky grains, gently rinse them in a colander with cold water, then drain thoroughly before refrigerating. This removes excess starch and helps prevent clumping.

Store cooled grains in a sealed container in the fridge for up to five days or freeze in portioned containers for longer-term use.

A Sample Week of Dinners (with leftovers for next day lunch)

These meal ideas are meant to inspire you—but feel free to create your own weekly themes to match your tastes, traditions, and schedule.

- **Multicolored Bowl Monday:** Bowls are versatile, satisfying meals that can be endlessly varied (page 304). Begin with a base of whole grains. Top with steamed or roasted vegetables, add protein choices, such as baked tofu cubes, edamame, chickpeas, or kidney beans, and flavor with a delicious sauce such as Tasty Peanut Sauce (page 273). Top with avocado cubes, nuts, seeds, sprouts, fresh herbs, or sliced green onions.
- **Taco Tuesday:** Tacos for All (page 295) is always a crowd-pleaser. Try classic refried black or pinto beans. Serve with

chopped tomatoes, grated carrots, thinly sliced lettuce, avocado, salsa, and a squeeze of fresh lime.

- **Wrap Wednesday:** Wraps are a quick, satisfying meal perfect for busy midweek dinners. Try our Mediterranean Hummus Wrap (page 287), the zesty Fiesta Refried Bean Wrap (page 289), or the savory Asian Tofu and Veggie Wrap with Peanut Sauce (page 291). Pair with a soup if you like.
- **Global Flavors Thursday:** Explore a different world cuisine each week. Try Mexican-inspired Easy Peasy Chili (page 297), Roasted Cauliflower with Chickpeas and Olives (page 302), or French-inspired Marvelous Mushroom Ragout (page 307). The options are endless, and ethnic dishes are intensely flavorful and naturally plant-forward!
- **Pasta Friday:** A warm, comforting bowl of pasta is the perfect end to the week. Use whole grain or legume-based noodles and top with Red Lentil Pasta Sauce (page 305) or a store-bought marinara enhanced with sautéed mushrooms, spinach, and grated cashew cheese. To boost protein add lentils, soy curls, or veggie crumbles.
- **Soup and Salad Saturday:** A nourishing bowl of lentil or bean-based soup (pages 276–285) plus a fresh salad (pages 262–269) loaded with greens, colorful vegetables, nuts or seeds, and a simple dressing makes a perfect meal.
- **Family and Friends Sunday:** Gatherings are a wonderful time to prepare a special dish, like Tofu Cacciatore (page 309). For dessert, serve Apple Pear Crisp (page 317) or chocolate pudding (page 312) and fresh fruit. Or host a plant-based potluck and bring your favorite dish.

Find Community and Inspiration

Here are some great ways to connect with like-minded plant-based diet folks and stay inspired:

- **Join local plant-based cooking classes:** Often available through community centers, wellness clinics, or continuing education programs.
- **Explore virtual learning:** Online communities, videos, and expert-led classes (such as those at bravopb.com) offer flexible support and learning.
- **Check out plant-based cookbooks and magazines:** Your local library is a treasure trove of new recipes and ideas.
- **Visit farmers' markets:** Chat with growers, discover new produce, and find ideas for seasonal cooking.
- **Consider a local produce delivery service:** Many regions offer weekly boxes of organic or local fruits and vegetables.
- **Find a cooking buddy:** Share recipes, prep together, or swap meals.
- **Connect with like-minded groups:** Look for plant-based meetups, potlucks, or discussion groups in your area through social media, senior centers, or places of worship.

Finding Community Tip: Don't hesitate to check local natural food stores, community or senior centers, or online for plant-based groups, classes, and events. Many communities host small but valuable gatherings—you just need to know where to look.

Smart Shopping for Plant-Based Living

Whenever possible, choose a variety of fruits and vegetables that are fresh, affordable, and appealing to you—whether organic or conventionally grown. Pesticides are used in agriculture to control insects, weeds, and fungi. While high levels of exposure can pose health risks, the amounts found on produce are typically very low and regulated to remain well within established safety limits.

You may come across resources such as the Shopper's Guide to Pesticides in Produce from the Environmental Working Group, which ranks fruits and vegetables based on pesticide residues. While these lists can be helpful for those who prefer to prioritize organic purchases, they reflect the *presence* of residues, not the level of risk. In most cases, even the highest levels detected are far below safety thresholds set by regulatory agencies.

The most important message is this: The health benefits of eating a wide variety of fruits and vegetables far outweigh the potential risks from pesticide residues. Avoiding produce because of these concerns may do more harm than good.

If choosing organic fits your preferences, it can be a meaningful option. Some people choose organic to reduce pesticide exposure or to support environmental sustainability and farming practices they value. However, if cost or access is a concern, conventionally grown produce remains a safe, nutritious, and accessible choice.

If you're working within a budget, consider these practical strategies:

- Prioritize organic for items you eat with the skin or don't peel.
- Choose conventional options for produce with skins that will be removed, such as bananas, avocados, mangoes, melons, oranges, and pineapples.
- Shop local. Farmers' markets and small farms may use fewer or no synthetic pesticides, even if not certified organic.
- Wash all produce thoroughly. Rinse under running water, use a produce brush for firm items, and dry with a clean towel. While washing doesn't remove all residues, it can reduce them.

Whether organic or conventional, fruits and vegetables are among the most nutrient-dense foods you can eat. Focus on variety, color, and consistency—enjoying the full spectrum of plant foods in whatever form is most accessible to you.

How Can We Ensure That the Items We Buy Are Free of Animal Products?

If you're striving to avoid animal products, label reading is essential but not always straightforward. Many animal-derived ingredients appear under unfamiliar names or are used in small amounts as additives or processing aids.

Common hidden animal ingredients include:

- Gelatin (from animal collagen, often in gummy candies or marshmallows)
- Carmine or cochineal (a red dye made from crushed insects)
- Casein and whey (milk proteins found in some "nondairy" creamers or cheese alternatives)
- Lard or tallow (animal fat; used in some baked goods or traditional piecrusts)
- Anchovy paste or fish sauce (found in dressings, sauces, and some condiments)
- Rennet (an enzyme from animal stomachs, used in cheese making)

Resource Tip: For a more comprehensive list, visit the *Vegetarian Journal's Guide to Food Ingredients* online at vrg.org/ingredients. This excellent resource breaks down common food additives and identifies whether they're animal or plant-derived.

Food Sleuth Tip: When in doubt, choose products with a certified vegan or organic label.

PLANT-POWERED SHOPPING LIST

Use this list as a guide. Some examples are provided in brackets—adapt to your preferences.

LEGUMES: BEANS, LENTILS; SOY

- ☐ Dried legumes (lentils, beans)
- ☐ Frozen legumes (peas, edamame)
- ☐ Canned lentils, chickpeas, or beans
- ☐ Prepared bean or lentil soups
- ☐ Canned chili, baked, or refried beans
- ☐ Tofu, tempeh, seitan
- ☐ Hummus
- ☐ Plant-based meat alternatives

GRAIN PRODUCTS

- ☐ Oats (rolled, steel cuts, or groats)
- ☐ Brown rice
- ☐ Barley
- ☐ Quinoa
- ☐ Whole grain bread, wraps, crackers
- ☐ Pasta (whole grain or legume-based)
- ☐ Flour (whole wheat or other)

VEGETABLES AND FRUITS

- ☐ Fresh greens (kale, lettuce, broccoli)
- ☐ Garlic (whole or minced)
- ☐ Onions
- ☐ Seasonal vegetables
- ☐ Seasonal fruits

- ☐ Canned tomato products
- ☐ Canned water-packed fruits
- ☐ Dried fruits (raisins, dates, prunes)
- ☐ Frozen vegetables
- ☐ Frozen fruit

PLANT-BASED DAIRY ALTERNATIVES

- ☐ Fortified soy, pea, or oat milk
- ☐ Cultured nut cheese
- ☐ Plant-based yogurt

NUTS, SEEDS, AND BUTTERS

- ☐ Nuts (almonds, cashews, walnuts)
- ☐ Nut butters (peanut, almond)
- ☐ Seeds (hemp, flax, chia, pumpkin)
- ☐ Seed butters (tahini, sunflower)

SWEETENERS

- ☐ Maple or date syrup
- ☐ Blackstrap molasses

OTHER BEVERAGES

- ☐ Teas (herbal, green, black)
- ☐ Coffee

FATS AND OILS

- ☐ Canola or olive oil spray
- ☐ Oils (olive, avocado, canola, sesame)

SEASONINGS, CONDIMENTS, AND OTHER

- ☐ Nutritional yeast
- ☐ Seaweed (kelp, wakame, nori, agar)

- ☐ Miso, tamari, soy, and other sauces
- ☐ Vegetable stock or broth
- ☐ Vinegar (balsamic, rice, apple cider)
- ☐ Lemon or lime juice
- ☐ Curry paste
- ☐ Ketchup, mustard, relish, pickles

HERBS AND SPICES

- ☐ Fresh herbs (parsley, cilantro, basil)
- ☐ Fresh ginger
- ☐ Dried herbs (basil, oregano, thyme)
- ☐ Spices (cinnamon, nutmeg, cumin)
- ☐ Salt, pepper
- ☐ Mixed herb/spice blend

KEY TAKEAWAYS

Learning how to cook simple meals can become a rewarding part of your plant-powered journey.

Any previous experience in the kitchen is valuable, and you can find easy ways to create more healthy meals, even with minimal equipment.

Stocking a few essential ingredients, and making time to prepare food once or twice a week can set you up for success.

Over time, you will develop more confidence and identify dishes you love to cook and eat!

Bringing Your Kitchen to Life: Recipes for Joyful, Plant-Powered Living

Now that your kitchen is stocked and you've explored strategies for planning, shopping, prepping, and cooking with ease, you're ready for the heart of the journey: the recipes! In the next chapter, you'll find a collection of nourishing, flavorful, and satisfying plant-based dishes designed with older adults in mind. They are easy to prepare, budget-friendly, and endlessly adaptable. Whether you're cooking for one, sharing with family, or hosting a special gathering, these recipes make plant-based eating both joyful and delicious.

CHAPTER 9

RECIPES FOR JOYFUL, PLANT-POWERED LIVING

Chapter at a Glance

Now that you've explored foundations of plant-based eating, it's time to bring those skills to life with nourishing, delicious meals. Whether you're cooking for one, sharing meals with loved ones, or hosting a gathering, these recipes were crafted to satisfy and inspire.

In the pages ahead, you'll discover:

- Simple, senior-friendly recipes organized by meal type: breakfasts, lunches, salads, sauces, soups, entrées, and wholesome desserts
- Nutritional analyses to guide meal planning
- Practical tips that save time, reduce effort, and support health
- Flexible options for ingredient swaps and additions

Bringing Your Kitchen to Life

Food is more than fuel; it's comfort, connection, and celebration. In the pages ahead, you'll find recipes that the three of us turn to daily—dishes that are fun, flavorful, and easy to prepare. They reflect the vibrant, plant-powered lifestyle we've come to love. All have been tested (and given high ratings!) by volunteers, including seniors, to ensure they work beautifully in real-world kitchens.

We've included nutritional analyses for each recipe, to help you make informed choices and meet your nutritional needs with confidence. We listed most but not the full long list of vitamins and minerals; for more on this topic, see Chapter 5. To get the most out of this information, here are a few notes on how to interpret the analyses we provide:

- Many *basic* recipes include optional add-ins or variations. All nutritional analyses are done using the *basic* recipe without the optional add-ins or variations.
- When a recipe includes ingredient choices (e.g., water, broth, or wine for sautéing), the analysis is based on the first-listed option, which is typically the simplest or most health-promoting.

Each recipe lists a yield in cups and/or number of servings. As we've shared earlier in the book, batch cooking can be an effective strategy for supporting a healthy, sustainable lifestyle. Preparing meals in advance means you'll always have something nourishing on hand when time or energy is short. Over time, it also simplifies daily cooking and builds habits that support long-term well-being.

We also encourage batch cooking staples like legumes, hearty vegetables, and whole grains. Having these prepared makes it easy to assemble nourishing meals on the fly—think grain bowls with beans and greens, topped with a flavorful sauce. Cooking larger quantities of dishes like soups, stews, or salads takes only a bit more effort and yields multiple meals. Whether you're cooking for yourself, a household, or a gathering, this strategy saves time and energy. Extra portions store well in the refrigerator or freezer for quick, healthy meals when you need them.

Refrigerating cooked starchy foods, like potatoes, rice, and pasta, can even improve their health benefits by increasing resistant starch, which supports blood sugar balance, gut health, and satiety. If you're trying a recipe for the first time, feel free to start small. Over time, you'll build a go-to collection of "keeper" recipes you'll want to return to again and again.

In the pages that follow, you'll find ideas for breakfasts, salads, dressings and sauces, soups, entrées, and even desserts. Yes, sweets can absolutely be part of a plant-powered lifestyle—when they're made with wholesome ingredients and enjoyed in moderation. For quick reference, here are the recipes that we have included:

BREAKFASTS

Loaded Overnight Oats
Breakfast Oats Five Ways
Cashew French Toast
Golden Scrambled Tofu
Power-Packed Blueberry Smoothie
Pink Cadillac with Protein

SALADS

Full-Meal Salad
Colorful Bean and Vegetable Salad
Calcium-Rich Greens
Rainbow Quinoa Salad
Sweet and Crunchy Coleslaw

DRESSINGS AND SAUCES

Creamy Coleslaw Dressing
Tahini-Balsamic Dressing
Ginger Lime Miso Dressing
Perfect Peanut Sauce

SOUPS

Savory Black Bean Soup
Easy Minestrone Soup
Luscious Cream of Pea Soup
Middle Eastern Lentil Soup
Lentil Tomato Kale Soup
White Bean and Mushroom Soup

ENTRÉES

Mediterranean Hummus Wrap
Fiesta Refried Bean Wrap
Asian Tofu and Veggie Wrap with Peanut Sauce
Best Black Bean Burgers
Tacos for All
Easy Peasy Chili
Tasty Tofu with Two Marinades
Roasted Cauliflower with Chick-peas and Olives
The Multicolored Bowl
Red Lentil Pasta Sauce
Marvelous Mushroom Ragout
Tofu Cacciatore

DESSERTS AND BAKED GOODS

Easy Chocolate Pudding
Creamy Chia Pudding
Simple Stewed Fruit
Apple Pear Crisp
Cashew-Pear Cream
Cranberry Pecan Muffins
Double Corn Muffins
Molasses Ginger Cookies
No-Bake Chocolate Clusters
Nutty Date Cookies
Seedy Cinnamon Crunch Cookies

Breakfast: A Powerful, Plant-Based Fresh Start to Your Day!

Breakfast is more than just the first meal of the day; it sets the tone for everything that follows. A nourishing, balanced breakfast helps stabilize blood sugar, boosts energy and concentration, and supports healthy weight management. And the best part? Making it plant-based is simple, satisfying, and delicious.

Today, plant-based alternatives are widely available and easy to use. Dairy products like milk and yogurt can be swapped for calcium and protein-rich plant-based options. Eggs? Try our Golden Scrambled Tofu, a savory, satisfying dish that's quick to prepare. Craving something sweet? Our Cashew French Toast, topped with Simple Stewed Fruit or fresh bananas and maple syrup, is a comforting choice that doesn't compromise on nutrition.

Busy mornings? We've got you covered. Blend up a Power-Packed Blueberry Smoothie. It's ready in minutes and full of nutrients. Prep Loaded Overnight Oats the night before. Breakfast Oats Five Ways offers many options, depending on your preferences.

Looking for more quick ideas? Keep it simple with:

- Avocado toast topped with sliced tomato and smoked tofu
- A multigrain bagel or toast with peanut butter and banana
- A whole grain wrap filled with hummus and veggies
- A hearty muffin served with plain plant-based yogurt and fruit
- A colorful yogurt parfait layered with fruit and granola

When breakfast is built on whole plant foods, you're not just filling your plate, you're fueling your body, mind, and day with intention.

LOADED OVERNIGHT OATS

Makes 2 cups (before addition of fruit)

This creamy, comforting breakfast is assembled the night before and ready to enjoy by morning, with no cooking required. Prepared overnight oats will keep for up to three days, refrigerated, though the texture will soften over time. Soaking the grains enhances their digestibility and improves mineral absorption. This recipe delivers plant-based protein, calcium, vitamin B_{12}, vitamin D, zinc, and omega-3 fatty acids. Customize with your favorite fruits, nuts, or spices, such as nutmeg, cardamom, allspice, or cloves. You can also replace some of the milk with unsweetened, plant-based yogurt for extra creaminess.

1 cup old-fashioned rolled oats or other rolled grains

2 tablespoons chopped prunes, raisins, or other dried fruit

2 tablespoons hempseeds

1 tablespoon chia seeds

2 tablespoons chopped walnuts, almonds, or other nuts

¼ teaspoon ground cinnamon (see Chef's Tip on page 331)

1½ cups unsweetened, fortified soy milk or other plant-based milk

1½–2 cups fresh fruit (e.g., sliced bananas, berries, chopped or grated apple, apricot, mango, peach, or pear)

1. Place the oats, dried fruit, hempseeds, chia seeds, nuts, cinnamon, and plant-based milk in a bowl or container and stir well.
2. Cover and refrigerate overnight (or for at least 6 hours).
3. Just before serving, stir in fresh fruit.

OPTIONAL TOPPINGS:

- Your favorite plant-based milk
- Ground flaxseeds

Per half recipe: Calories: 444, Protein: 17 g, Fat: 18 g, Carbohydrate: 61 g, Fiber: 10 g

Minerals: Calcium: 307 mg, Iron: 4 mg, Magnesium: 189 mg, Potassium: 829 mg, Sodium: 67 mg, Zinc: 3 mg

Vitamins: A: 11 mcg, C: 11 mg, E: 1 mg, Folate: 30 mg DFE

Percent of calories from: Protein 13%, Fat 32%, Carbohydrate 55%

BREAKFAST OATS FIVE WAYS

Discover how versatile and satisfying oats can be! This recipe collection takes you from Quick Oats (1) all the way to Oat Groats (4)—the whole, unprocessed form of oats. You'll also find a high-protein option (5) featuring quinoa and lentils for added variety and staying power. All forms of oats are rich in soluble fiber, which supports blood sugar balance and heart health. Though oat groats require longer cooking, their intact structure slows digestion and helps you stay fuller longer, making them a particularly satisfying and sustaining option.

To save time, consider soaking groats ahead of time. If oats are a regular part of your morning routine, feel free to double, triple, or quadruple any of these recipes. Cooked oats keep well in the refrigerator for four to six days. Batch cooking can make breakfast quicker and easier throughout the week. Personalize your bowl with the optional add-ins and toppings listed at the end of this section. While salt is optional, even a small pinch can enhance the flavor of these nourishing dishes.

1 Quick Oats Makes 1 cup

STOVETOP METHOD

1. Place 1 cup of water in a saucepan with a lid and bring to a boil.
2. Stir in ½ cup quick oats and set heat to low.
3. Cover and simmer for 1 minute or until most of the water is absorbed, stirring occasionally.

MICROWAVE METHOD

1. Place 1 cup of water and ½ cup of quick oats in a microwave-safe bowl and microwave on high for 1½ to 2 minutes. Stir and serve.

2 Old-Fashioned Rolled Oats Makes 1 cup

1. Place 1 cup of water in a saucepan with a lid and bring to a boil.
2. Stir in ½ cup of rolled oats and set heat to low.
3. Cover and simmer for 5 to 10 minutes or until most of the water has been absorbed, stirring occasionally.

3 Steel-Cut Oats Makes 1½ cups

1. Place 1½ cups of water in a saucepan with a lid and bring to a boil.
2. Stir in ½ cup of steel-cut oats and set heat to low.
3. Cover and simmer for about 35 minutes, or until most of the water has been absorbed, stirring occasionally. Add a little plant-based milk or water to thin, if needed. (This also can be cooked in an Instant Pot or Pressure Cooker; decrease water to 1 cup.)

4 Oat Groats (Whole Oats) Makes 3 cups

INSTANT POT OR PRESSURE COOKER METHOD

1. Rinse 1 cup of oat groats.
2. Place 2 cups of water and the oat groats in an Instant Pot or pressure cooker and cook for 30 minutes on high pressure and allow to release naturally. Drain any excess water.

STOVETOP METHOD

1. Rinse 1 cup of oat groats.
2. Bring 3 cups of water to a boil in a saucepan with a lid.
3. Add the oat groats, lower heat, cover, and simmer for 60 minutes or until groats are tender, stirring occasionally.

Oat groats can be eaten warm or cold. If reheating, add a little plant-based milk or water, as well as toppings listed below.

5 Hearty Oat Groat Porridge Plus Makes about 3 cups

INSTANT POT OR PRESSURE COOKER METHOD

1. Rinse ½ cup of groats and ¼ cup each of quinoa and small brown or red lentils.
2. Place oat groats, quinoa, lentils, and 2 cups of water in an Instant Pot or pressure cooker and cook on high pressure for 20 minutes. Add plant-based milk or water to achieve desired consistency.

STOVETOP METHOD

1. Rinse ½ cup oat groats, and ¼ cup each of quinoa and lentils.
2. Bring 2½ cups of water to a boil in a saucepan with a lid.
3. Add oat groats, quinoa, and lentils.
4. Cover and simmer until the water has been absorbed (about an hour), stirring occasionally. Add plant-based milk or water to achieve desired consistency.

Per cup of Quick and Regular Rolled Oats: Calories: 166, Protein: 5 g, Fat: 4 g, Carbohydrate: 28 g, Fiber: 4 g
Minerals: Calcium: 21 mg, Iron: 2 mg, Magnesium: 63 mg, Potassium: 164 mg, Sodium: 1 mg, Zinc: 2 mg
Vitamins: A: 0 mcg, C: 0 mg, E: 0.3 mg, Folate: 26 mcg DFE
Percent of calories from: Protein 13%, Fat 15%, Carbohydrate 72%

Per cup of Hearty Oat Groat Porridge Plus: Calories: 205, Protein: 10 g, Fat: 3 g, Carbohydrate: 36 g Fiber: 6 g,
Minerals: Calcium: 31 mg, Iron: 3 mg, Magnesium: 83 mg, Potassium: 301 mg, Sodium: 7 mg, Zinc: 2 mg
Vitamins: A: 0.4 mcg, C: 0.7 mg, E: 0.4 mg, Folate: 117 mcg DFE
Percent of calories from: Protein 19%, Fat 12%, Carbohydrate 69%

OPTIONAL ADD-INS FOR ALL VERSIONS

These can be added to water at the same time as the oats.

- Salt–add 1/8 teaspoon salt for rolled and steel-cut oats or ¼ teaspoon for oat groats or hearty oat groat porridge plus
- Fortified plant-based milk—use instead of water (or use part water, part milk) for a nutrition boost
- Dried fruit–blueberries, cherries, cranberries, currants, blueberries, or chopped apricots, dates, figs, peaches, or prunes
- Seeds–chia, ground flax, hemp, pumpkin, or sunflower
- Nuts–chopped almonds, hazelnuts, pecans, pistachios, or walnuts
- Unsweetened, shredded coconut
- Nut or seed butter
- Allspice, cardamom, cinnamon, cloves, nutmeg, ginger, or pumpkin pie spice
- Vanilla extract (¼ teaspoon) or a pinch of vanilla bean powder

TOPPINGS FOR ALL VERSIONS

Add to the bowl before eating.

- Fresh berries or other chopped fresh fruit
- Fortified soy milk or other plant-based milk
- Fruit compote
- Seeds or chopped nuts
- Nondairy yogurt
- A sprinkle of cinnamon or nutmeg.
- Brown, date, or coconut sugar; maple syrup or molasses—use sparingly!

CASHEW FRENCH TOAST

Makes 6 slices

This healthy version of French toast is easy, delicious, and rich in minerals such as calcium, iron, magnesium, and zinc as well as protein. Serve it hot with fresh fruit, fruit sauce, or maple syrup.

½ cup fortified soy milk or other plant-based milk

¼ cup cashew nuts

¼ teaspoon vanilla

½ tablespoon maple syrup (optional)

6 slices whole grain bread or gluten-free bread

1. Place soy milk, cashews, vanilla, and maple syrup, if using, in a blender and blend on high speed to make a smooth cashew cream.
2. Pour the cashew cream into a shallow dish.
3. Lightly oil or spray a nonstick skillet and warm it over medium heat.
4. Dip each slice of bread into the cashew mixture, coating both sides.
5. Place 2 or 3 slices on the skillet, depending on skillet size. Avoid overlapping and leave a little space between slices. Cook on medium heat until golden brown, then flip each slice and cook on the other side.

Per half recipe (3 slice serving): Calories: 395, Protein: 18 g, Fat: 12 g, Carbohydrate: 55 g, Fiber: 7 g
Minerals: Calcium: 259 mg, Iron: 4 mg, Magnesium: 136 mg, Potassium: 439 mg, Sodium: 527 mg, Zinc: 3 mg
Vitamins: A: 38 mcg, C: 0 mg, E: 0.8 mg, Folate: 57 mcg DFE
Percent of calories from: Protein 17%, Fat 28%, Carbohydrate 55%

GOLDEN SCRAMBLED TOFU

Makes 3 to 4 cups

A hearty, protein-packed alternative to scrambled eggs, this savory dish is both nourishing and satisfying. It's rich in high-quality plant protein, calcium, and iron—key nutrients for supporting muscle strength, bone health, and sustained energy in older adults. Feel free to customize with your favorite seasoning blends, herbs, or extra veggies to suit your taste. Serve warm with toast or roasted potatoes, if desired.

⅓ cup unsweetened fortified soy milk or other plant-based milk

1 tablespoon tahini

1½ tablespoons nutritional yeast

½ teaspoon turmeric powder

1 teaspoon jarred fresh garlic or minced garlic, or ½ teaspoon garlic powder

½ teaspoon onion powder

½ teaspoon salt (or use black salt—Kala Namik—for an eggy flavor)

1 block (14–16 oz, 1 pound) firm or medium firm tofu, drained

1–2 cups chopped vegetables (e.g., green onions, mushrooms, peppers, zucchini)

1–2 cups spinach, coarsely chopped

Fresh ground black pepper to taste

1. In a small bowl, whisk the plant-based milk, tahini, nutritional yeast, turmeric, garlic, onion powder, and salt.
2. In a medium-sized bowl, crumble the tofu into bite-sized pieces using your hands or a fork.
3. Heat a large pan over medium heat. Put in the chopped vegetables (except spinach) and sauté until just tender, adding a splash of water, broth, or olive oil as needed to prevent sticking.
4. Add the tofu to the vegetables and cook for another 3 to 4 minutes.
5. Pour the milk mixture over the tofu and stir gently to coat. Cook for 5 minutes, stirring occasionally.
6. Add the spinach and cook for a minute or until spinach is wilted.
7. Finish with black pepper, to taste.

Per cup (1/3 recipe)*: Calories: 168, Protein: 16 g, Fat: 9 g, Carbohydrate: 10 g, Fiber: 3 g

Minerals: Calcium: 330 mg, Iron: 3 mg, Magnesium: 70 mg, Potassium: 464 mg, Sodium: 434 mg, Zinc: 2 mg

Vitamins: A: 75 mcg, C: 27 mg, E: 0.5 mg, Folate: 361 mcg DFE

Percent of calories from: Protein 35%, Fat 44%, Carbohydrate 21%

*Protein and calcium levels can vary with tofu selected. Check labels.

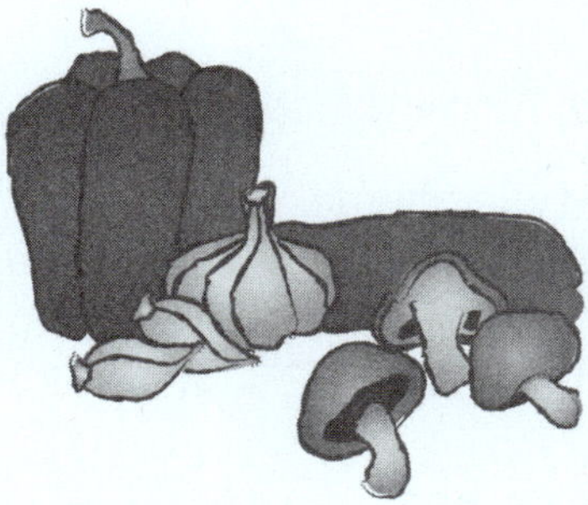

POWER-PACKED BLUEBERRY SMOOTHIE

Makes 2 cups

This smoothie makes a winning breakfast or snack, delivering many of the key nutrients your body needs to start the day strong. Blueberries are rich in antioxidants, kale provides calcium, hempseeds supply omega-3 fatty acids, and fortified soy milk adds protein, calcium, and vitamin D. Using frozen fruit creates a thicker texture. For bigger appetites, feel free to double the recipe. Don't miss the Optional Add-Ins—you might find you enjoy them all!

1 cup fortified soy milk

1 cup blueberries

1 cup kale, packed

2 tablespoons hempseeds

½ banana, fresh or frozen

Place soy milk, blueberries, kale, hempseeds, and banana in a blender and process until smooth.

OPTIONAL ADD-INS:

1. Swap the soy milk for another plant-based milk or orange juice; add extra for a thinner smoothie.
2. Use other mild greens such as spinach or bok choy.
3. Boost the protein with 2–3 ounces soft tofu, ¼ cup cooked beans, or ½ scoop protein powder.
4. For extra sweetness and fiber, blend in 2 pitted dates, a half or one peeled orange, strawberries, pineapple chunks, a whole banana, or other fruit.
5. For a wider range of protective phytochemicals, add veggies such as frozen peas, a few carrot slices, or sunflower sprouts.

6. For antioxidant and anti-inflammatory action, add ¼ teaspoon of ground cinnamon, ¼ teaspoon of dried ginger (or 1–2 tablespoons of fresh, grated ginger), ½ teaspoon matcha (green powdered tea), or ⅛ teaspoon of dried cardamom, cloves, nutmeg, or allspice.
7. For more calcium and vitamin E, add 1 tablespoon of almond butter.
8. For extra flavor, add ¼ teaspoon vanilla.

Per 2 cups (whole recipe): Calories: 333, Protein: 16 g, Fat: 15 g, Carbohydrate: 41 g, Fiber: 7 g
Minerals: Calcium: 365 mg, Iron: 3.5 mg, Magnesium: 209 mg, Potassium: 920 mg, Sodium: 97 mg, Zinc: 3 mg
Vitamins: A: 86 mcg, C: 35 mg, E: 1 mg, Folate: 53 mcg DFE
Percent of calories from: Protein 18%, Fat 36%, Carbohydrate 46%

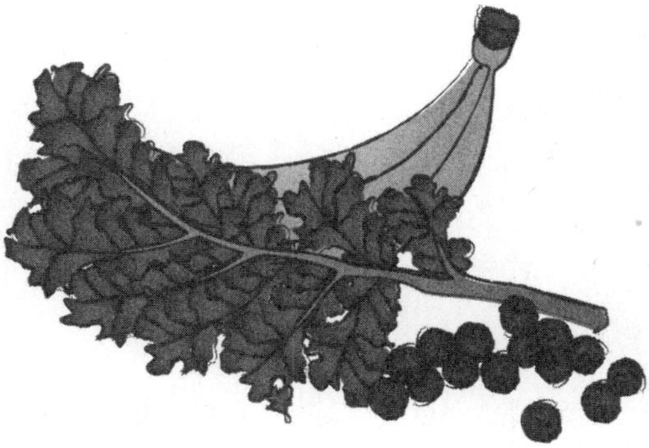

PINK CADILLAC WITH PROTEIN

Makes 2 cups

This refreshing and antioxidant-rich smoothie delivers about 22 grams of protein. Vitamin C in the fruit increases the absorption of iron in tofu. Hempseeds are an outstanding source of omega-3 fatty acids, as well as protein. Fruit can be fresh or frozen. Ripe or overripe bananas can be peeled, bagged, and frozen. For a higher fiber meal, enjoy it alongside a slice of high-fiber, whole grain toast with avocado and tomato slices or nut butter.

Juice of 2 oranges (¾ cup orange juice)

½ cup strawberries

½ cup mango or ½ banana

½ (5–6-oz) package soft or silken tofu

3 tablespoons hempseeds

Place juice, strawberries, mango, tofu, and hempseeds in a blender and process until smooth.

OPTIONAL ADD-INS OR VARIATIONS:

- Replace mango or strawberries with raspberries, pitted cherries, or other fruit.
- Include a half or one scoop of protein powder.
- Replace juice with 1 large, peeled orange plus ⅓ cup of plant-based milk.

Per smoothie (whole recipe): Calories: 512, Protein: 22 g, Fat: 21 g, Carbohydrate: 42 g, Fiber: 3 g

Minerals: Calcium: 219 mg, Iron: 5 mg, Magnesium: 286 mg, Potassium: 1151 mg, Sodium: 16 mg, Zinc: 4 mg

Vitamins: A: 64 mcg, C: 166 mg, E: 1 mg, Folate: 171 mcg DFE

Percent of calories from: Protein 20%, Fat 42%, Carbohydrate 38%

Salads, Dressings, and Sauces

Salads can be so much more than a side dish! A well-composed salad can be the centerpiece of a nourishing, satisfying meal. They're an easy and versatile way to load up on fiber, antioxidants, and essential nutrients. Leafy greens provide folate, vitamin K, and calcium. Brightly colored vegetables and fruits supply vitamins such as A and C, potassium, and powerful phytochemicals like carotenoids and flavonoids. Whether you're tossing together fresh greens or building a hearty grain-and-bean bowl, salads offer an abundance of health benefits in every bite. Adding beans, nuts, seeds, or whole grains boosts protein, iron, zinc, and healthy fats.

Homemade dressings take things to the next level. Unlike most store-bought versions, which are often heavy on oils, sodium, added sugars, and preservatives, the dressings and sauces featured here are made from whole-food ingredients like nuts, seeds, tahini, and peanut butter. While many fat-free dressings rely heavily on added sugars for flavor, a small amount of healthy fat helps the body absorb fat-soluble vitamins and beneficial phytochemicals from salads. Our dressings provide healthy fats, plant protein, and extra fiber, without sacrificing flavor or convenience.

To save time, prep a few dressing or sauce favorites ahead of time and store them in the fridge. They keep well for a week or so and can quickly transform a simple bowl of greens, steamed veggies, grains, or legumes into something crave-worthy.

From zesty to creamy, these recipes will help you mix and match flavors, boost nutrition, and keep meals exciting throughout the week.

FULL-MEAL SALAD

This salad can be as large or as small as you like, and can last for one or for several days, adding some ingredients just before serving.

If you would like to have salad available at a moment's notice, chop a base of leafy greens. This can last up to four days, stored and refrigerated in a big bowl with a lid. When you are ready to eat, add some of the vegetables and protein foods listed below. Then add any of the dressings on pages 270 to 272. You will have an instant feast that is rich in protective phytochemicals. Alternatively, this can be a hearty salad for a group.

Leafy Greens: Your base can be 8 or more cups of chopped mixed greens, including any of the following: lettuce, spinach, kale, (stems removed and sliced matchstick thin), thinly sliced cabbage, or other greens. For a flavor boost, mix in a little dill, parsley, basil, or other herbs.

Green Veggies: Add 1 or more cups of prepared (chopped or sliced) green vegetables such as broccoli florets, broccolini, asparagus, snow peas, zucchini, or celery. For broccoli or asparagus, lightly steam if desired, then plunge into an ice bath to preserve color and crispness.

White-Beige Veggies: Add thin strips of kohlrabi or jicama, or cauliflower florets (steam, if desired).

Red, Orange, Yellow Veggies and Avocado: Just before serving, add sliced tomatoes, cherry or grape tomatoes, sweet peppers, radishes, red onions, and avocado.

Plant Protein Foods: Choose one or two of the following cooked high protein foods, providing ½ to 1 cup per person: marinated tofu cubes (page 299), tempeh, edamame, chickpeas, other beans, lentils, or falafel balls. For the entire salad (not per person), add ¼ to ½ cup of peanuts, pumpkin or sunflower seeds, or other nuts or seeds.

Starchy Additions: To make the meal even more satisfying, include ½ to 1 cup per person of any of the following: steamed and cubed sweet potato, potato, squash, or beets; cooked quinoa, Kamut, spelt, wild rice, or corn (sliced from a cob or niblets).

Chef's Notes

1. If saving some salad for meals later in the week, add the Red, Orange, and Green Veggies, the Plant Protein Foods, and the Starchy Additions to your leafy green base just before serving on each occasion. Serve with a dressing of your choice (pages 270–272).
2. If the salad will be eaten by a group at one meal, add a variety of veggies to the base of leafy greens. The Plant Protein Foods and Starchy Additions can be added to this mix or served separately, along with a dressing of your choice (pages 270–272).

COLORFUL BEAN AND VEGETABLE SALAD

Makes 6 cups

This vibrant bean and veggie salad is a delicious way to add protein, fiber, B vitamins, and essential minerals to your meals. Make a batch and keep it in the fridge for up to five days. It's perfect for quick lunches, hearty sides, or a satisfying snack that keeps you energized between meals. Use any colorful beans you enjoy: black, chickpeas, cannellini, pinto, red, Anasazi, lima, or navy beans all work beautifully.

MARINADE

¼ cup balsamic or cider vinegar or lemon or lime juice (or a mix)

2 tablespoons olive oil, avocado oil, or toasted sesame oil (optional)

1–2 teaspoons Dijon mustard

2 tablespoons chopped fresh dill, 2 teaspoons dried dill

1–2 teaspoons minced garlic

¼ teaspoon each of salt and pepper, or to taste

BEANS

3 cups cooked or canned beans, rinsed and drained

VEGETABLES: (a total of 3 cups), such as:

1 cup diced bell pepper

1 cup canned corn niblets, drained

1 cup halved cherry tomatoes

1. Place the marinade ingredients: vinegar, oil, mustard, dill, garlic, salt, and pepper in a small jar with a lid. Shake well.
2. Place beans, vegetables, and marinade in a large bowl and gently toss to mix.

OPTIONAL ADD-INS:

For veggies: Consider chopped artichoke hearts, asparagus, avocado, celery, Napa cabbage, snow peas, zucchini, cooked or raw broccoli or cauliflower florets, or steamed green beans.

Bold flavor boosters: Mix in a handful of chopped olives or sun-dried tomatoes for added richness and depth.

A hint of sweetness: Add 1 tablespoon of maple syrup to the dressing.

More tang: Increase vinegar or lemon/lime juice by an additional 2 tablespoons.

A bit of heat: Add hot sauce to taste.

Per cup: Calories: 175, Protein: 9 g, Fat: 1 g, Carbohydrate: 30 g, Fiber: 9 g

Minerals: Calcium: 42 mg, Iron: 2 mg, Magnesium: 63 mg, Potassium: 504 mg, Sodium: 375 mg, Zinc: 1 mg

Vitamins: A: 51 mcg, C: 36 mg, E: 1 mg, Folate: 157 mcg DFE

Percent of calories from: Protein 22%, Fat 6%, Carbohydrate 72%

CALCIUM-RICH GREEN SALAD

Makes 3½ cups

Kale is a good source of calcium, and this mineral is absorbed twice as efficiently as that from dairy products and tofu. Napa cabbage (also known as Chinese cabbage or siu choy) and broccoli also rank well for calcium availability. The broccoli can be steamed to make it easier to chew, or eaten raw. For bonus points, add other calcium-rich ingredients such as sliced figs, orange or mandarin sections, toasted almonds, or sesame seeds. Leftover salad can be covered and refrigerated for up to four days.

1 cup broccoli florets, steamed or raw

1 cup kale, thinly sliced

1 cup Napa cabbage, chopped

½ –1 red bell pepper, chopped

1. Place broccoli florets in a steamer over water and steam, or place in a saucepan with water and boil, until they are soft when pierced with a fork.
2. Fold kale leaf in half, remove the stem; then slice leaves matchstick thin.
3. Cut Napa cabbage leaves in half lengthwise and slice into ½-inch strips.
4. Place broccoli, kale, Napa cabbage, and red pepper in a bowl and mix.

Per cup: Calories: 27, Protein: 2 g, Fat: 0.3 g, Carbohydrate: 5 g, Fiber: 2 g

Minerals: Calcium: 48 mg, Iron: 0.6 mg, Magnesium: 18 mg, Potassium: 241 mg, Sodium: 34 mg, Zinc: 0.3 mg

Vitamins: A: 130 mcg, C: 64 mg, E: 1 mg, Folate: 73 mcg DFE

Percent of calories from: Protein 23%, Fat 10%, Carbohydrate 67%

Figure 3.1 Your Plant-Powered Day

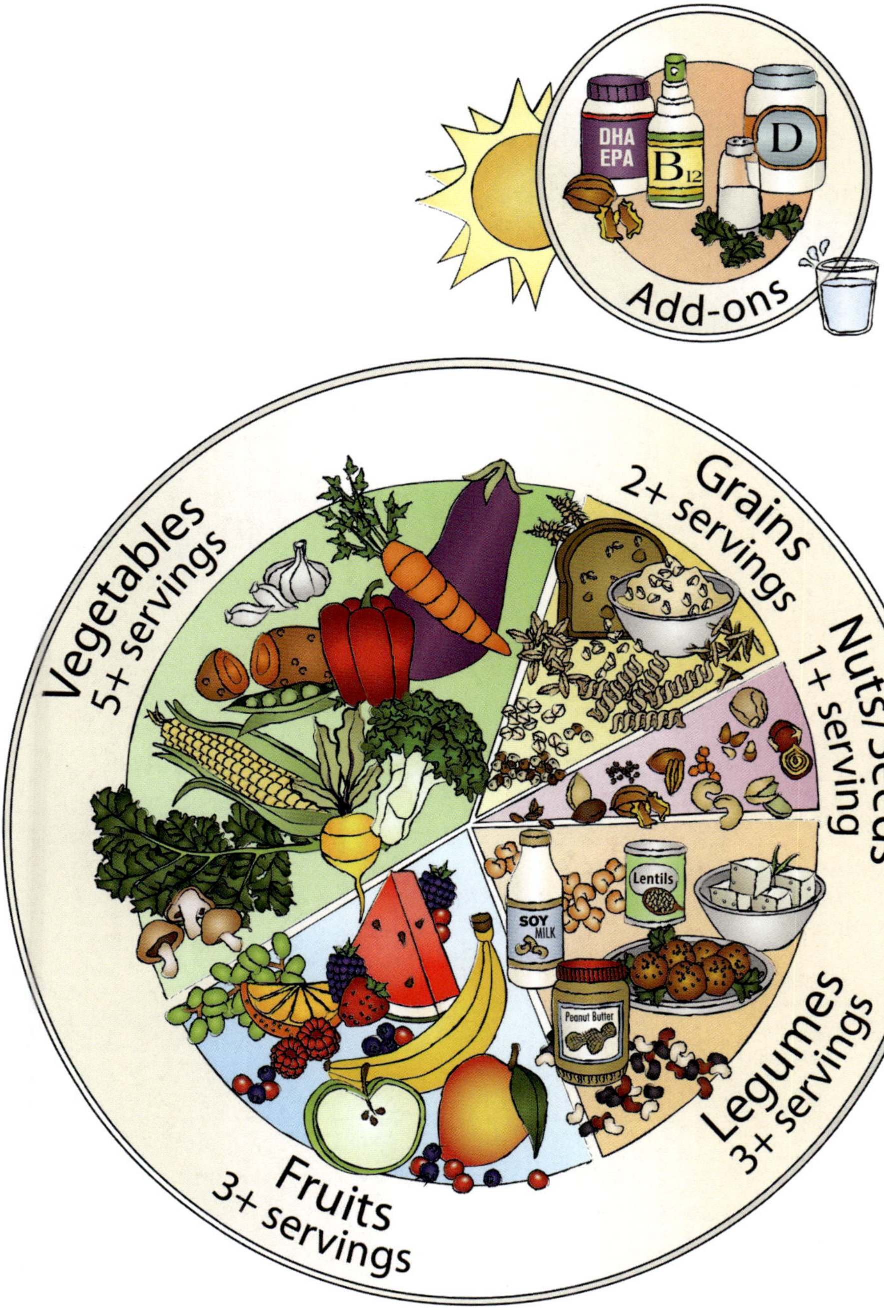

Table 3.1 Your Plant-Based Day: A Daily Guide to Major Food Groups
(Simplified version—see the full version on pp. 43-44)

FOOD GROUP **# Servings Suggested**	**FOODS INCLUDED** **Serving Sizes**	**CALCIUM-RICH CHOICES** **Within each food group**	**PROTEIN-RICH CHOICES** **Protein/ Serving (Grams)**
Vegetables (5 or more servings) Choose a rainbow of colors!	½ cup raw or cooked vegetables 1 cup raw leafy vegetables ½ cup vegetable juice	Bok choy, broccoli, collard greens, kale, mustard greens, napa cabbage, or okra Calcium-fortified juice	Fresh peas (4 g) Hubbard squash (3 g) Spinach, cooked (2.7 g) Corn (2.4 g)
Fruits (3 or more servings) Go for variety!	1 medium fruit ½ cup fruit juice ¼ cup dried fruit	Dried figs Oranges Calcium-fortified juice	Guava, durian, mango (2 g) Avocado (1.5 g)
Legumes (3 or more servings) Include with meals and snacks.	½ cup cooked beans, peas, lentils, tofu 1 cup peas 1 cup soy or pea milk ¼ cup peanuts 2 Tbsp peanut butter 2 oz veggie meat	Calcium-fortified soy or pea milk Soy or pea-based yogurt Edamame, soybeans, black beans, or white beans Calcium-set tofu	Tofu or tempeh (10-20 g) Soybeans, cooked (17 g) Veggie meat (15 g) Edamame (11 g) Peanuts (10 g) Lentils, split peas (9 g) Other beans (7-8 g)
Grains (2 or more servings) Choose mostly whole grains.	3 oz seitan ½ cup cooked pasta ½ cup sprouted grains 1 oz ready-to-eat cereal, bread, crackers	Calcium-fortified oat milk Calcium-fortified cereal Calcium-fortified tortilla	Seitan (16 g) Amaranth (5 g) Quinoa (4 g) Pasta (4-5 g) Other grains (2-3 g)
Nuts & Seeds (1 or more servings) Include an omega-3-rich choice.	¼ cup nuts or seeds 2 Tbsp nut or seed butter	Calcium-fortified nut or seed milk Almonds, almond butter Chia seeds Sesame seeds, tahini	Hempseeds/hearts (13-14g) Pumpkin seeds (10 g) Almonds (8 g) Nut or seed butter (6-7 g) Other nuts or seeds (5-7 g)

Loaded Overnight Oats (p. 250)

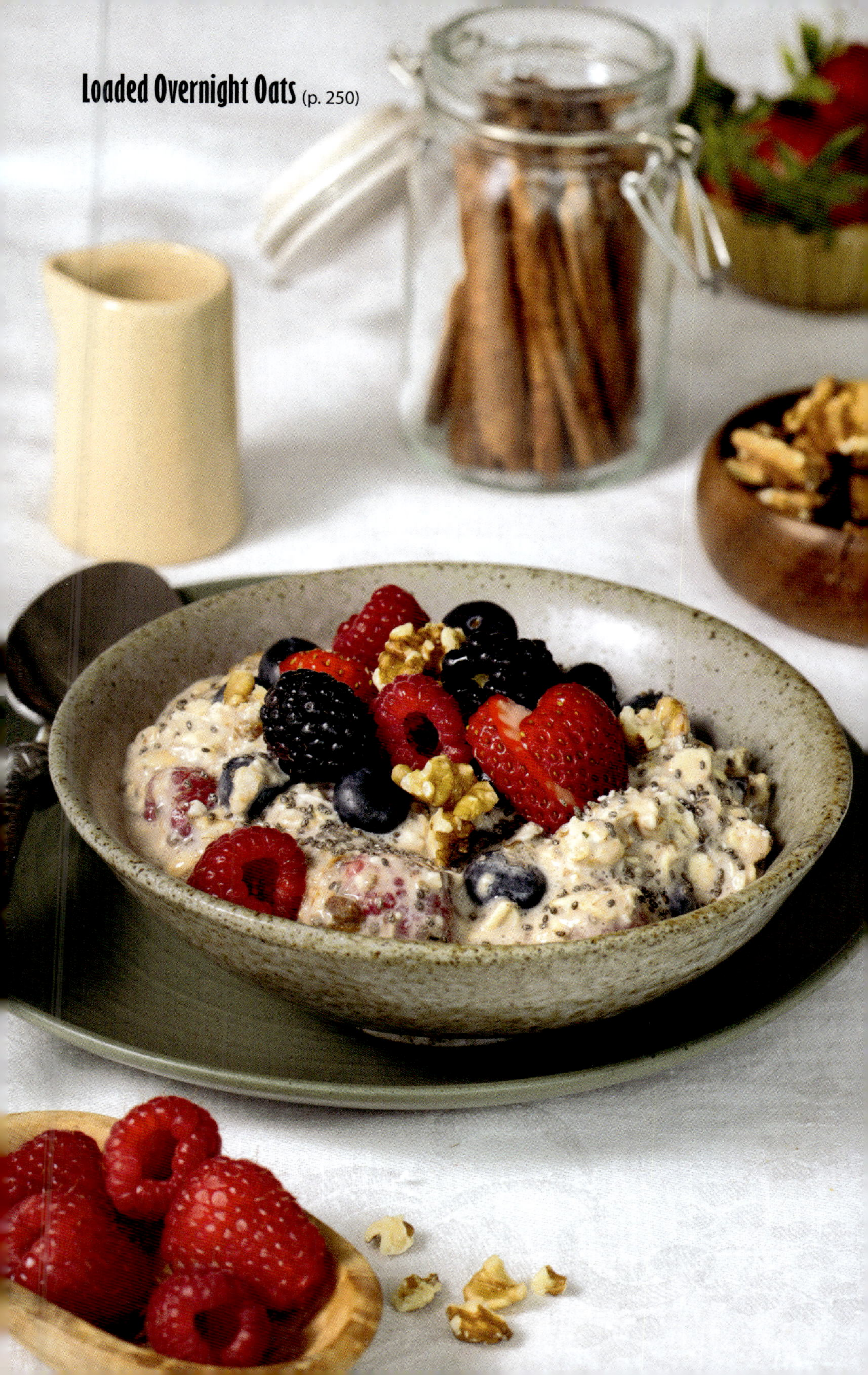

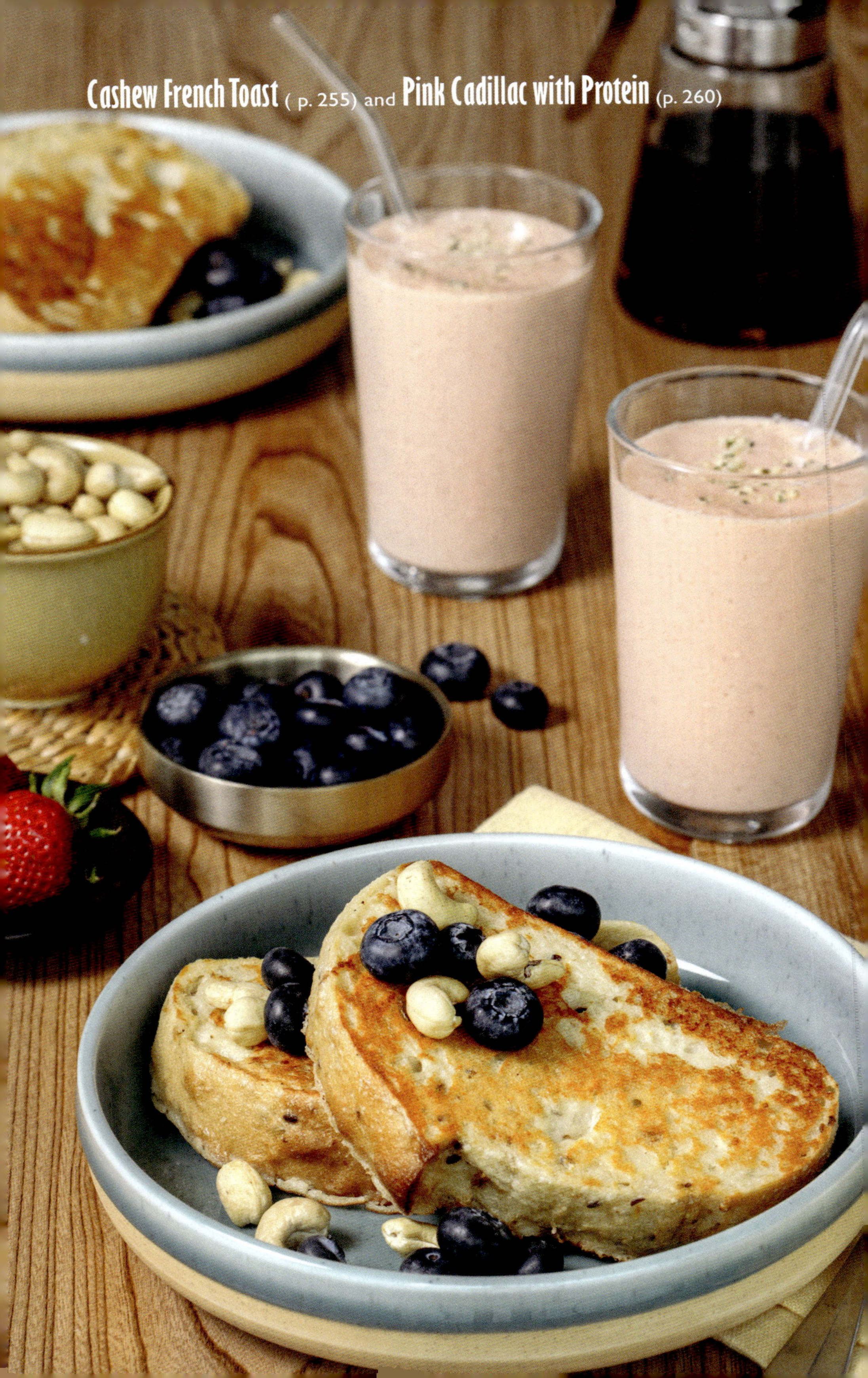

Cashew French Toast (p. 255) and **Pink Cadillac with Protein** (p. 260)

Golden Scrambled Tofu (pp. 256–257)

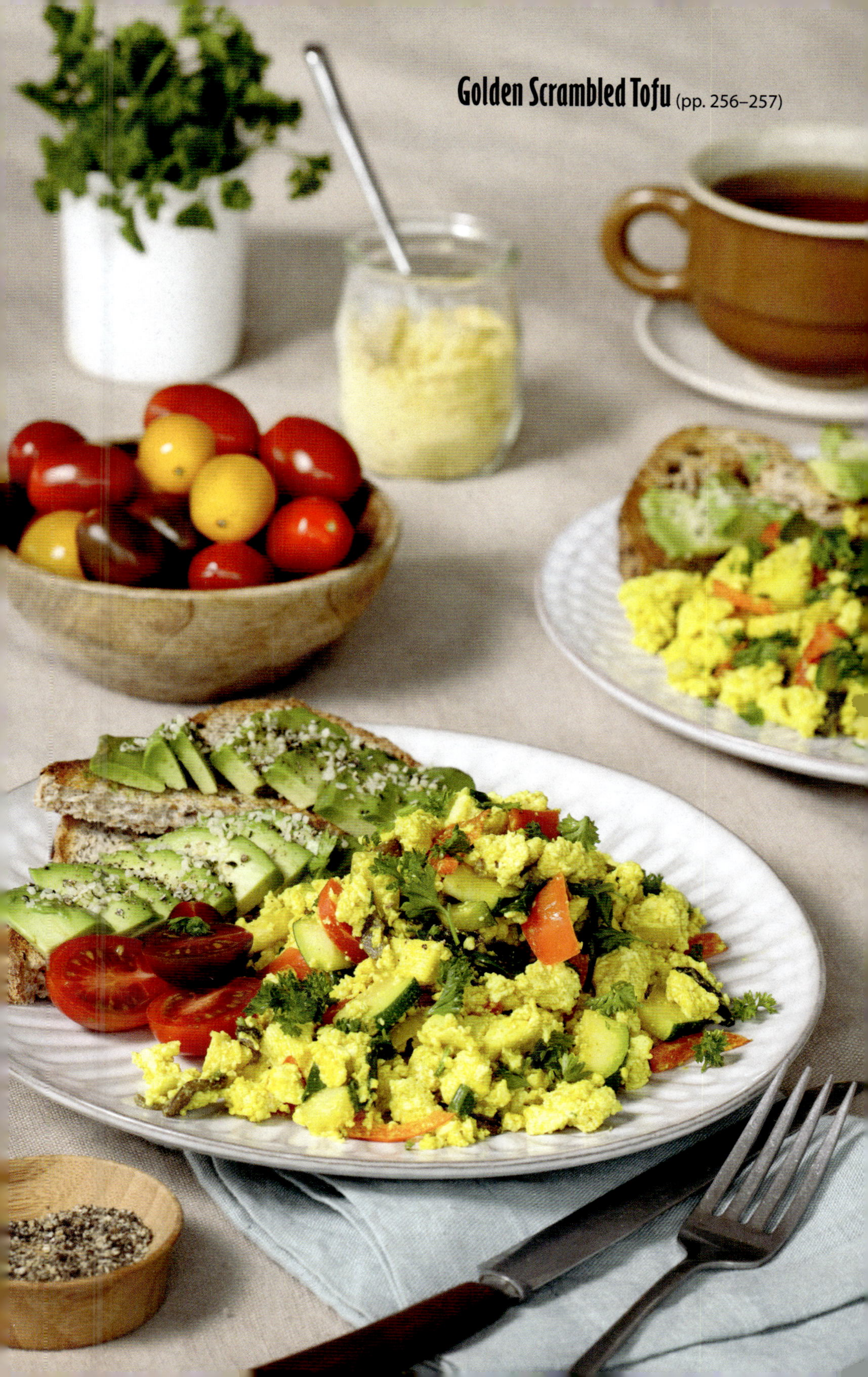

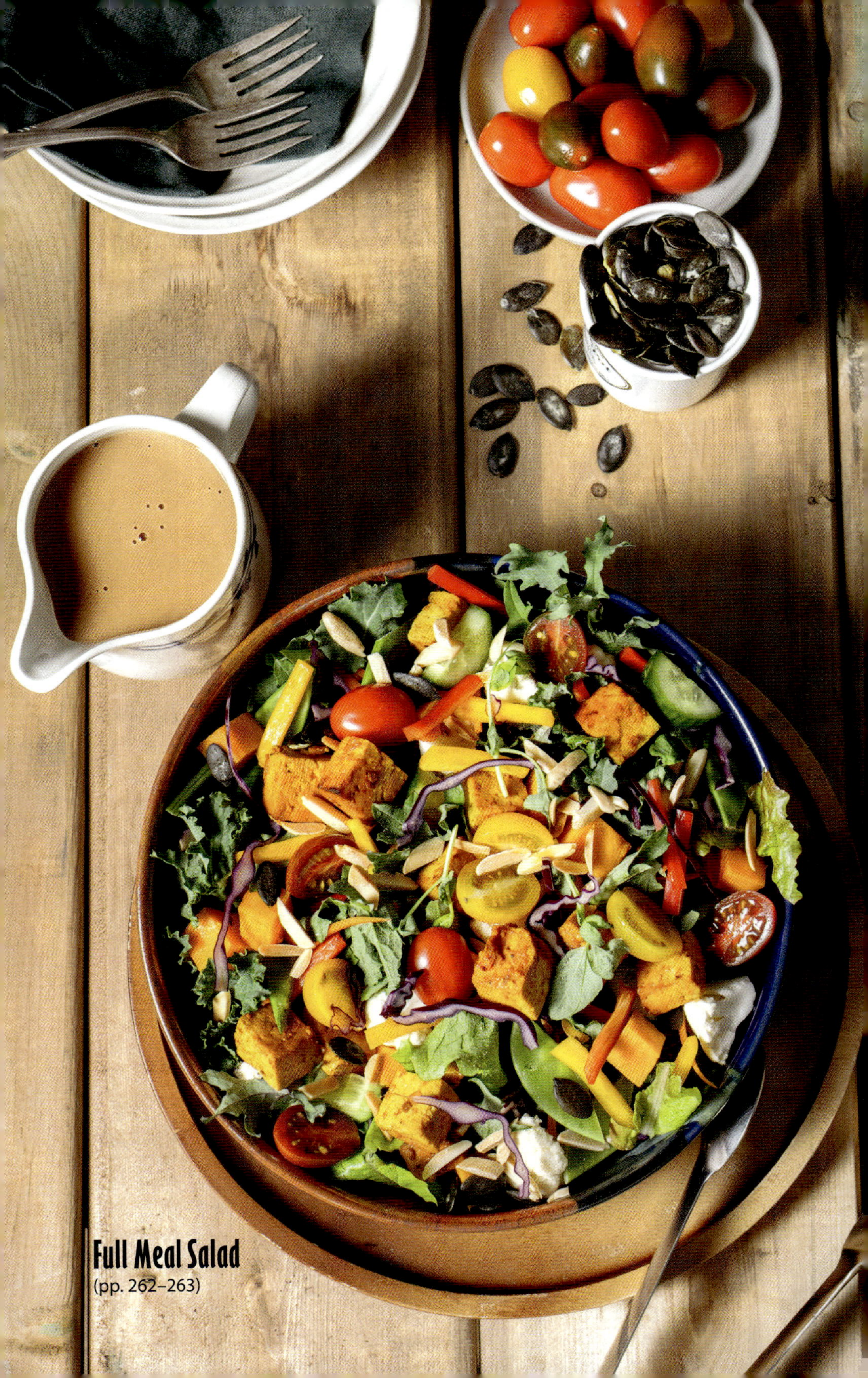

Full Meal Salad
(pp. 262–263)

Rainbow Quinoa Salad (pp. 267–268)

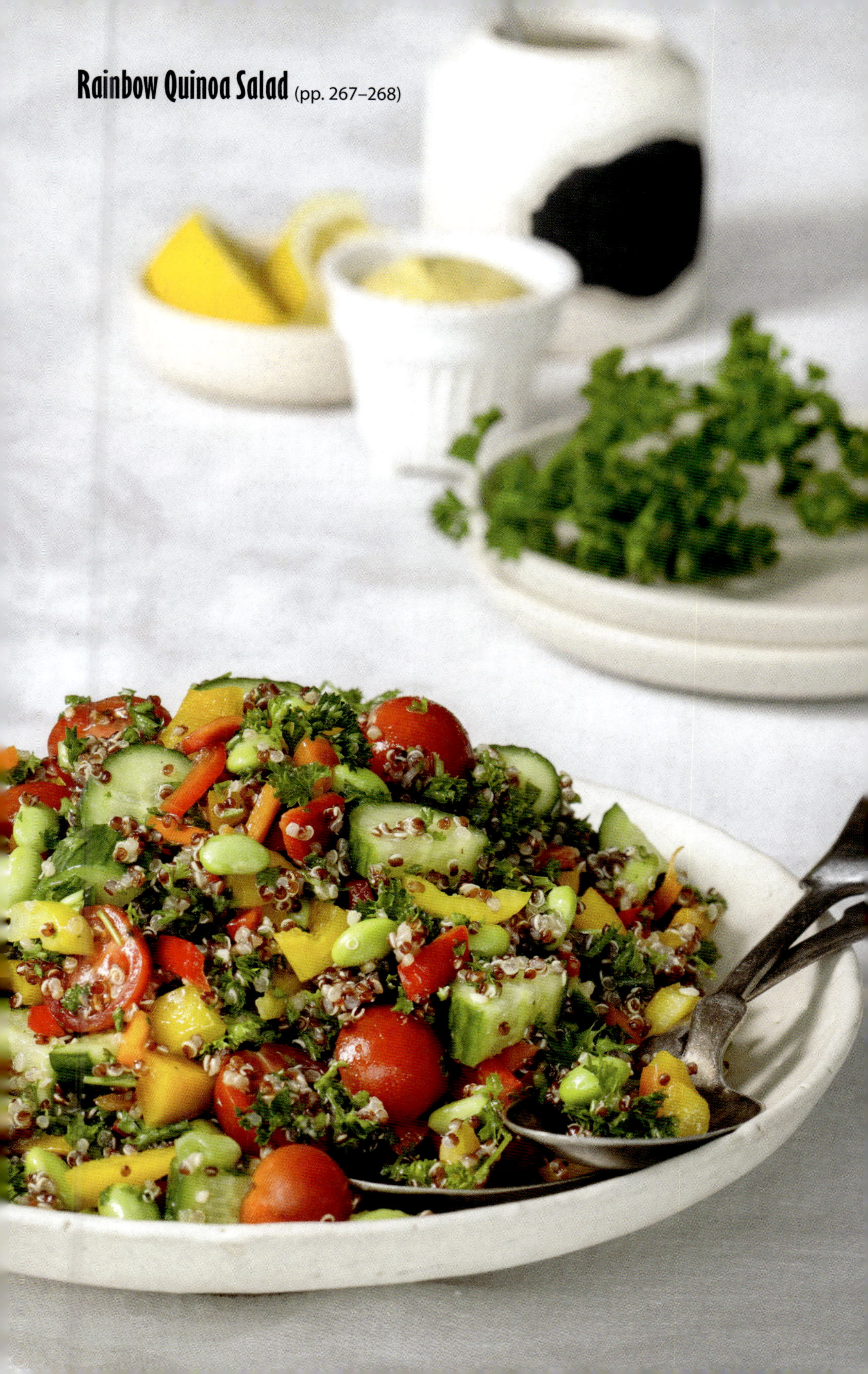

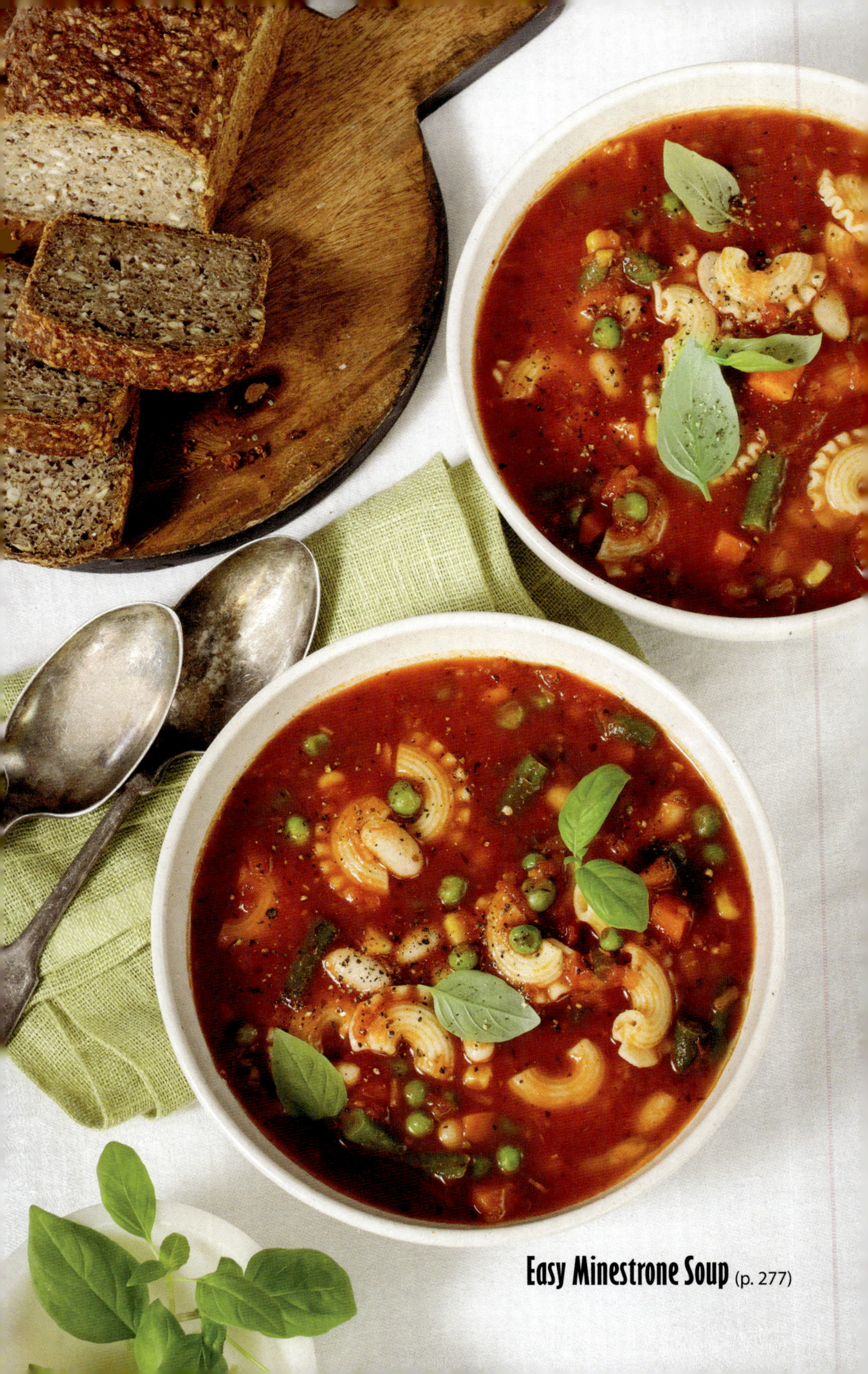

Easy Minestrone Soup (p. 277)

Middle Eastern Red Lentil Soup

(pp. 280–281)

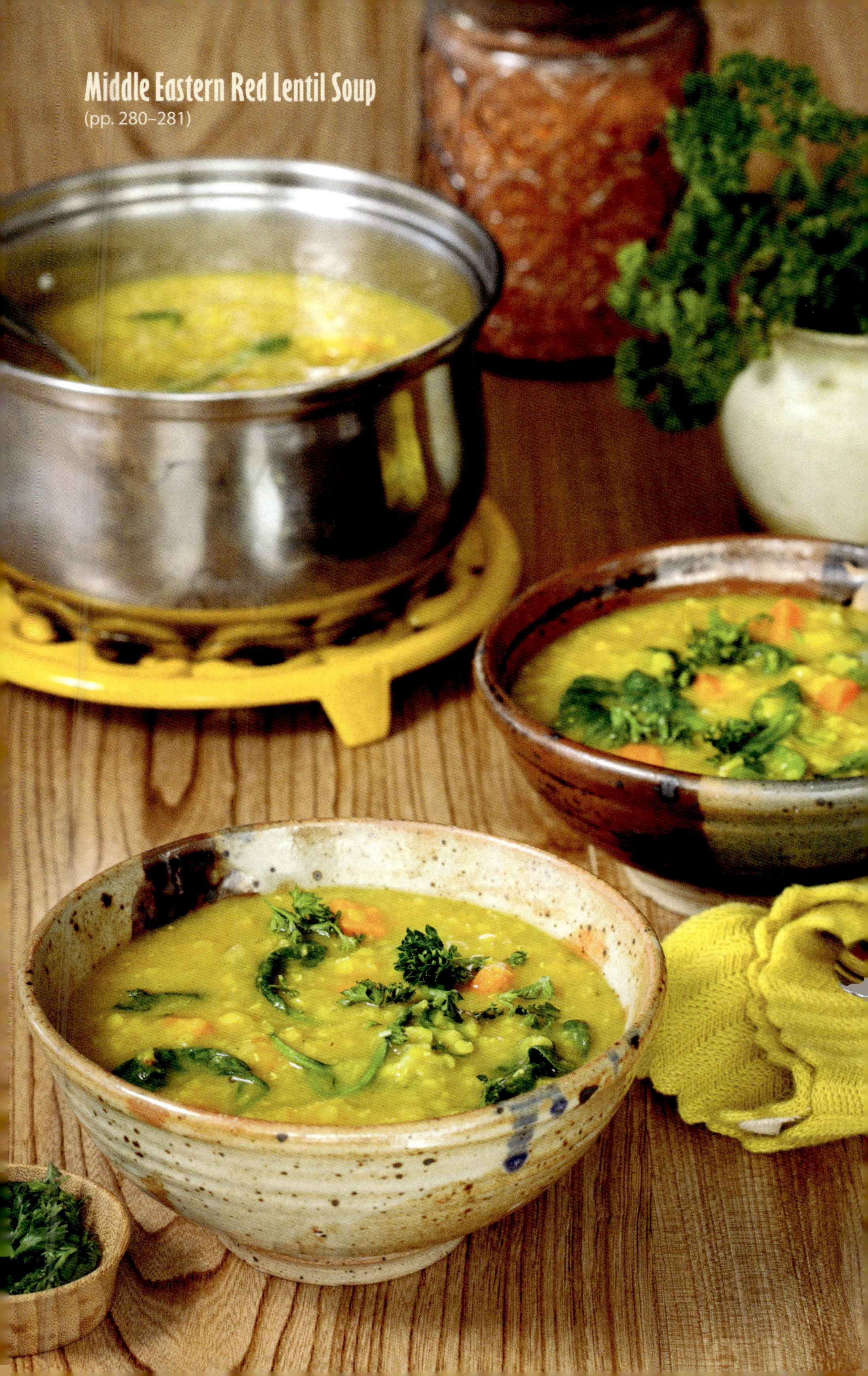

Best Black Bean Burgers (pp. 292–294)

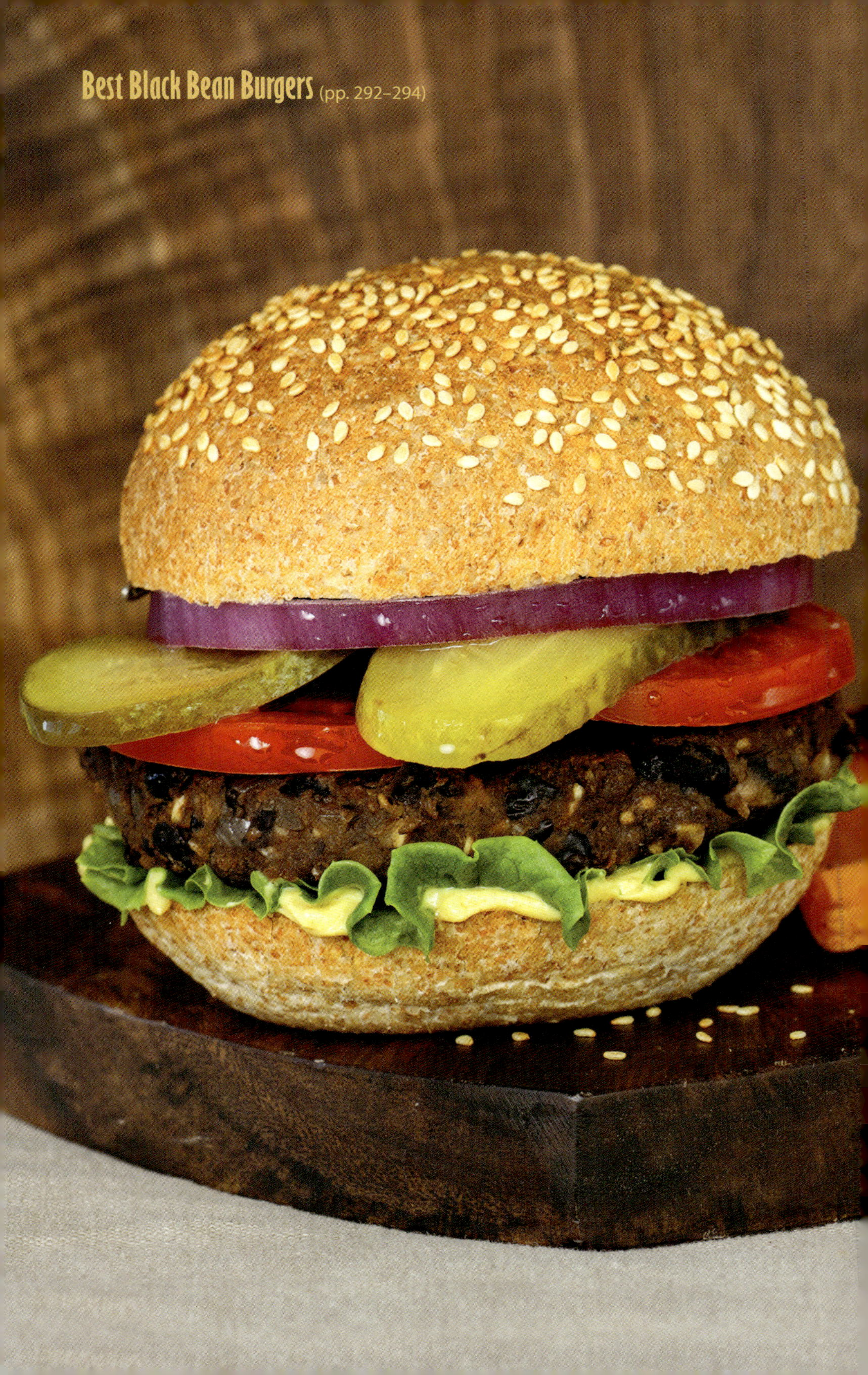

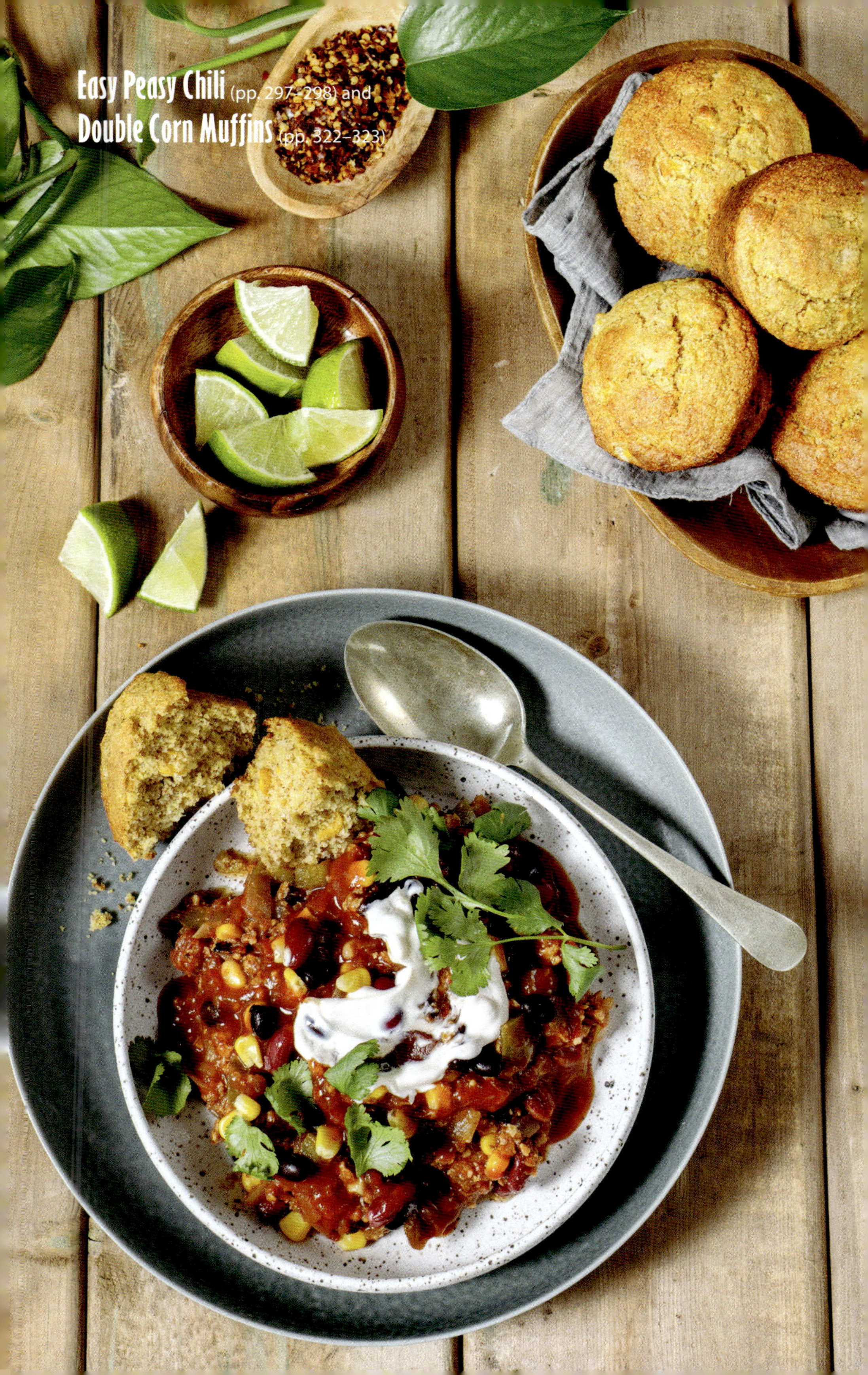

Easy Peasy Chili (pp. 297–298) and
Double Corn Muffins (pp. 322–323)

The Multicolored Bowl (p. 304)

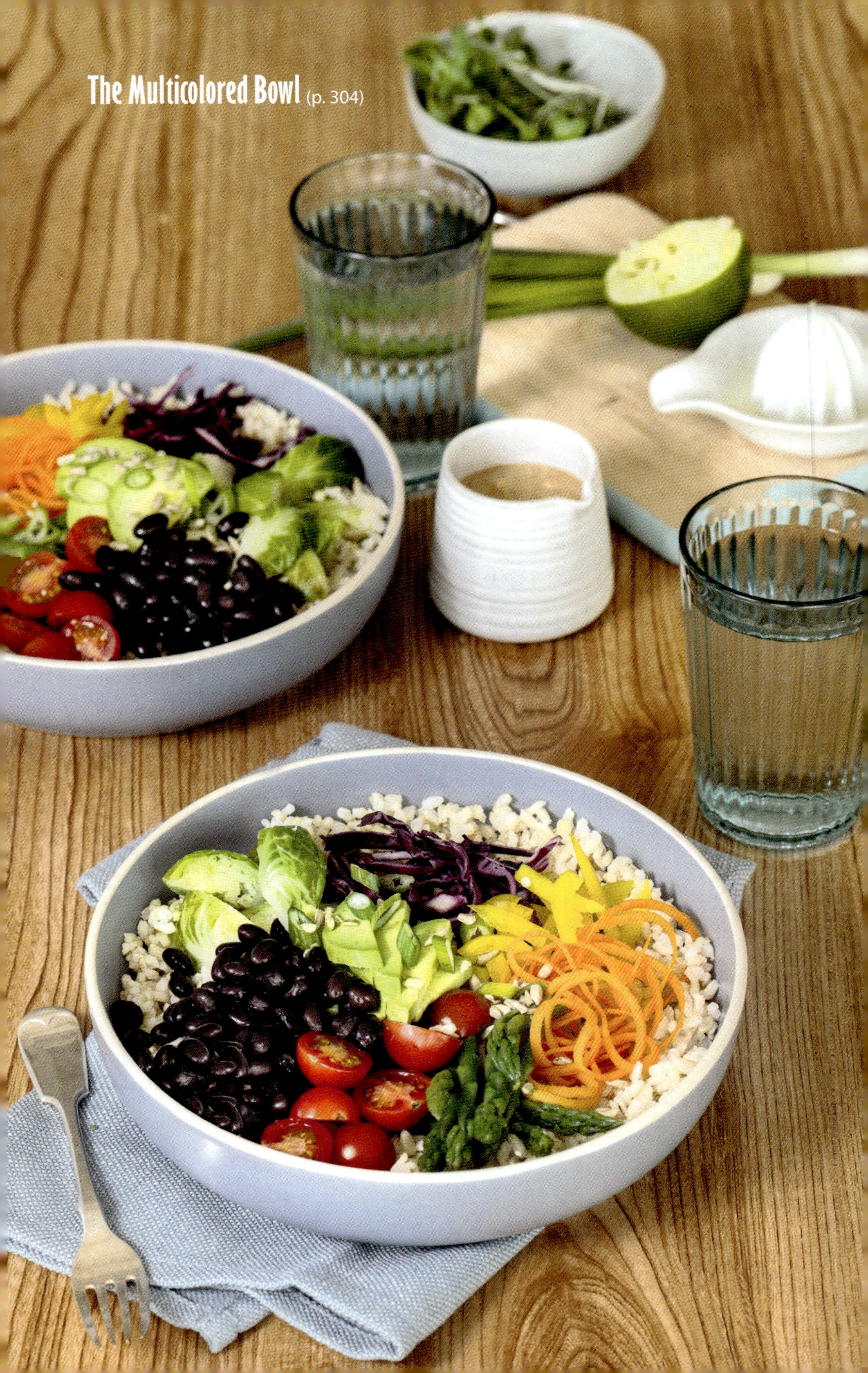

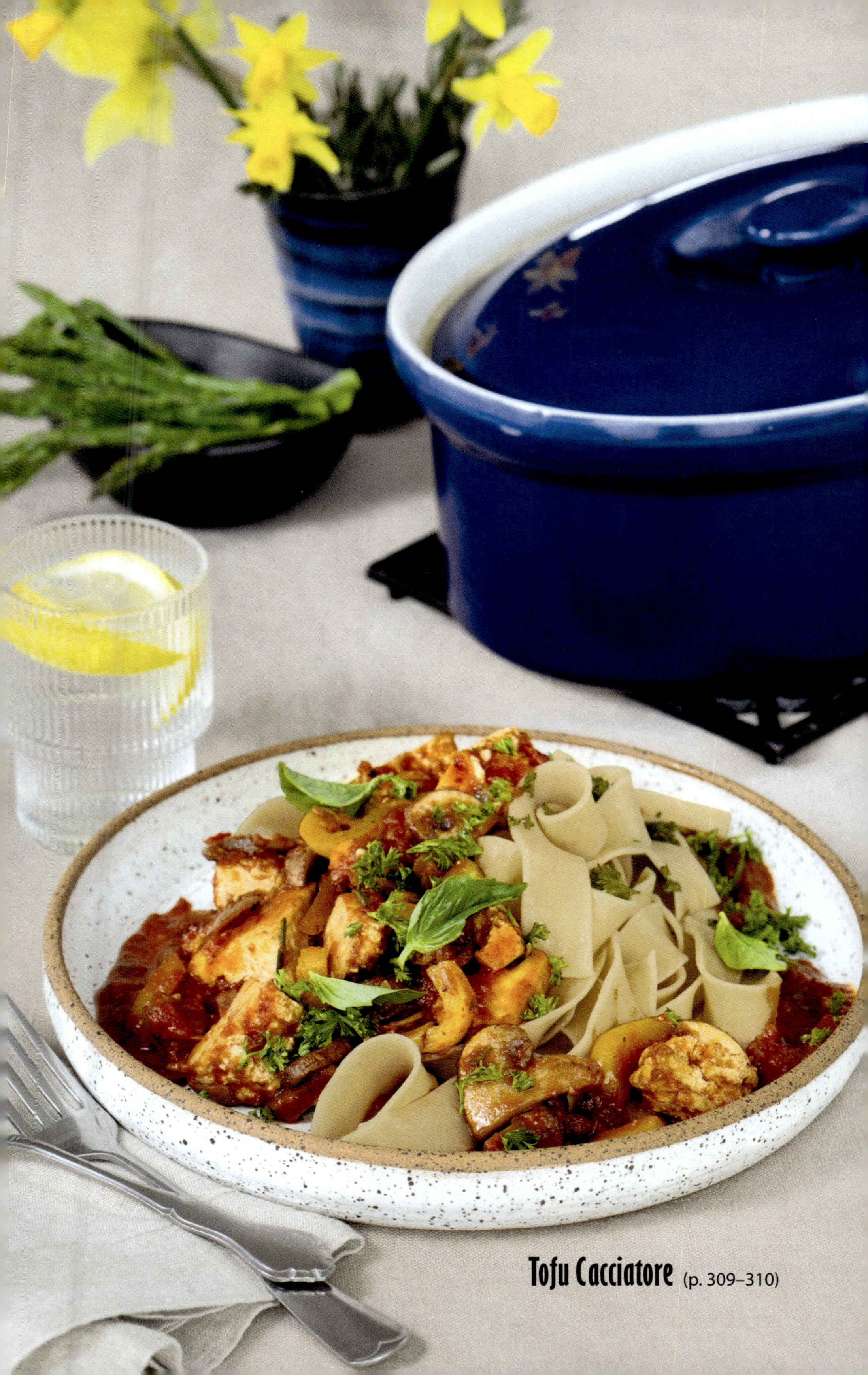

Tofu Cacciatore (p. 309–310)

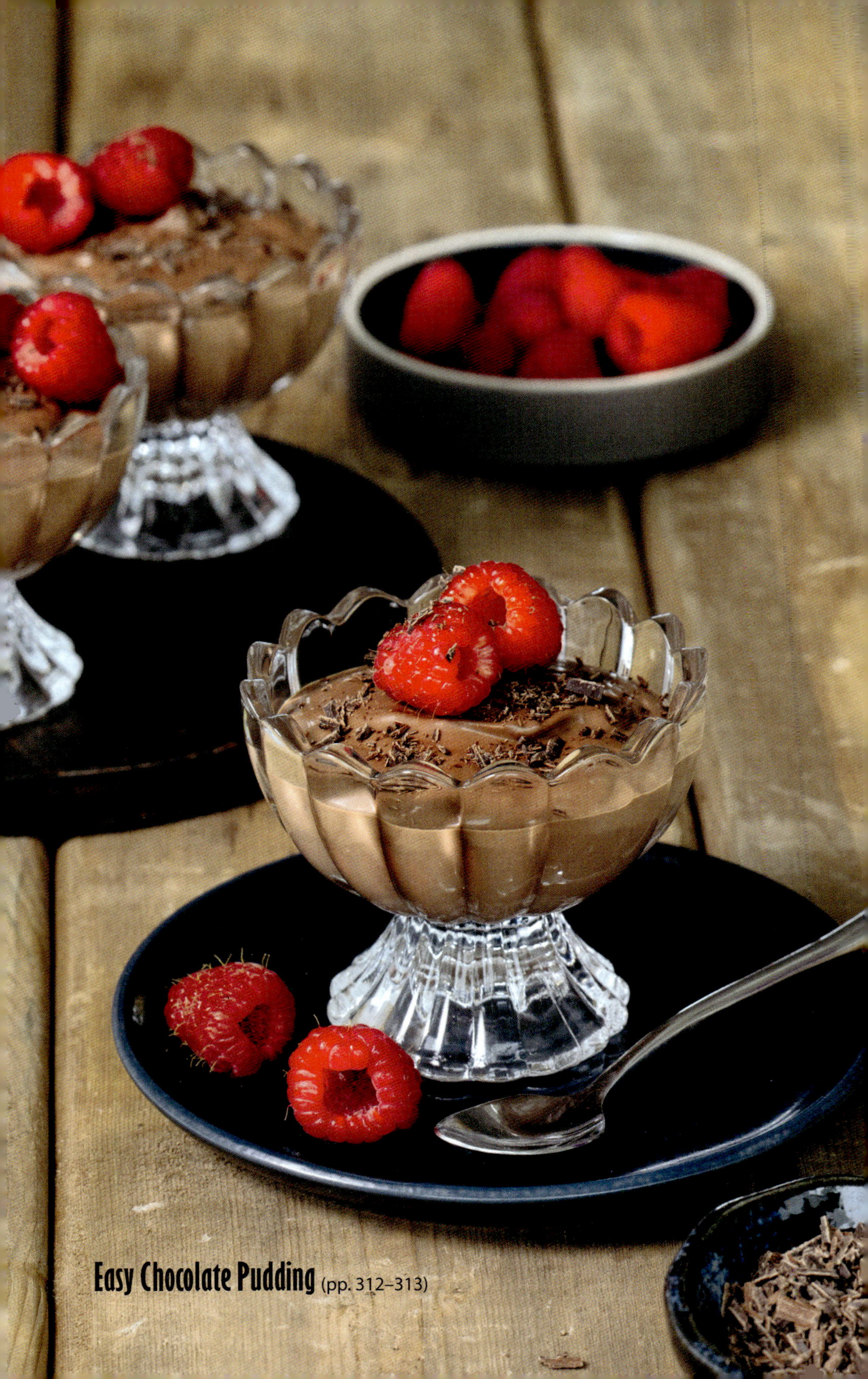

Easy Chocolate Pudding (pp. 312–313)

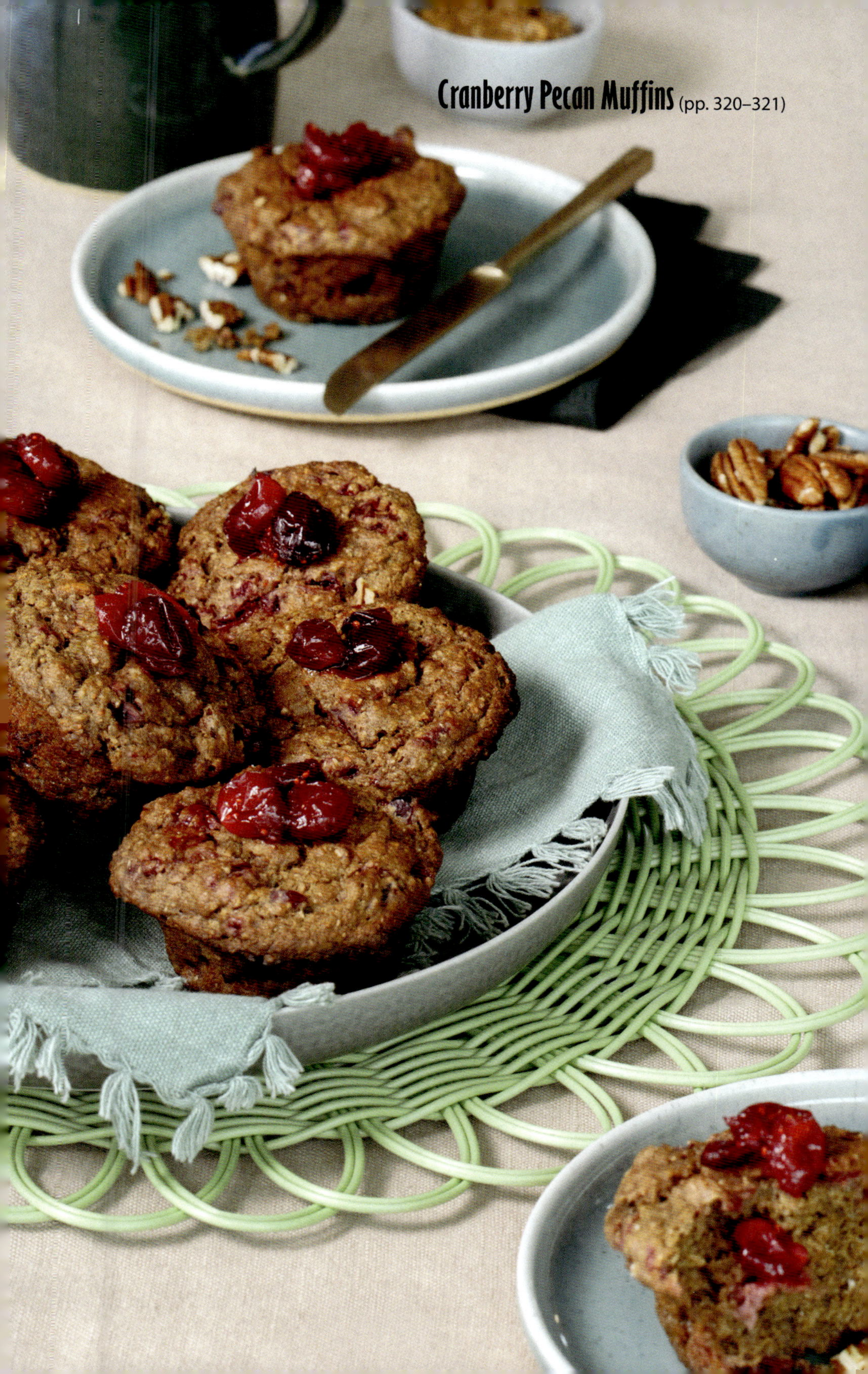

Cranberry Pecan Muffins (pp. 320–321)

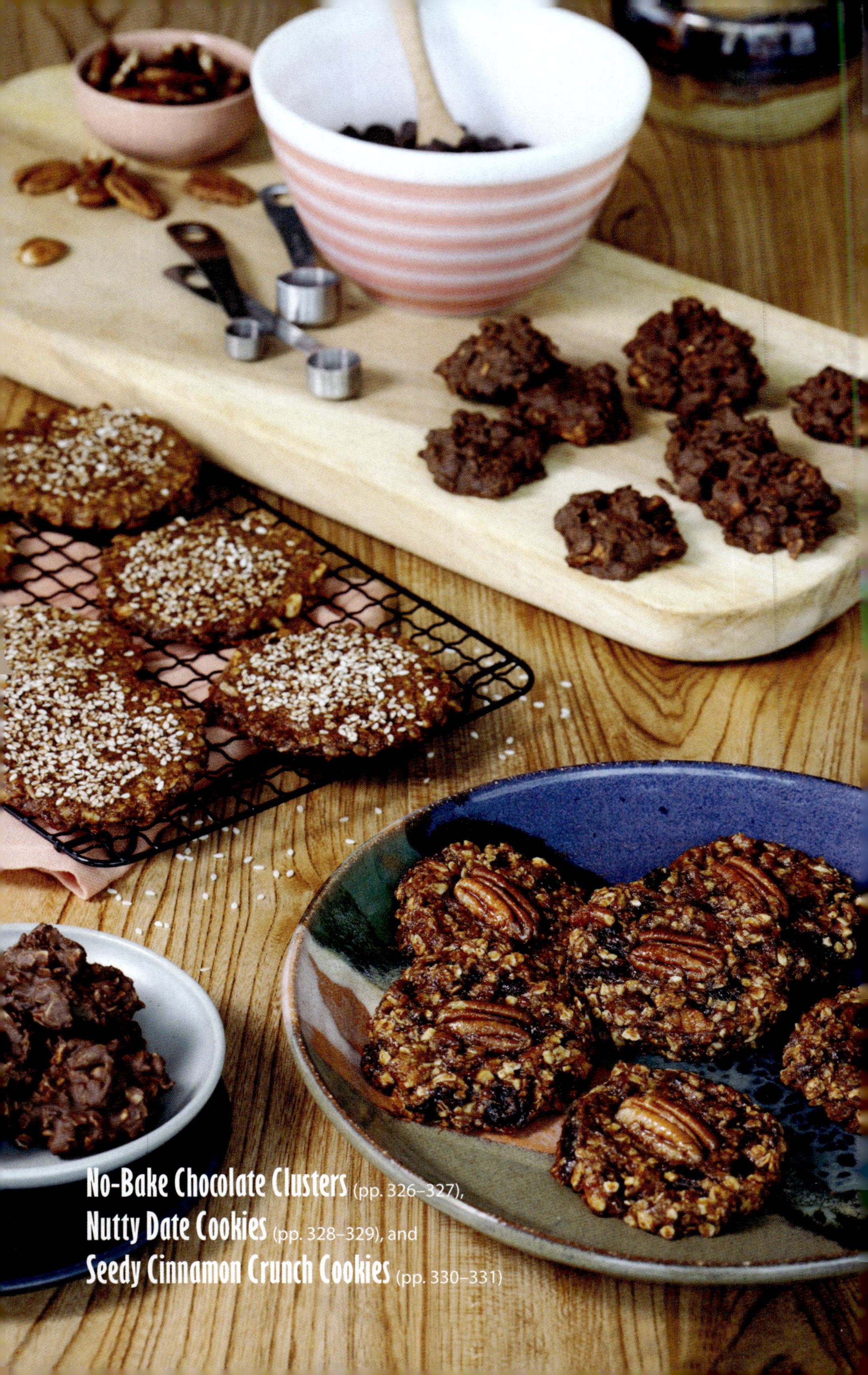

No-Bake Chocolate Clusters (pp. 326–327),
Nutty Date Cookies (pp. 328–329), and
Seedy Cinnamon Crunch Cookies (pp. 330–331)

RAINBOW QUINOA SALAD

Makes 8 cups (4 generous servings)

This colorful, nutrient-rich salad is a perfect portable meal. Packed with fiber, plant protein, and a medley of antioxidants, it's satisfying and endlessly adaptable. Swap the edamame or chickpeas for baked tofu, tempeh, or another legume of your choice. For an even more vibrant dish, feel free to increase the parsley and other vegetables to suit your taste. Top with diced avocado just before serving, or for added crunch, sprinkle on toasted pumpkin seeds, sunflower seeds, or sliced almonds.

SALAD

3 cups cooked and cooled quinoa (see page 234 for instructions)

1 cup edamame beans, cooked and cooled

1 cup chopped parsley

1 cup chopped orange and yellow peppers

1 cup chopped cucumbers

1 cup halved cherry tomatoes

2 green onions, sliced (optional)

DRESSING

2 tablespoons extra virgin olive oil (optional)

3 tablespoons fresh lemon or lime juice (about 1 lemon or 2 limes)

2 cloves garlic, minced (1 teaspoon jarred)

1 tablespoon Dijon mustard

2 teaspoons maple syrup

1 tablespoon low-sodium or regular tamari, Bragg's Liquid Aminos, or coconut aminos

1. In a large bowl, mix quinoa, edamame, parsley, peppers, cucumber, tomatoes, and green onions (if using).
2. In a small bowl or jar, whisk together the olive oil (if using), lemon juice, garlic, Dijon mustard, maple syrup, and tamari.
3. Pour the dressing over the salad and toss gently to combine.
4. Refrigerate for 1 to 3 hours before serving to allow the flavors to meld.

Per 2 cups of salad with dressing: Calories: 265, Protein: 13 g, Fat: 6 g, Carbohydrate: 43 g, Fiber: 8 g

Minerals: Calcium: 92 mg, Iron: 4.4 mg, Magnesium: 137 mg, Potassium: 745 mg, Sodium: 435 mg, Zinc: 2.5 mg

Vitamins: A: 149 mcg, C: 82 mg, E: 2 mg, Folate: 236 mcg DFE

Percent of calories from: Protein 19%, Fat 19%, Carbohydrate 62%

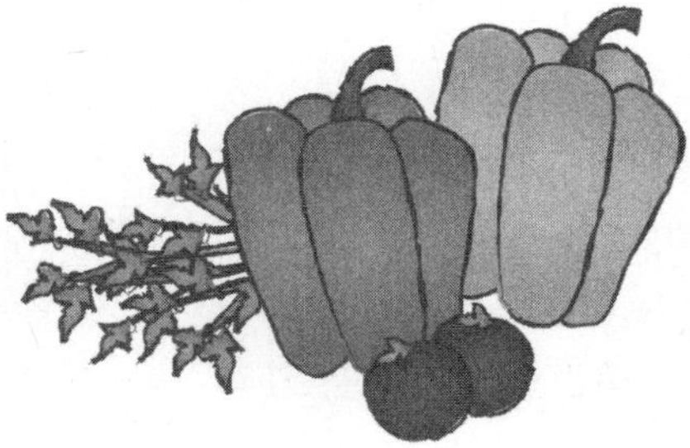

SWEET AND CRUNCHY COLESLAW

Make 4 cups

This colorful coleslaw delivers a satisfying mix of crunch and natural sweetness. Cabbage is an excellent source of vitamin C and potassium, while carrots add fiber, antioxidant-rich carotenoids, and a boost for eye health. Apples and raisins contribute natural sweetness, making this slaw both nourishing and delicious. Stored in the fridge with dressing, it stays crisp and flavorful for up to five days.

1½ cups green cabbage, thinly sliced

½ cup red cabbage, thinly sliced (or use more green cabbage)

1 cup grated carrot

¾–1 cup chopped apple

½ cup raisins or currants

1. In a large bowl, combine green and red cabbage, carrots, apples, and raisins. Toss well.
2. Add 1 cup (or desired amount) of Creamy Coleslaw Dressing (page 270) and mix until evenly coated.

OPTIONAL ADD-INS:

More crunch and color: Add chopped bell pepper, cauliflower, celery, fresh fennel, pineapple, or steamed broccoli.

A little bite: Stir in ¼ cup finely chopped green or red onion, sliced red radish, or a dash of hot sauce.

Fresh herbs: Add 2–4 tablespoons of chopped fresh cilantro, parsley, or dill.

Per cup, without dressing: Calories: 97, Protein: 1.5 g, Fat: 0.2 g, Carbohydrate: 25 g, Fiber: 3 g

Minerals: Calcium: 39 mg, Iron: 0.7 mg, Magnesium: 17 mg, Potassium: 351 mg, Sodium: 30 mg, Zinc: 0.2 mg

Vitamins: A: 238 mcg, C: 22 mg, E: 0.3 mg, Folate: 23 mcg DFE

Percent of calories from: Protein 6%, Fat 2%, Carbohydrate 92%

CREAMY COLESLAW DRESSING

Makes 1 cup

This rich, tangy dressing pairs beautifully with coleslaw and also works well on leafy green salads, grain bowls, or baked potatoes. It keeps for up to five days in a covered container in the refrigerator.

½ cup cashews

2 tablespoons plant-based milk or water

1–2 tablespoons apple cider vinegar

1–2 tablespoons lemon juice

1 tablespoon maple syrup

1 tablespoon Dijon mustard

½ teaspoon onion powder

1. Soak cashews in hot water for at least 30 minutes, then drain.
2. Place drained cashews, milk, vinegar, lemon juice, maple syrup, mustard, and onion powder in a blender. Blend until smooth and creamy.

OPTIONAL ADD-INS AND VARIATIONS:

Blender-free: Use ⅓ cup vegan mayo instead of cashews. Combine all ingredients in a jar and shake or whisk until smooth.

Tofu swap: Replace cashews with ½ cup soft tofu and blend until creamy.

Customize flavor: Adjust lemon juice or vinegar to your liking. Add salt and pepper if desired.

Add texture or spice: Add 1 tablespoon poppy seeds or ¼ teaspoon celery seeds for extra flavor and crunch.

Per ¼ cup: Calories: 120, Protein: 3 g, Fat: 8 g, Carbohydrate: 10 g, Fiber: 1 g

Minerals: Calcium: 23 mg, Iron: 1 mg, Magnesium: 47 mg, Potassium: 123 mg, Sodium: 97 mg, Zinc: 1 mg

Vitamins: A: 4 mcg, C: 1 mg, E: 0.2 mg, Folate: 13 mcg DFE

Percent of calories from: Protein 9%, Fat 59%, Carbohydrate 32%

TAHINI-BALSAMIC DRESSING

Makes 1½ cups

This creamy, tangy dressing brings both flavor and nutrition. Thanks to sesame tahini, it delivers calcium, protein, iron, and zinc, and is more nutrient dense than oil-based dressings. It's perfect for leafy salads, steamed vegetables (like broccoli or cauliflower), or baked potatoes. Keeps in the fridge for up to three weeks in a covered container.

½ cup water

½ cup tahini

⅓ cup balsamic vinegar, lemon juice, or lime juice

1–2 tablespoons low-sodium or regular tamari or soy sauce

1 tablespoon maple syrup or 2–4 dates (optional)

1 teaspoon minced garlic (fresh or jarred) or ⅛ teaspoon garlic powder

1. **Jar method:** Place the water, tahini, vinegar, tamari, maple syrup, and garlic in a jar and stir or shake until well combined.
2. **Blender method:** If using dates or you prefer a smoother consistency, place ingredients in a blender and process for 30 seconds or until smooth.

OPTIONAL ADD-INS AND VARIATIONS:

Boost protein and omega-3s: Add ⅓ cup of hempseeds and blend.

Add depth and nutrition: Mix in ¼ cup of nutritional yeast for a cheesy flavor.

Spice it up: Add 1–2 tablespoons of Dijon mustard or a pinch of cayenne.

Enhance flavor: Add 1 teaspoon of cumin.

Adjust consistency: Add a little water for a thinner dressing.

Per ¼ cup: Calories: 143, Protein: 4 g, Fat: 11 g, Carbohydrate: 9 g, Fiber: 1 g

Minerals: Calcium: 37 mg, Iron: 1 mg, Magnesium: 22 mg, Potassium: 117 mg, Sodium: 128 mg, Zinc: 1 mg

Vitamins: A: 1 mcg, C: 0 mg, E: 0.1 mg, Folate: 20 mcg DFE

Percent of calories from: Protein 11%, Fat 25%, Carbohydrate 64%

GINGER LIME MISO DRESSING

Makes 1¾ cups

This bold and zesty dressing is perfect for grain bowls (like the Multicolored Bowl on page 304), salads, and stir-fries. It delivers a tangy kick with savory depth and a touch of natural sweetness, along with vitamin E from the seed or nut butter.

⅓ cup fortified soy milk, other plant-based milk, or water

¼ cup sunflower butter, almond butter, or cashew butter

2 tablespoons miso

2 tablespoons low-sodium or regular tamari or soy sauce

¼ cup rice vinegar or other vinegar

2 tablespoons lime juice

1–2 medjool pitted dates, or 3–6 regular pitted dates or 1 tablespoon maple syrup.

2 tablespoons grated fresh ginger

2 cloves garlic

1. **Blender method:** Combine all ingredients in a blender and process until smooth.
2. **Jar method (no blender):** Use maple syrup instead of dates. Place all ingredients in a jar with a lid, and whisk or shake until smooth.

Per ¼ cup: Calories: 89, Protein: 3 g, Fat: 5 g, Carbohydrate: 8 g, Fiber: 1 g

Minerals: Calcium: 28 mg, Iron: 0.8 mg, Magnesium: 34 mg, Potassium: 113 mg, Sodium: 391 mg, Zinc: 0.6 mg

Vitamins: A: 0.1 mcg, C: 2 mg, E: 2 mg, Folate: 23 mcg DFE

Percent of calories from: Protein 14%, Fat 53%, Carbohydrate 33%

PERFECT PEANUT SAUCE

Makes 10 tablespoons (about 2/3 cup)

This flavorful peanut sauce is a winner! It's a versatile staple to keep on hand for tossing with salads; drizzling over grain bowls, noodles, and steamed vegetables; or serving as a dipping sauce. Brightened with ginger and lime, it strikes a delicious balance of nutty, salty, tangy, and sweet. The sauce can be stored in an airtight container in the refrigerator for up to two weeks; stir before using. If it is too thick, add 1 tablespoon of hot water at a time and mix until the desired consistency is reached.

¼ cup smooth peanut butter

1½–2 tablespoons low-sodium or regular tamari or soy sauce

1 tablespoon maple syrup (optional, for sweetness)

1 tablespoon rice vinegar

1 teaspoon toasted sesame oil

1–2 teaspoons grated fresh ginger

Juice of 1 lime (about 1½ tablespoons)

Pinch red pepper flakes or a few drops of hot sauce (optional)

1. In a small bowl, whisk together the peanut butter and tamari until smooth. If the mixture is thick, microwave it for 20 to 30 seconds to soften, or place the bowl in a larger bowl or saucepan of hot water.
2. Add the maple syrup, rice vinegar, sesame oil, ginger, lime juice, and red pepper flakes (if using). Whisk until smooth.

Per 2 tablespoons: Calories: 97, Protein: 3 g, Fat: 7.5 g, Carbohydrate: 4 g, Fiber: 0.7 g

Minerals: Calcium: 7 mg, Iron: 0.2 mg, Magnesium: 22 mg, Potassium: 80 mg, Sodium: 196 mg, Zinc: 0.3 mg

Vitamins: A: 1 mcg, C: 1 mg, E: 1 mg, Folate: 12 mcg DFE

Percent of calories from: Protein 14%, Fat 70%, Carbohydrate 16%

Soups

Soups are a cornerstone of health-supportive, whole-food, plant-based eating, offering nourishment, versatility, and comfort in every bowl. Their soft consistency makes them especially accessible for individuals with dental or digestive challenges while their high water and fiber content supports satiety and overall health.

From a nutritional perspective, soups provide an ideal vehicle for incorporating legumes—a foundation of most plant-based diets and a rich source of protein, iron, zinc, and soluble fiber. For those who are new to plant-based eating or who experience difficulty digesting legumes, soups offer a gentle, well-tolerated introduction. (In such cases, begin with much smaller amounts of legumes; then gradually increase amounts.) The combination of thorough cooking, hydration, and blending can reduce any intestinal discomfort while preserving nutritional value.

Soups also invite culinary creativity. Home cooks and professionals can adapt these recipes in many ways. With less liquid, they may be closer to stews (or "stoups!"). Recipes can include added whole grains, leafy greens, cruciferous vegetables, herbs, and spices, making each batch an opportunity to expand variety and nutrient density. They can be prepared in large quantities, stored easily, and adapted to diverse cultural flavor profiles, making them both practical and globally inspired.

Whether served as a light entrée or a hearty main dish, soups remain one of the easiest and most impactful ways to elevate daily nutrition using whole-plant foods.

What Is the Difference Between Vegetable Broth, Stock, and Bouillon?

Vegetable Broth is a ready-to-use liquid base for soups, stews, and sauces, as well as for cooking grains. It is made by simmering vegetables in water, often with herbs and spices.

Vegetable Stock is made by simmering vegetables for a long time for a richer, more concentrated flavor than broth. In plant-based cooking, the terms *broth* and *stock* are often used interchangeably.

Bouillon is a convenient, concentrated form of broth or stock that comes in cubes, powder, or paste. It is dissolved in water to make broth or stock. Any of the above can be high in sodium, so check labels.

To prepare your own broth or stock, simmer aromatic vegetables, such as chopped onions, carrots, celery, and garlic, along with vegetable trimmings and herbs, in water for 45 to 60 minutes, then strain. This yields a rich, clean base without excess sodium.

To prepare your own bouillon powder, mix one cup of nutritional yeast, ½ cup dried onion flakes (or 3 tablespoons onion powder), 2 tablespoons dried garlic flakes (or 1 tablespoon garlic powder), 1 tablespoon each of salt, dried oregano, and dried parsley flakes, and 1 teaspoon each of black pepper, paprika, dried thyme, and ground turmeric. Add other seasonings as desired.

SAVORY BLACK BEAN SOUP

Makes 7 to 8 cups

This hearty black bean soup delivers rich, comforting flavor with a bright lift from fresh lime juice stirred in just before serving. It's packed with fiber, protein, and colorful vegetables, and it freezes beautifully. To keep sodium intake low, select low-sodium or salt-free vegetable stock and canned beans.

½ to 1 onion, diced
4 cups low-sodium or regular vegetable stock or broth, divided
1 or more garlic cloves, minced
1 cup thinly sliced carrot
1 cup diced celery
2 cups kale, stem removed and chopped
¼ cup tomato paste
1½ teaspoons cumin
1 teaspoon oregano
1 teaspoon thyme
3 cups canned or cooked black beans (no added salt or regular)
Salt and pepper to taste
2 teaspoons lime juice

1. In a large saucepan over medium heat, sauté the onion in 2–4 tablespoons of vegetable stock until softened.
2. Add garlic, carrot, celery, and kale. Continue to cook for about 5 minutes or until vegetables soften, adding more stock if necessary.
3. Stir in tomato paste, cumin, oregano, thyme, beans, and remaining stock, cover, and simmer for 30 minutes or until vegetables are cooked.
4. Adjust the seasoning and add lime juice just before serving.

Per cup: Calories: 124, Protein: 8 g, Fat: 0.7 g, Carbohydrate: 24 g, Fiber: 8 g

Minerals: Calcium: 62 mg, Iron: 2.4 mg, Magnesium: 61 mg, Potassium: 480 mg, Sodium: 168 mg, Zinc: 1 mg

Vitamins: A: 162 mcg, C: 8 mg, E: 0.6 mg, Folate: 52 mcg DFE

Percent of calories from: Protein 23%, Fat 5%, Carbohydrate 72%

EASY MINESTRONE SOUP

Makes about 6 cups

This soup comes together in under thirty minutes and delivers a nourishing and tasty meal. Use whole grain pasta for a fiber boost or make it gluten-free with gluten-free pasta or potatoes. Marinara sauce and cannellini beans are rich in vitamin E. Leftover soup can be stored in mason jars and refrigerated or frozen.

2 cups low-sodium or regular vegetable stock or broth

1 (14–15-oz) can marinara or pasta sauce

1 (14–15-oz) can beans (any types), drained and rinsed (or 1½ cups cooked beans)

½ cup uncooked pasta

1 tablespoon minced garlic

2 tablespoons onion flakes or 1 teaspoon onion powder

1½ cups mixed frozen vegetables or other chopped vegetables

1–2 tablespoons Italian seasoning

1. In a large saucepan, combine the vegetable stock, marinara sauce, beans, uncooked pasta, garlic, onion flakes, frozen vegetables, and Italian seasoning.
2. Bring to a boil, then lower heat and simmer for about 20 minutes or until the pasta and vegetables are tender.
3. Taste and adjust the seasoning before serving.

OPTIONAL ADD-INS AND VARIATIONS:

- Replace uncooked pasta with 1 cup cooked pasta or cooked, cubed potato.
- Replace Italian seasoning with 2–3 tablespoons each of fresh basil and oregano.
- Replace the vegetable stock and marinara sauce with 4 cups of tomato juice.
- Add hot sauce or pepper to taste.

Per cup: Calories: 211, Protein: 10 g, Fat: 3 g, Carbohydrate: 37 g, Fiber: 8 g
Minerals: Calcium: 97 mg, Iron: 3 mg, Magnesium: 69 mg, Potassium: 682 mg, Sodium: 624 mg, Zinc: 1 mg
Vitamins: A: 126 mcg, C: 6 mg, E: 3 mg, Folate: 115 mcg DFE
Percent of calories from: Protein 18%, Fat 12%, Carbohydrate 70%

LUSCIOUS CREAM OF PEA SOUP

Makes 6 to 6½ cups (3–4 servings)

This is not your grandmother's pea soup. Instead of the dense texture of traditional split pea soup, this version is lighter and a more vibrant green. Green split peas and sweet green peas form the silky base while smoked paprika adds a subtle depth. A finishing touch of lemon brightens every spoonful. This soup is nourishing enough for a main course and sufficiently elegant to serve as a starter.

1 medium onion, diced

1 celery rib, including leaves, diced

3 cups water

3 garlic cloves, chopped, or 1 tablespoon minced garlic

2/3 cup green split peas, soaked in 2 cups water for 2 hours (or soaked in boiling water for at least 15 minutes), then drained

1 tablespoon light miso

2 bay leaves or ½ teaspoon dried thyme

1 teaspoon smoked paprika

½ teaspoon salt or to taste (optional)

Freshly ground black pepper, to taste

2 cups frozen green peas

1 cup unsweetened soy, oat, or other plant-based milk

2 tablespoons fresh parsley, chopped (optional)

Juice of ½ lemon (about 2 tablespoons lemon juice) or to taste

1. In a large pot over medium heat, put in the onion and celery. Dry sauté for 2 to 3 minutes, stirring frequently. If the vegetables begin to stick or brown, add 1 to 2 tablespoons of water as needed to deglaze the pot and continue cooking, adding more water if

necessary. Sauté until softened, about 8 to10 minutes. Add garlic and miso and cook 1 to 2 minutes more.

2. Stir in the split peas, 3 cups water, bay leaves, smoked paprika, salt, and black pepper.
3. Bring to a boil, then reduce heat. Cover and simmer for 1 to 1½ hours, stirring occasionally, until the split peas are soft. Add a splash of water only if needed.
4. Add the frozen peas and cook for 2 minutes. Stir in the plant-based milk and parsley (if using). Remove the bay leaves. Turn the burner off and let the soup cool slightly before blending.
5. Purée the soup in a blender until smooth and velvety.
6. Stir in the lemon juice. Taste and adjust seasoning as needed. Serve warm.

OPTIONAL ADD-INS

Boost flavor:

- Add 1–2 tablespoons fresh dill or parsley, chopped or 1 teaspoon dried.
- Add ½ teaspoon ground coriander for gentle citrus-like depth.
- Add a pinch of cayenne (⅛ teaspoon or less) for subtle warmth.
- Add ⅓ cup raw cashew pieces (soaked or rinsed) for a richer version. Add the cashews at the same time as the peas.

Garnish:

- Fresh dill or mint
- Toasted pumpkin seeds
- Dried sweet peppers

Per serving (~2 cups): Calories: 290, Protein: 19 g, Fat: 4 g, Carbohydrate: 48 g, Fiber: 16 g

Minerals: Calcium: 164 mg, Iron: 4 mg, Magnesium: 74 mg, Potassium: 746 mg, Sodium: 327 mg, Zinc: 3 mg

Vitamins: A: 117 mcg, C: 24 mg, E: 0.4 mg, Folate: 190 mcg DFE

Percent of calories from: Protein 25%, Fat 12%, Carbohydrate 63 %

MIDDLE EASTERN RED LENTIL SOUP

Makes 6 cups (3–4 servings)

The comforting lentil stews of the Middle East inspire this hearty, golden soup. Red lentils simmer quickly with onions, carrots, and seasonings, and are brightened with lemon and a handful of fresh greens. The result is aromatic, deeply satisfying, and perfect with a slice of whole grain bread. Leftovers taste even better the next day and freeze beautifully for future meals.

2 tablespoons vegetable stock or broth or water, or 2 teaspoons olive oil

1 small onion, diced

1 medium carrot, diced

2 cloves garlic, finely chopped

1 tablespoon Middle Eastern spice blend*

½ teaspoon ground turmeric

1¼ cups red lentils, rinsed and drained

4½ cups water, vegetable stock, or broth

2 tablespoons fresh parsley, chopped

2 cups baby spinach or other tender greens such as baby kale, coarsely chopped

Juice of ½ lemon (about 1½ tablespoons), or to taste

½ teaspoon of salt, or to taste (optional)

Freshly ground black pepper, to taste

Chef's Shopping Tip *You can purchase a Middle Eastern spice blend or prepare your own using 1½ teaspoons cumin and ¾ teaspoon each of coriander and smoked paprika. Add a pinch of cinnamon and/or cayenne, if you like.

1. In a large soup pot or Dutch oven, heat the water, over medium heat.
2. Add onion and carrots and sauté until softened, for about 10 minutes.
3. Stir in garlic, spice blend, and turmeric. Cook for 1 to 2 minutes more, until fragrant.
4. Add lentils and the 4½ cups water. Bring to a boil, then lower heat, cover, and simmer for 30 to 40 minutes, stirring occasionally, until lentils have broken down and the soup is thick.
5. Remove from heat. Stir in parsley and spinach until just wilted. If using tougher greens such as mature kale, chop more finely and add during the last 5 to 10 minutes of cooking.
6. Add lemon juice and season with salt and black pepper to taste. Serve warm.

Per serving (~2 cups): Calories: 323, Protein: 21 g, Fat: 2 g, Carbohydrate: 58 g, Fiber: 11 g
Minerals: Calcium: 103 mg, Iron: 8 mg, Magnesium: 81 mg, Potassium: 829 mg, Sodium: 51 mg, Zinc: 3 mg
Vitamins: A: 291 mcg, C: 16 mg, E: 1 mg, Folate: 216 mcg DFE
Percent of calories from: Protein 25%, Fat 6%, Carbohydrate 69%

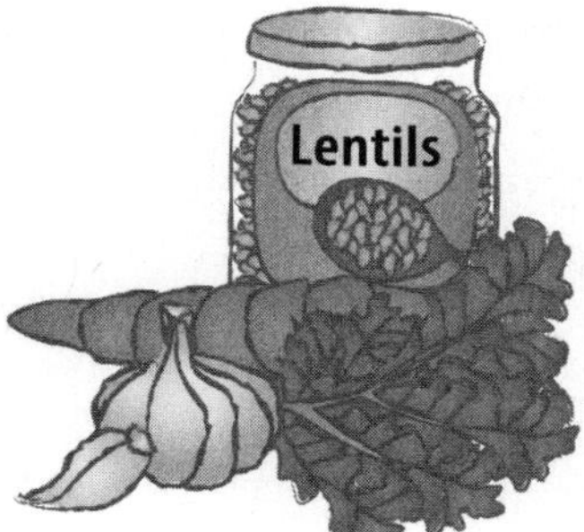

LENTIL TOMATO KALE SOUP

Makes 7 cups

This hearty, one-pot soup is a warming and nutrient-packed meal featuring protein-rich lentils, whole grain brown rice, and vibrant, calcium-rich kale. Fragrant with curry spices and full of fiber and plant-based goodness, it's as satisfying as it is simple to prepare. Not a fan of Indian spices? Swap in 1 tablespoon of Italian seasoning or your favorite herb blend. Finish with fresh cilantro or parsley or a squeeze of lemon for added brightness. This soup freezes well.

1 small onion, chopped

3 large cloves garlic, minced

1 medium-sized carrot, chopped

½ cup brown/green lentils, uncooked, rinsed

⅓ cup brown rice, uncooked, rinsed

3 cups vegetable stock or broth

1 (28-oz) can diced tomatoes

2 tablespoons tomato paste*

1–2 tablespoons Italian seasoning

Pinch of cayenne (optional)

Salt and pepper to taste

2 cups chopped kale

Chef's Tip * Tomato paste in a tube is a game changer! Unlike canned versions, it stays fresh longer and lets you use just what you need, without waste.

1. In a large soup pot, combine the onion, garlic, carrot, lentils, rice, and vegetable stock. Bring to a boil, then lower heat and simmer for 45 minutes, or until the rice and lentils are tender.
2. Stir in the diced tomatoes, tomato paste, Italian seasoning, cayenne (if using), salt, and pepper. Simmer for another 10 minutes to allow the flavors to meld.
3. Add the kale and cook for 2 to 3 minutes, just until wilted.
4. Serve hot.

Per 1¾ cup serving: Calories: 213, Protein: 10 g, Fat: 2 g, Carbohydrate: 43 g, Fiber: 8 g

Minerals: Calcium: 120 mg, Iron: 3.5 mg, Magnesium: 64 mg, Potassium: 765 mg, Sodium: 497 mg, Zinc: 1.5 mg

Vitamins: A: 211 mcg, C: 36 mg, E: 2 mg, Folate: 146 mcg DFE

Percent of calories from: Protein 18%, Fat 6%, Carbohydrate 76%

VARIATION:

Replace Italian seasoning with 1–2 tablespoons yellow curry powder or curry paste.

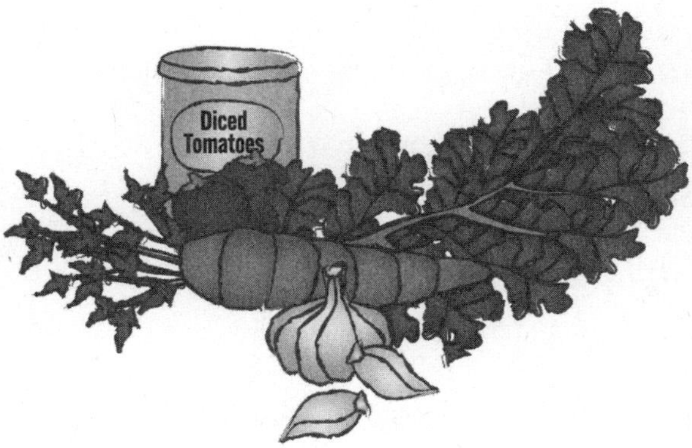

WHITE BEAN AND MUSHROOM SOUP

Makes 6½ cups (4 servings)

Hearty and comforting, this fiber-rich soup is loaded with white beans, earthy mushrooms, and leafy greens in a creamy, plant-based broth. Cashews and miso add richness and umami, while simple ingredients make it easy to prepare.

3 cups sliced mushrooms

1 medium onion, chopped

3 cloves garlic, minced (about 1½ teaspoons)

2¼ cups low-sodium or regular vegetable stock or broth

1–2 tablespoons vegetable broth, white wine, or water for deglazing

1 (14–15 oz) can white beans (e.g., Great Northern), rinsed and drained (1½ cups)

1 tablespoon French herb mix (e.g., Herbes de Provence)

1 cup unsweetened soy, oat, or other plant-based milk

⅓ cup raw cashews, rinsed and drained (soak 2–4 hours for smoother blending)

1 tablespoon light miso paste (or tamari)

Freshly ground black pepper to taste

1. In a medium soup pot or large skillet, dry sauté the mushrooms, onion, and garlic over medium heat for about 10 minutes, stirring occasionally. If they begin to stick, deglaze with 1 to 2 tablespoons broth, white wine, or water.
2. Add the stock, white beans, and French herb mix. Bring to a gentle boil, then lower heat and simmer for 10 minutes.
3. In a blender, combine the plant-based milk, cashews, and miso. Blend on high until completely smooth and creamy.

4. Pour the cashew mixture into the soup pot and stir to combine. Simmer gently for another 5 to 10 minutes until heated through and slightly thickened.
5. Season with freshly ground black pepper to taste. Serve warm.

OPTIONAL ADD-INS

- For added depth, replace ¼–½ cup of broth with white wine in step 2.
- Add 2 cups chopped spinach or kale (stem removed and finely chopped) during the last 10 minutes of cooking, just until wilted. The greens offer added nutrition and color.
- Make your own Herbes de Provence by combining 2 tablespoons each of rosemary and thyme, and 1 tablespoon each of oregano and marjoram. Mix well and store in an airtight container.

Per serving (~1½ cups): Calories: 266, Protein: 15 g, Fat: 10 g, Carbohydrate: 34 g, Fiber: 7 g

Minerals: Calcium: 174 mg, Iron: 5 mg, Magnesium: 114 mg, Potassium: 835 mg, Sodium: 524 mg, Zinc: 3 mg

Vitamins: A: 39 mcg, C: 4 mg, E: 1 mg, Folate: 92 mcg DFE

Percent of calories from: Protein 21%, Fat 31%, Carbohydrate 48%

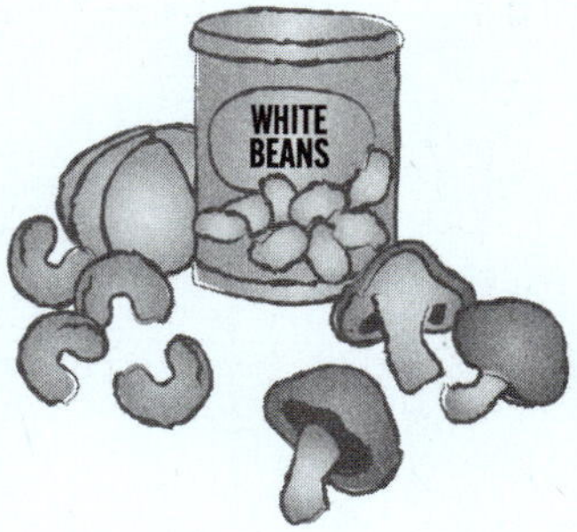

Entrées

Transitioning from meat-centered meals to plant-centered entrées can feel unfamiliar at first, but it is, in fact, an invitation to reimagine nourishment, eating satisfaction, and culinary enjoyment. Our entrée collection is designed to support that shift with recipes that are bold in flavor, rich in texture, and grounded in evidence-based nutrition.

Each dish demonstrates how whole-plant foods, such as legumes, tofu, whole grains, nuts, seeds, and an abundance of vegetables, can provide hearty textures and deep flavors that satisfy without compromise.

Far from being restrictive, plant-based entrées open the door to a broader range of global flavors and culinary creativity. From umami-forward Tofu Cacciatore and Best Black Bean Burgers to the vibrant Multicolored Bowl, Easy Peasy Chili, and globally inspired wraps, these recipes deliver both familiarity and adventure. Others, like Roasted Cauliflower with Chickpeas and Olives or Marvelous Mushroom Ragout, showcase the elegance of minimalism in whole-food cooking.

Plant-centered meals can meet, and often exceed, the nutrients traditionally provided by dishes based on animal products. Adequate protein is easily obtained through legumes, tofu, and tempeh; iron and zinc are present in beans, lentils, whole grains, nuts, and seeds. When paired with vitamin C–rich foods, plant-based iron becomes even more bioavailable. These meals also provide fiber, prebiotics, phytochemicals, and antioxidants, components associated with long-term health and chronic disease prevention.

Ideal for everyday meals, family dinners, or entertaining, these recipes empower both newcomers and seasoned plant-based eaters to enjoy food that is as nutritionally robust as it is deeply flavorful.

MEDITERRANEAN HUMMUS WRAP

Makes 1 large wrap

This Mediterranean-inspired wrap is bursting with creamy hummus, fresh veggies, and buttery avocado, all rolled into a hearty whole grain tortilla. It's rich in the fat-soluble vitamins A and E and fiber, heart healthy, and ready in minutes. Perfect for lunch, travel, or a light dinner!

1 large whole grain or sprouted-grain tortilla or wrap

⅓ cup hummus

⅓ cup grated carrots

⅓ cup chopped tomatoes or halved cherry tomatoes

1 cup baby spinach, mixed greens, or shredded lettuce

½ small ripe avocado, thinly sliced

Any add-ins desired

Squeeze lemon or lime juice (optional)

1. If your tortilla feels stiff or cold, warm it for 15 to 20 seconds in the microwave or a dry skillet. This makes it more pliable and easier to roll without tearing.
2. Spread the hummus evenly across the tortilla.
3. Layer the carrots, tomatoes, greens, avocado, and any optional additions.
4. Add a squeeze of lemon or lime juice, if desired.
5. Roll tightly, tucking in the sides as you go. Slice in half (if desired) and serve immediately!

OPTIONAL ADD-INS

- 2 ounces smoked or flavored tofu, cut into strips
- ¼ cup chopped cilantro, parsley, or basil
- A few slices of red onion or one chopped green onion
- 2 tablespoons sliced olives
- 2–3 tablespoons tzatziki*
- A sprinkle of lemon or lime juice

Chef's Tip * **Making Plant-Based Tzatziki**

Combine 1 cup plant-based plain yogurt with 1 cup grated or diced cucumber, 2 tablespoons chopped fresh dill, 1 clove minced garlic (or ¼ tsp garlic powder), juice of a half lemon, and a pinch of salt.

Per wrap: Calories: 457, Protein: 12 g, Fat: 27 g, Carbohydrate: 47 g, Fiber: 14 g

Minerals: Calcium: 131 mg, Iron: 4 mg, Magnesium: 126 mg, Potassium: 1121 mg, Sodium: 557 mg, Zinc: 2mg

Vitamins: A: 409 mcg, C: 27 mg, E: 4 mg, Folate: 178 mcg DFE

Percent of calories from: Protein 10%, Fat 51%, Carbohydrate 39%

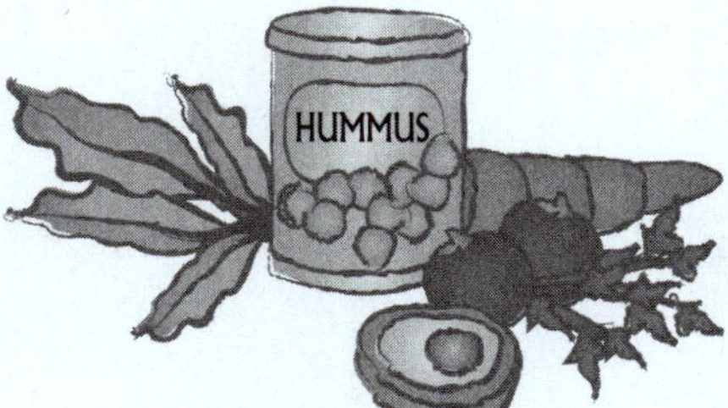

FIESTA REFRIED BEAN WRAP

Makes 1 wrap

Looking for a quick, hearty wrap that delivers big on flavor? This one's a winner. Soft refried beans, crunchy veggies, zesty salsa, guacamole, cilantro, and lime come together in a satisfying, protein-rich meal that's ready in minutes. If you don't have refried beans, you can mash and season black beans or pinto beans. Flexible, budget-friendly, and perfect for busy days, or anytime you want something with a little fiesta flair!

1 large whole grain or sprouted-grain tortilla, or corn wrap

⅔ cup low-sodium or regular vegetarian refried pinto or black beans (warmed slightly, if desired)

2 tablespoons salsa

½ small avocado, sliced, or 3 tablespoons guacamole

1 cup shredded lettuce or cabbage

¼ cup fresh chopped cilantro or parsley or to taste

Squeeze of fresh lime juice

Chef's Shopping Tip * Refried beans can be found in the Mexican or Latin section of the grocery store. Read the label, as some contain lard.

Make your own by mixing cooked or canned beans with cumin, chili powder, and optional salt—mash with a fork or potato masher.

1. If your tortilla feels stiff or cold, warm it for 15 to 20 seconds in the microwave or a dry skillet. This makes it more pliable and easier to roll without tearing.
2. Lay the tortilla flat and spread the refried beans evenly, leaving space at the edges for rolling.
3. Add salsa, avocado, shredded lettuce, cilantro, and any optional toppings. Add a squeeze of lime juice. Roll tightly, tucking in the sides as you go. Slice in half (if desired) and enjoy immediately!

OPTIONAL ADD-INS

- 1–2 tablespoons sliced green onions or chopped red onions
- ¼ cup tablespoons corn kernels
- ¼ cup grated carrots

Per wrap: Calories: 360, Protein: 16 g, Fat: 18 g, Carbohydrate: 65 g, Fiber: 16 g
Minerals: Calcium: 165 mg, Iron: 5 mg, Magnesium: 105 mg, Potassium: 1395 mg, Sodium: 710 mg, Zinc: 2 mg
Vitamins: A: 159 mcg, C: 12 mg, E: 2 mg, Folate: 113 mcg DFE
Percent of calories from: Protein 13%, Fat 33%, Carbohydrate 54%

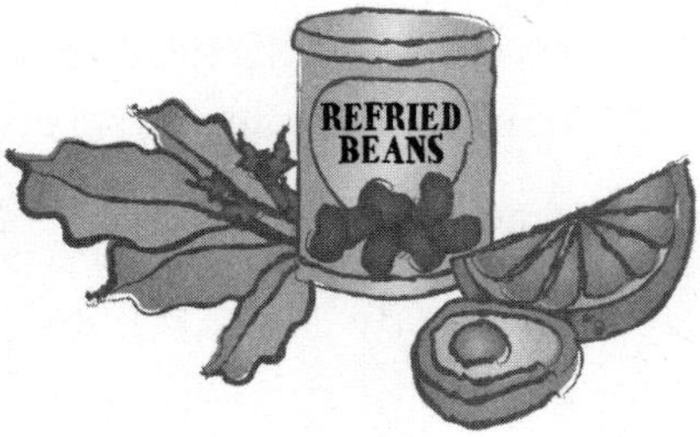

ASIAN TOFU AND VEGGIE WRAP WITH PEANUT SAUCE

Makes 1 large wrap

Colorful, crunchy, and full of flavor, this wrap combines crisp vegetables, aromatic herbs, and satisfying tofu with a creamy peanut sauce for a quick and nourishing meal. It's a great portable lunch and easy to customize with your favorite add-ins. To boost calcium, compare tofu labels, and select higher calcium varieties.

⅓ cup smoked or Asian-style flavored tofu, or firm or extra-firm tofu, sliced into strips

1 large whole grain or spinach tortilla wrap

2–3 tablespoons peanut sauce (page 273)

Splash of tamari

Pinch Chinese 5-Spice

½ cup carrot, shredded

½ cup red bell pepper, thinly sliced

½ cup cucumber, thin slices or strips

½ cup shredded red cabbage, Napa cabbage

A handful of Thai or regular basil (optional)

1. If using unflavored tofu, lightly pan sear the slices in a dry or lightly oiled nonstick pan over medium heat until golden on both sides. Add a splash of tamari and a little Chinese 5-Spice to boost flavor (optional).
2. If your tortilla feels stiff or cold, warm it for 15 to 20 seconds in the microwave or a dry skillet. This makes it more pliable.
3. Spread a generous layer of the peanut sauce over the tortilla.
4. Layer tofu, carrots, red pepper, cucumber, shredded cabbage, and basil (if using) in the center of the wrap.
5. Roll tightly, tucking in the sides as you go. Slice in half (if desired) and enjoy immediately!

Per wrap: Calories: 289, Protein: 14 g, Fat: 10 g, Carbohydrate: 39 g, Fiber: 7 g
Minerals: Calcium: 270 mg, Iron: 3.5 mg, Magnesium: 92 mg, Potassium: 733 mg, Sodium: 411 mg, Zinc: 2 mg
Vitamins: A: 599 mcg, C: 121 mg, E: 2 mg, Folate: 111 mcg DFE
Percent of calories from: Protein 19%, Fat 30%, Carbohydrate 51%

BEST BLACK BEAN BURGERS

Makes 3 patties

These hearty burgers are flavorful, moist, and satisfying. Black beans provide a protein-rich base while onion and mushrooms add sweetness, umami, and tenderness. A blend of warm spices ties everything together, and a flax "egg" helps bind the patties. Bake for ease or finish with a quick pan sear for a crisp exterior. Using whole grain breadcrumbs produces a lighter, more traditional texture, while oats can provide a heartier gluten-free option.

1 tablespoon ground flaxseed plus 2½ tablespoons warm water (flax "egg")

½ cup finely diced onion

½ cup finely diced mushrooms

1 (15-oz) can low-sodium or regular black beans, drained and rinsed

1 tablespoon low-sodium or regular tamari or soy sauce

1 teaspoon smoked paprika

1 teaspoon garlic powder

1 teaspoon onion powder

1 teaspoon chili powder

1 teaspoon ground cumin

¼ cup whole grain breadcrumbs or ¼ cup oats (regular, quick, or gluten-free)

Freshly ground black pepper, to taste

1. Preheat oven to 375°F.
2. In a small bowl, mix ground flaxseed with warm water to make a flax "egg." Let it sit for 10 minutes to thicken.
3. Dry sauté the onion and mushrooms in a nonstick skillet over medium heat until softened and most of the liquid has evaporated, 6 to 8 minutes. Use a splash of water or broth if needed to prevent sticking.

4. Place the black beans in a large bowl and microwave for 1 minute to soften. Mash with a potato masher or fork until mostly smooth, leaving some chunks for texture.
5. Add the flax egg, sautéed onion and mushrooms, tamari, smoked paprika, garlic powder, onion powder, chili powder, cumin, and breadcrumbs. Mix until well combined. If the mixture is too wet, add more breadcrumbs; if too dry, add a splash of water or broth.
6. Season with black pepper.
7. Form the mix into 3 patties. Patties can be cooked in a frying pan or baked in the oven.
    - **Pan Cooked:** Heat a nonstick skillet over medium heat. Lightly coat the pan with cooking spray or add a small amount of oil. Place the burgers in the pan and cook for 4 to 5 minutes per side, until heated through and lightly browned. Adjust the heat as needed to prevent sticking.
    - **Baked:** Line a baking sheet with parchment paper or a silicone mat. Place patties on the prepared baking sheet. Bake for 15 minutes, flip, and bake another 15 to 20 minutes until firm. For best texture, sear patties in a lightly oiled nonstick skillet for 2 to 3 minutes per side before serving.

OPTIONAL ADD-INS AND VARIATIONS

- Add 2 tablespoons of finely chopped walnuts, sunflower seeds, or hemp-seeds.
- Add 1 tablespoon of tomato paste or barbecue sauce.
- Make a double batch and freeze extras between parchment layers. They reheat beautifully for quick, healthy meals.

SERVING SUGGESTIONS

- Serve on a whole grain bun with avocado, tomato, and lettuce.
- Top with mushroom gravy or salsa.
- Crumble into tacos, wraps, or grain bowls for a quick meal.

Per patty (1/3 recipe): Calories: 203, Protein: 12 g, Fat: 2 g, Carbohydrate: 36 g, Fiber: 13 g

Minerals: Calcium: 93 mg, Iron: 4 mg, Magnesium: 78 mg, Potassium: 637 mg, Sodium: 443 mg, Zinc: 1 mg,

Vitamins: A: 14 mcg, C: 7 mg, E: 2 mg, Folate: 107 mcg DFE

Percent of calories from: Protein 23%, Fat 10%, Carbohydrate 67%

Why Make Your Own Veggie Burgers?

Homemade veggie burgers can offer advantages over many store-bought versions:

- **No additives or preservatives:** Just whole-food ingredients you recognize.
- **Customizable nutrition:** Add vegetables for extra fiber and antioxidants, use oats or whole grain breadcrumbs for heart-healthy carbs, or boost protein with beans, lentils, or tofu.
- **Better flavor and texture:** Fresh spices, herbs, and vegetables give more complexity and moisture than many frozen patties.
- **Budget-friendly:** Beans, oats, and vegetables are inexpensive staples, making homemade burgers a fraction of the cost of packaged ones.

At the same time, note that commercial veggie burgers can be significant providers of iron and protein and can be based on whole-plant foods. If you'd like to use these, check labels to find brands that are low in saturated fat and avoid ingredients such as palm oil.

TACOS FOR ALL

Makes 3 or more tacos

This meal works beautifully for families and gatherings where dietary preferences vary. Double or triple ingredients as needed. Simply chop the veggies, warm the beans and taco shells (soft or hard), and set out the colorful fillings in pretty bowls. This way, everyone can assemble their own taco to suit their tastes. Use cashew cheese to increase the content of zinc and other minerals. Avocados contribute potassium and aid in the absorption of fat-soluble nutrients.

1 cup shredded lettuce
2 ripe tomatoes, chopped
1–2 green onions, finely diced
¼–½ cup grated nondairy cheese
1 ripe avocado, peeled and sliced or mashed
1 teaspoon lemon juice
1 (14–15-oz) can refried beans
¼–½ cup salsa
3 or more tortillas or taco shells
½ cup pitted olives, chopped (optional)
Chopped cilantro (optional)

1. Chop lettuce, tomatoes, and onions and place in bowls, along with the grated cheese.
2. Add the avocado and sprinkle on lemon juice to keep it from browning.
3. Warm the refried beans in a microwave, small saucepan, or vegetable steamer, and if too thick, stir in a tablespoon or more of salsa.

4. Warm the taco shells in oven or microwave (optional).
5. Set all ingredients out in individual bowls. Allow each person to build their taco with their preferred combination of fillings.

OPTIONAL ADD-INS AND VARIATION

- Add 1 large carrot, grated.
- Replace the refried beans with 1½ cups of mashed black beans or pinto beans or with 1 package of vegetarian ground round.
- For a gluten-free option, use corn tortillas.

Per 1/3 recipe: Calories: 349, Protein: 12 g, Fat: 19 g, Carbohydrate: 38 g, Fiber: 14 g

Minerals: Calcium: 99 mg, Iron: 3 mg, Magnesium: 89 mg, Potassium: 1074 mg, Sodium: 539 mg, Zinc: 2 mg

Vitamins: A: 91 mcg, C: 21 mg, E: 2 mg, Folate: 77 mcg DFE

Percent of calories from: Protein 13%, Fat 46%, Carbohydrate 41%

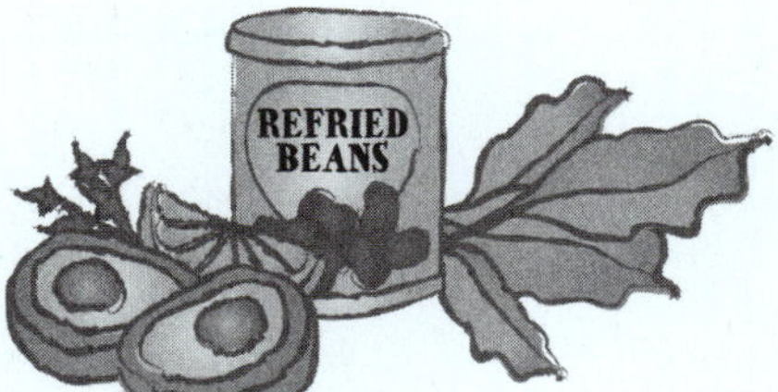

EASY PEASY CHILI

Makes 9 cups

This satisfying, flavor-packed chili is a perfect crowd-friendly meal. Some veggie crumbles provide significantly more iron and zinc than others, so be sure to compare labels. Spice your chili up with diced jalapeño and finish with fresh toppings. Pair with Double Corn Muffins (page 322). Leftovers taste even better the next day and freeze well!

1 medium onion, chopped

1 green pepper, diced

4 cloves garlic, minced

¼ cup low-sodium or regular vegetable stock or broth or water

1 (28-oz) can low-sodium or regular diced tomatoes (or 4 cups chopped fresh tomatoes)

1 (8–10-oz) package veggie crumbles (burger replacement)

2 cups cooked or 1 (19-oz) can kidney, black, or pinto beans (or a combination of these), rinsed and drained

1 cup frozen corn

1 cup mild, medium, or hot salsa

1–2 teaspoons chili powder, or to taste

1 teaspoon oregano

½ teaspoon cumin

1. In a large saucepan, sauté the onion, pepper, and garlic in broth over medium heat for about 10 minutes, or until softened.
2. Stir in the diced tomatoes, veggie crumbles (or tofu or tempeh, as in the Variation on the next page), beans, corn, salsa, chili powder, oregano, and cumin.

3. Bring to a simmer and cook for 5 minutes to heat through. Then lower heat, cover, and simmer gently for 40 to 45 minutes, stirring occasionally.
4. If the chili thickens too much, add an extra ½ cup of broth or water.

OPTIONAL TOPPINGS

- Avocado cubes, thinly sliced green onion, chopped cilantro, shredded veggie cheese, veggie sour cream, and lime wedges

TOFU OR TEMPEH VARIATION

- Replace veggie crumbles with 10 to 12 ounces of crumbled extra-firm tofu or tempeh. Bake crumbled tofu or tempeh at 400°F for 15 to 20 minutes until lightly browned for extra texture.

SAUCY VARIATION:

- Add 1–1½ cups of tomato marinara sauce at the same time as the diced tomatoes.

Per 1½-cup serving: Calories: 241, Protein: 17 g, Fat: 7g, Carbohydrate: 31 g, Fiber: 8 g
Minerals: Calcium: 137 mg, Iron: 6 mg, Magnesium: 49 mg, Potassium: 755 mg, Sodium: 382 mg, Zinc: 1 mg
Vitamins: A: 59 mcg, C: 40 mg, E: 1.5 mg, Folate: 101 mcg DFE
Percent of calories from: Protein 27%, Fat 23%, Carbohydrate 50%

TASTY TOFU WITH TWO MARINADES

Makes 4 servings (3–4 ounces each)

Tofu is a highly versatile protein food that readily absorbs flavor through marination. This recipe offers two distinct and delicious marinades: an Asian-inspired ginger-garlic blend and a savory tomato-based option. Both are rich in flavor and adaptable.

Marinated tofu can be sprinkled on a salad, included in a stir-fry, enjoyed as a snack, or prepared in slices and used in a sandwich. The protein, iron, and calcium per serving can vary slightly with the type of tofu selected, and the variations are significant!

Though freshly chopped ginger and garlic are great, pre-minced and jarred versions are available in supermarkets and online and can make preparation simpler! Leftover marinades can be reused or become a light salad dressing or be served over brown rice.

Choosing the Right Tofu

Firm, extra-firm, or super-firm tofu works best for marinated tofu cubes because they hold their shape well and develop a crisp exterior when baked or air-fried. Pressing firm tofu before marinating removes excess moisture, allowing it to absorb more flavor and achieve a meatier texture. Extra- or super-firm tofu often requires little or no pressing.

TOFU

- One block of firm or extra-firm tofu (such as 12–16 oz), cut into 1/3-inch cubes or 1/3 x 1/3 x 1-inch fingers.

ASIAN GINGER-GARLIC MARINADE #1

Makes 1 cup

¼ cup low-sodium or regular tamari or soy sauce

¼ cup (or more) finely chopped fresh ginger

2 tablespoons rice vinegar or cider vinegar

1–2 tablespoons toasted sesame oil

1 tablespoon minced garlic

Place ingredients in a wide, flat-bottomed container and stir.

TOMATO-BASED MARINADE #2

Makes 1½ cups

1 cup fresh or canned tomatoes or tomato sauce

¼ cup low-sodium or regular tamari, soy sauce, or Bragg's Liquid Aminos

2–4 tablespoons apple cider vinegar or rice vinegar

1 tablespoon toasted sesame oil

1 tablespoon (or more) peeled, minced ginger root

1 clove garlic, minced, or 1 teaspoon minced garlic

½ teaspoon turmeric

Place the tomatoes, tamari, vinegar, sesame oil, ginger, garlic, and turmeric in a blender and puree for 15 seconds or until smooth; then pour into a wide, flat-bottomed container. If using tomato sauce, blending is not necessary.

TO MARINATE AND COOK TOFU

1. Place tofu cubes in either marinade #1 or #2, ensuring all pieces are coated.
2. Marinate tofu for at least an hour; overnight or longer deepens the flavor.

3. With a slotted spoon, lift the tofu from the marinade. Leftover marinade can be refrigerated and reused.
4. Use one of the following cooking methods:
   - **Air Fryer:** Cook tofu at 375°F to 400°F for 10 minutes until golden and lightly crisped. If you like, shake halfway through and adjust cooking time.
   - **Oven:** Place tofu on a lined baking sheet (silicone mat or parchment). Bake at 400°F (375°F convection) for 20 to 25 minutes until nicely browned.
   - **Stovetop:** Place tofu on a nonstick or lightly oiled skillet and cook over medium heat until browned on all sides, for 8 to 10 minutes.

OPTIONAL ADD-INS AND VARIATIONS

- **For heat:** Add ½–1 teaspoon sriracha or other chili sauce to the marinade.
- **For sweetness:** Stir in 1 teaspoon maple syrup.
- **For texture:** Toss marinated tofu in nutritional yeast or whole grain breadcrumbs before baking or air frying.
- **For no-blender prep:** Use tomato sauce in Marinade #2 and whisk all ingredients in a bowl or jar.
- **To enhance marinade absorption:** Press tofu before slicing by placing it between clean kitchen towels with a weight (e.g., cutting board + canned goods) for 30 to 60 minutes.
- **To reduce prep time:** Skip the marinade. Place tofu on a lined cookie sheet. Sprinkle with tamari, soy sauce, or Bragg's Liquid Aminos. Sprinkle on seasonings of your choice (e.g., turmeric, pepper, onion powder, garlic powder, dried herbs, seasoning blends) and optional nutritional yeast. Bake as directed above or sauté in a nonstick pan until browned.

ROASTED CAULIFLOWER WITH CHICKPEAS AND OLIVES

Makes about 6 cups (serves 6 as a side dish, or 3–4 as a main dish)

This Mediterranean-inspired dish is as nourishing as it is flavorful. Cauliflower roasts to golden perfection alongside chickpeas, garlic, and briny olives, creating a satisfying balance of textures and tastes. It's delicious as a side dish, or you can serve it as a hearty main with a salad, soup, or hummus and bread. The leftovers keep beautifully, making it a great make-ahead option.

1 medium head cauliflower (about 1 pound or 5½–6 cups florets)

1 (15-oz) can chickpeas (about 1½ cups cooked), rinsed and drained, patted dry

¾ cup pitted green or black olives (about 24 olives), halved

8 garlic cloves, coarsely chopped

1–2 tablespoons extra-virgin olive oil

½ teaspoon crushed red pepper flakes (optional, for heat)

¼ teaspoon salt or to taste

Freshly ground black pepper to taste

3 tablespoons chopped, fresh flat-leaf parsley

Zest and juice of ½ fresh lemon

1. Preheat the oven to 450°F.
2. In a roasting pan or rimmed baking sheet, lined with parchment paper or a silicone mat, combine cauliflower florets, chickpeas, olives, and garlic. Drizzle with olive oil, sprinkle with red pepper flakes (if using), salt and black pepper, and toss well to coat.
3. Spread the mixture in a single layer.
4. Roast for 20 to 25 minutes, stirring once halfway through, until cauliflower is golden brown and tender-crisp and chickpeas are lightly crisped.
5. Remove from the oven. Add parsley, lemon zest, and lemon juice. Toss gently and serve warm.

OPTIONAL ADD-INS AND VARIATIONS

- **For a spiced version:** Add 1 teaspoon smoked paprika or ground cumin with the oil and spices.
- **For added color and complexity:** Add 1 sliced red bell pepper or 1 small red onion (cut into wedges) to the roasting pan.
- **For a low-oil option:** Use 1 tablespoon olive oil and 1 tablespoon aquafaba (liquid drained from canned chickpeas) to reduce calories while maintaining moisture.

Per cup: Calories: 119, Protein: 6 g, Fat: 6 g, Carbohydrate: 14 g, Fiber: 5 g

Minerals: Calcium: 55 mg, Iron: 1 mg, Magnesium: 31 mg, Potassium: 348 mg, Sodium: 500 mg, Zinc: 0.7 mg

Vitamins: A: 11 mcg, C: 41 mg, E: 1 mg, Folate: 62 mcg DFE

Percent of calories from: Protein 15%, Fat 41%, Carbohydrate 44%

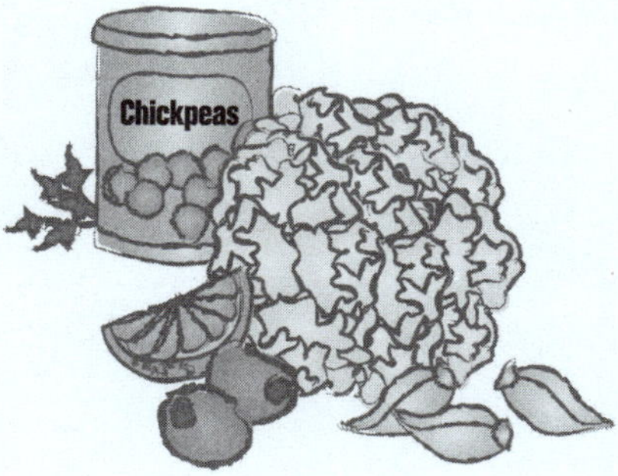

THE MULTICOLORED BOWL

Makes 2 generous servings (2 cups of cooked grain, 4 cups of cooked vegetables, and 1–1½ cups of cooked beans)

Bowls are very trendy, and for good reason! This colorful, build-your-own bowl delivers plant-based protein, essential minerals, and a wide array of phytochemicals from vibrantly hued vegetables. It's meal-prep friendly, endlessly adaptable, and nutritionally robust. Serve it with Ginger Lime Miso Dressing (page 272) or another favorite dressing.

5–6 cups chopped vegetables (such as asparagus, broccoli, Brussels sprouts, bok choy, cauliflower, carrots, red or yellow pepper, and purple cabbage)

2 cups cooked brown rice, quinoa, or other whole grain

1 (15–19-oz) can or 1½–2 cups cooked, rinsed, and drained beans such as edamame, garbanzo (chickpeas), kidney, white, or black beans

1. Arrange the vegetables in a steamer basket over boiling water. Place the denser vegetables (e.g., Brussel sprouts, cauliflower and carrots) in the bottom layer and the more delicate ones (e.g., asparagus, bok choy, and bell pepper) on top. Steam until all are tender-crisp or about 5 to 10 minutes.
2. Place cooked grains into bowls.
3. Warm beans in microwave or saucepan.
4. Top each bowl with steamed vegetables and beans.

OPTIONAL ADD-INS:

- Top with toasted almonds, sunflower, sesame, or pumpkin seeds, sprouts, sliced green onions, or avocado.
- For vegetables, replace those listed with celery, green peppers, kale or other greens, onions, and snow peas.
- Instead of beans, choose cooked marinated tofu (page 299), tempeh, or veggie beef or chicken.
- Add hot sauce, if desired.

RED LENTIL PASTA SAUCE

Makes about 7 cups

Red lentils are the fastest cooking of all legumes and are ready in just 20 minutes. They dissolve beautifully into sauces, adding body, protein, iron, and fiber. You may use most, or all of the vegetables listed here, substitute others that you prefer, or use even more. Serve with your favorite pasta, or spaghetti squash. For more protein, use chickpea, edamame, or lentil pasta. Top with a grated plant-based cheese if desired.

1 onion, chopped

2–4 cups thinly chopped vegetables such as mushrooms, carrots, celery, and bell pepper

2 ½ cups water or vegetable stock

1–3 teaspoons minced garlic (to taste)

1 cup dry red lentils

1 (24-oz) can or jar tomato sauce

1 tablespoon of Italian herbs or ¼ cup mix of fresh basil, oregano, and rosemary

Salt and pepper to taste

STOVETOP METHOD

1. In a large pot with a lid over medium heat, place onion, vegetables, ½ cup of water, and garlic, cover, and cook until the onion and vegetables soften, adding water as needed.
2. Add lentils and 2 cups of water. Bring to a boil, then lower heat. Cover and simmer for 20 minutes or until lentils are soft.
3. Add tomato sauce and warm through.
4. Adjust seasonings to taste.

CROCK-POT METHOD

Place all ingredients in a Crock-Pot and cook on high heat for 1 hour.

OPTIONAL ADD-INS AND VARIATIONS:

- For vegetables, choose broccoli, leeks, or others that you prefer or have on hand.
- Use precooked or canned lentils and skip step 2.
- Use a different size jar of tomato sauce.
- Add any of these at the same time as the tomato sauce:
  - 2–3 teaspoons of miso or tamari
  - ¼–½ cup of red cooking wine
  - ⅓ can or more of tomato paste

Per cup: Calories: 170, Protein: 9 g, Fat: 2 g, Carbohydrate: 30 g, Fiber: 6 g

Minerals: Calcium: 68 mg, Iron: 3 mg, Magnesium: 41 mg, Potassium: 644 mg, Sodium: 466 mg, Zinc: 1 mg

Vitamins: A: 118 mcg, C: 18 mg, E: 3 mg, Folate: 80 mcg DFE

Percent of calories from: Protein 20%, Fat 12%, Carbohydrate 68%

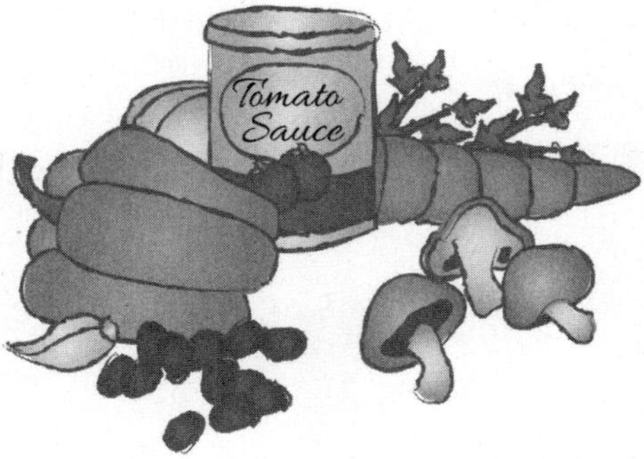

MARVELOUS MUSHROOM RAGOUT

Makes 5 cups (4 servings)

A comforting, umami-rich creamy sauce featuring mushrooms, white beans, garlic, and onions in a luscious plant-based sauce—no blender required. This versatile dish pairs beautifully with mashed potatoes, whole grain pasta, quinoa, or brown rice. Serve with a green vegetable. Replace thyme with other herbs, if desired.

VEGETABLE BEAN BASE

1 medium sweet onion, finely chopped

4 cups sliced cremini or white button mushrooms (10–12 oz)

3 cloves garlic, minced

2 cups cooked (19-oz can) white beans (cannellini or Great Northern), drained and rinsed

1 tablespoon fresh thyme (1 teaspoon dried)

NO-BLENDER CREAMY SAUCE

1½ tablespoons cornstarch (for thickening)

3 tablespoons cold water

1½ cups unsweetened, unflavored soy, oat, or cashew milk

2 tablespoons nutritional yeast

1 tablespoon tahini

2 teaspoons light miso

¾ teaspoon onion powder

¼–½ teaspoon salt, or to taste

1 tablespoon lemon juice (juice from ½ lemon)

Fresh ground black pepper, to taste

1. In a large skillet over medium heat, dry sauté the onion and mushrooms for 10 to 12 minutes, stirring occasionally. Add a splash of wine, broth, water, or a little oil as needed to prevent sticking.
2. Add the garlic and cook for 1 more minute. Lower the heat to low, then stir in the white beans and thyme.
3. In a small bowl or cup, whisk together the cornstarch and cold water until smooth. Set aside.
4. In a small saucepan (off heat), whisk together the plant-based milk, nutritional yeast, tahini, miso, onion powder, and salt.
5. Stir in the cornstarch slurry and place over medium-low heat. Cook, whisking constantly, for about 5 minutes, or until the sauce thickens to a smooth, creamy consistency.
6. Remove from heat and stir in the lemon juice and black pepper to taste.
7. Pour the sauce over the bean mixture and stir gently to combine.
8. Simmer on low heat for about 5 minutes, stirring occasionally to blend flavors.
9. Taste and adjust seasonings as needed. Serve hot over your favorite pasta, grain, or mashed potatoes.

Per 1¼-cup serving: Calories: 267, Protein: 16 g, Fat: 4 g, Carbohydrate: 44 g, Fiber: 8 g

Minerals: Calcium: 227 mg, Iron: 3 mg, Magnesium: 102 mg, Potassium: 1039 mg, Sodium: 478 mg, Zinc: 2 mg

Vitamins: A: 2 mcg, C: 9 mg, E: 1 mg, Folate: 126 mcg DFE

Percent of calories from: Protein 23%, Fat 14%, Carbohydrate 63%

TOFU CACCIATORE

Makes about 7 cups (4 servings)

A hearty, plant-powered take on a classic Italian dish, this Tofu Cacciatore features tender, savory tofu simmered in a rich tomato sauce with mushrooms, peppers, and herbs. It's deeply satisfying and perfect served over your favorite pasta or whole grain—making it a wonderful meal for company as well as everyday enjoyment.

TOFU

1 (14–16-oz) package firm or extra-firm tofu, drained and pressed

1–2 tablespoons low-sodium or regular tamari, soy sauce, or Bragg's Liquid Aminos

Fresh ground pepper

SAUCE

1 large onion, diced

2 cups mushrooms (cremini or button), trimmed and sliced (or cut into quarters or halves for smaller mushrooms)

1 green, yellow, or orange bell pepper, sliced into strips (or a mix of colors)

3 garlic cloves, minced (1½ teaspoons)

3 ripe tomatoes, coarsely chopped

½ cup dry red wine or vegetable broth

3 cups low-sodium or regular chunky or other marinara or tomato sauce

1 tablespoon fresh rosemary, chopped

½ teaspoon red pepper flakes or to taste (optional)

Fresh ground pepper, or to taste

TOPPINGS

Fresh basil leaves or parsley, chopped (optional)

1. Preheat the oven to 400°F.
2. Prepare the tofu. Tear tofu into craggy 1-inch pieces (or cut into ¾-inch cubes) and place on a parchment- or silicone-lined baking sheet. Drizzle with tamari and sprinkle with pepper.
3. Place the pan on the middle rack and bake for 25 minutes, flipping halfway through, until tofu is lightly browned and crispy.
4. Prepare the sauce. In a large 12" skillet or a Dutch oven, dry sauté the onions and mushrooms for about 10 minutes or until nicely browned. If necessary, add a little broth or oil to prevent sticking.
5. Add the peppers, garlic, and fresh tomatoes, and cook for an additional 5 to 7 minutes, stirring occasionally.
6. Add the red wine and continue simmering for 10 minutes.
7. Stir in the marinara sauce, rosemary, and red pepper flakes (if using). Add the tofu and stir gently. Simmer for another 10 minutes.
8. Spoon the tofu cacciatore over your favorite pasta, rice, quinoa, or other whole grain.
9. Garnish with fresh basil, if desired.

Per ¼ recipe: Calories: 252, Protein: 15 g, Fat: 7 g, Carbohydrate: 30g, Fiber: 7 g

Minerals: Calcium: 280 mg, Iron: 4 mg, Magnesium: 95 mg, Potassium: 1232 mg, Sodium: 196 mg, Zinc: 2 mg

Vitamins: A: 107 mcg, C: 45 mg, E: 5 mg, Folate: 74 mcg DFE

Percent of calories from: Protein 24%, Fat 26%, Carbohydrate 47%, Alcohol 3%

Desserts and Sweet Treats

Dessert can be more than an indulgence; it can contribute to your nutritional needs. A sweet bite at the end of a meal can signal to the body and mind that the dining experience is finished, creating a sense of satisfaction and closure. This ritual need not be abandoned in a health-supportive lifestyle; it can be thoroughly enjoyed with whole-food ingredients.

In this collection, we celebrate sweet treats that honor both flavor and function, using ingredients that satisfy the palate while supporting overall well-being. Instead of refined sugars and processed fats, these recipes feature dried fruits, pure maple syrup, and molasses for natural sweetness. These ingredients offer micronutrients, antioxidants, and, in the case of dried fruits, dietary fiber. We've used nut butters in place of butter, margarine, shortening, or oil, providing richness, plant-based protein, and healthy fats that contribute to satiety and metabolic health.

From no-bake confections to warm fruit crisp to creamy puddings, each recipe invites you to experience pleasure without compromising your commitment to healthy plant-based eating. Whether enjoyed as a daily ritual or a festive treat, these creations provide snacks or round out a meal in a way that is beautifully aligned with whole-food, plant-based living.

EASY CHOCOLATE PUDDING

Makes 2 cups (4 servings)

Silky, rich, and deeply chocolatey, this effortless pudding comes together in minutes with just two or three core ingredients. It's perfect as a quick dessert, snack, or even a wholesome sweet for guests. It delivers calories and protein for those who are underweight. Thanks to soft or silken tofu, this treat offers a smooth, mousse-like texture along with flavonoid-rich dark chocolate.

Leftovers (if there are any!) will keep in the refrigerator for three to four days.

3½ ounces dark chocolate, chopped, or ⅔ cup of dark chocolate chips

1 (10–12-oz) package soft tofu or silken tofu at room temperature, drained

2 tablespoons maple syrup (optional)

Melt the chocolate:

STOVETOP METHOD

- Place chocolate in a double boiler over simmering water until fully melted.

MICROWAVE METHOD

- Place chocolate in a microwave-safe bowl with high sides. Microwave in 30-second intervals, stirring after each, until melted.

1. **Blend the pudding:** Add the tofu, maple syrup, and any Optional Add-Ins to the melted chocolate. Blend using an immersion blender or transfer to a high-speed blender. Process until smoothly mixed and glossy, scraping down the sides as needed.
2. **Chill and serve:** Spoon the pudding into 4 small bowls or ramekins. Chill for at least 30 minutes to set. Serve with Optional Add-Ins or Toppings.

OPTIONAL ADD-INS:

- For added protein, blend or stir in some peanut butter (warmed slightly or at room temperature) and/or yogurt based on pea or soy protein to taste.
- Add ¼ teaspoon salt.
- Add ½ teaspoon vanilla.
- For an even more chocolatey flavor, blend in 2–3 tablespoons of cocoa powder.

OPTIONAL TOPPINGS:

- Chocolate shavings
- Berries
- Fresh mint
- Chopped toasted nuts (hazelnuts are divine)
- Cashew-Pear Cream (page 319)

Per ½ cup: Calories: 188, Protein: 7 g, Fat: 11 g, Carbohydrate: 16 g, Fiber: 2 g

Minerals: Calcium: 109 mg, Iron: 3 mg, Magnesium: 61 mg, Potassium: 243 mg, Sodium: 13 mg, Zinc: 1 mg

Vitamins: A: 1 mcg, C: 0 mg, E: 0.1 mg, Folate: 37 mcg DFE

Percent of calories from: Protein 15%, Fat 52%, Carbohydrate 33%

CREAMY CHIA PUDDING

Makes 2¼ cups (3 servings)

This quick, make-ahead dish works equally well for breakfast or as a light dessert or snack. Rich in omega-3s, calcium, and fiber, it's also endlessly customizable. Adjust the sweetness to taste, and top with fruit, nuts, or granola for added texture and flavor. For an added nutritional boost, try the whole-food blender variation using dates or prunes and hempseeds!

2 cups fortified, unsweetened soy, oat, or other plant-based milk

1 tablespoon of maple syrup (adjust to taste)

½ teaspoon vanilla extract

5 tablespoons chia seeds

1. Place the milk, maple syrup, and vanilla in a bowl or jar and stir well.
2. Add chia seeds and mix thoroughly with a fork or table knife until evenly distributed.
3. Refrigerate. After 30 minutes, stir again to prevent clumping and ensure a creamy texture.
4. Cover and refrigerate overnight (or for at least 4 hours), until thickened.
5. Before serving, stir again. If the pudding is too thick, add enough plant-based milk to achieve the desired consistency.

TOPPINGS

- Fresh or stewed fruit (e.g., berries, plums, peaches)
- A dash of cinnamon or other spices
- A spoonful of granola or chopped nuts/seeds

VARIATIONS

- **Chocolate Chia Pudding:** Add 3 tablespoons cocoa powder along with the milk, maple syrup, and vanilla. Increase the maple syrup to 1½–2 tablespoons depending on sweetness preference.
- **Whole-Food Blender Chia Pudding:** Blend 2 cups plant-based milk with 3 tablespoons hempseeds, 4 dried prunes or pitted dates, and ½ teaspoon vanilla extract. Process on high speed until smooth and creamy. Add 4 tablespoons chia seeds and pulse briefly. Stir after about 30 minutes to prevent clumping.

Per ¾ cup serving: Calories: 158, Protein: 8 g, Fat: 8 g, Carbohydrate: 15 g, Fiber: 7 g
Minerals: Calcium: 317 mg, Iron: 2 mg, Magnesium: 86 mg, Potassium: 286 mg, Sodium: 60 mg, Zinc: 1 mg
Vitamins: A: 100 mcg, C: 0.3 mg, E: 0.1 mg, Folate: 9 mcg DFE
Percent of calories from: Protein 19%, Fat 45%, Carbohydrate 36%

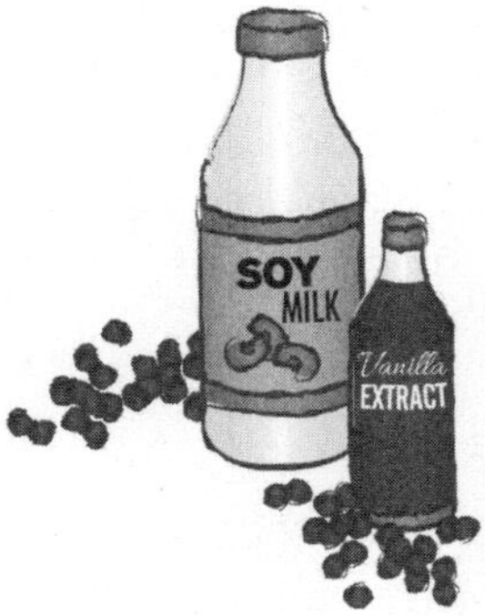

SIMPLE STEWED FRUIT

Makes about 2 cups

This simple, no-sugar-added fruit compote lets the natural sweetness of berries and stone fruits shine. It's perfect on chia pudding, breakfast bowls, plant-based yogurt or ice cream, pancakes, or French toast.

2 cups fresh or frozen fruit or berries (e.g., blueberries, raspberries, strawberries, chopped apples, pears, peaches, or a mix)

1–3 tablespoons water (optional)

2 teaspoons cornstarch

2 tablespoons cold water (for slurry)

Pinch of cinnamon or grated lemon zest (optional)

1. Combine fruit and water (if using) in a small saucepan over medium heat. If using very juicy fruit, you can omit the initial water or use only 1 tablespoon.
2. Stir occasionally until the fruit begins to release its juices and soften (5 to 15 minutes, depending on the fruit). Softer fruits, like berries, require less cooking time, while firmer fruits need more time.
3. Make the slurry. Place the cornstarch and 2 tablespoons cold water in a small bowl and whisk together until smooth.
4. Stir the slurry into the hot fruit mixture. Continue to cook, stirring constantly, until the liquid thickens and becomes glossy, for 1 to 2 minutes.
5. Add a pinch of cinnamon for extra flavor, if desired.
6. Cool slightly before serving warm or refrigerate and serve chilled. Keeps well in the fridge for 4 to 5 days.

Per ½ cup (¼ recipe): Calories: 47, Protein: 0.6 g, Fat: 0.2 g, Carbohydrate: 12 g, Fiber: 2 g

Minerals: Calcium: 5 mg, Iron: 0.2 mg, Magnesium: 5 mg, Potassium: 57 mg, Sodium: 1 mg, Zinc: 0.1 mg

Vitamins: A: 13 mcg, C: 7 mg, E: 0.4 mg, Folate: 4 mcg DFE

Percent of calories from: Protein 4%, Fat 4%, Carbohydrate 92%

APPLE PEAR CRISP

Makes 8 servings

This also can be done with either pears or apples (instead of both). It is best to use cooking apples such as Macintosh, Spartan, or Cortland. If using firmer apples such as Honeycrisp, Braeburn, or Granny Smith, cover the casserole dish for the first twenty to twenty-five minutes of cooking, then remove the lid to achieve a crispy topping. Add a dollop of Cashew-Pear Cream (page 319) to each bowl.

FRUIT LAYER

3 apples, cored and thinly sliced (about 4 cups)

3 ripe pears, cored and thinly sliced (about 3 cups)

1 teaspoon cinnamon

¼ teaspoon nutmeg

1 tablespoon cornstarch

1–2 tablespoons maple syrup (optional)

2 tablespoons lemon juice

¼ cup raisins or currants

OAT TOPPING

3 tablespoons maple syrup or date syrup

¼ cup almond or other nut butter

Pinch of salt

1½ cups rolled oats

½ cup chopped walnuts or ¼ cup walnuts and ¼ cup sunflower seeds

1 teaspoon cinnamon

1. Preheat oven to 350°F (325°F convection).
2. Place apples, pears, cinnamon, nutmeg, cornstarch, maple syrup (if using), lemon juice, and raisins in a large bowl. Mix well, then place in an 8 x 8-inch baking dish or casserole dish.
3. In a medium bowl, combine the maple syrup, almond butter, vanilla, and salt (if using). Add the oats, walnuts, and cinnamon and mix well to combine.
4. Sprinkle the oat mixture evenly over the fruit.
5. Bake 35 to 45 minutes or until top is golden brown. Serve with Cashew-Pear Cream or other favorite topping.

VARIATION

Replace the apples and pears with one of the following:

- 6 cups of sliced peaches or nectarines.
- 3 cups of peaches or nectarines plus 3 cups of strawberries, blueberries, raspberries, blackberries. Increase cornstarch to 2 tablespoons.

Per 1/8 recipe: Calories: 270, Protein: 5 g, Fat: 11 g, Carbohydrate: 43 g, Fiber: 7 g

Minerals: Calcium: 63 mg, Iron: 1.4 mg, Magnesium: 60 mg, Potassium: 344 mg, Sodium: 21 mg, Zinc: 1 mg

Vitamins: A: 3 mcg, C: 7 mg, E: 3 mg, Folate: 19 mcg DFE

Percent of calories from: Protein 8%, Fat 33%, Carbohydrate 59%

CASHEW PEAR CREAM

Makes 2¼ cups

This is the healthiest and most delicious replacement for whipped cream. Use on fruit crisps or crumbles, breakfast bowls or pancakes, fruit salads, pumpkin or other pies, or other desserts. Soaking the cashews for two to four hours prior to blending makes this an even smoother cream.

1 (15-oz) can or jar of pears in water or juice

1¼ cups raw cashews, rinsed and drained

½ teaspoon vanilla

1. Blend pears (with their water or juice), cashews, and vanilla at high speed until very smooth.
2. Pour into a jar and refrigerate. Increase cashews to 1½ cup cashews for a thicker cream (more like whipping cream) and reduce cashews to 1 cup for a thinner cream.

Per ¼ cup: Calories: 133, Protein: 4 g, Fat: 8 g, Carbohydrate: 13 g, Fiber: 1 g

Minerals: Calcium: 10 mg, Iron: 1 mg, Magnesium: 58 mg, Potassium: 166 mg, Sodium: 4 mg, Zinc: 1 mg

Vitamins: A: 0 mcg, C: 0.6 mg, E: 0.2 mg, Folate: 5 mcg DFE

Percent of calories from: Protein 10%, Fat 53%, Carbohydrate 37%

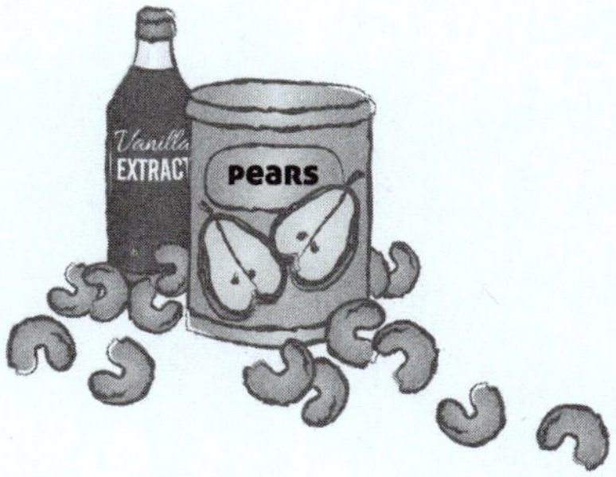

CRANBERRY PECAN MUFFINS

Makes 12 muffins

If you are a muffin lover, stock your freezer with cranberries, as you may want to make these often! Using small muffin tins, you may make eighteen small muffins and these may be a little lighter in texture. Cooking some of the cranberries with maple syrup and adding some uncooked cranberries, along with spices and orange, gives a variety and depth of flavor.

2½ cups cranberries, fresh or frozen, divided

¾ cup maple syrup, divided

2 cups whole wheat, spelt flour, or gluten-free flour

2 tablespoons ground flaxseed

2 teaspoons baking powder

1 teaspoon baking soda

2 teaspoons ground cinnamon

½ teaspoon allspice

½ teaspoon cloves

¾ teaspoon salt (optional)

1 (10–12-oz) package soft tofu

3 tablespoons tahini or oil such as avocado oil

⅔ cup fortified soy milk or other plant-based milk

3 tablespoons orange juice (juice from one small orange)

Grated rind from one orange (optional)

1 teaspoon vanilla extract

1 cup coarsely chopped pecans

1. Put 1½ cups of the cranberries and ½ cup of the maple syrup into a saucepan and cook over medium heat for about 10 minutes until

the cranberries have popped (or you can mash the cranberries). Remove from heat. Chop the remaining cranberries and add them to the mix.

2. Preheat oven to 400⁰ F (375⁰ F convection).
3. In a large bowl, combine flour, ground flaxseed, baking powder, baking soda, cinnamon, allspice, cloves, and salt (if using).
4. In a medium bowl, whisk together or mix with an immersion blender: tofu, tahini, the remaining ¼ cup of maple syrup, plant-based milk, orange juice, orange rind (if using), and vanilla.
5. Create a well in the dry ingredients, then add the wet ingredients, cranberries, and pecans. Stir gently to mix.
6. Spoon the dough into lightly sprayed muffin tins (or use paper liners).
7. Bake for 25 to 30 minutes, or until a toothpick inserted comes out clean.

Per small muffin: Calories: 165, Protein: 4 g, Fat: 7 g, Carbohydrate: 23 g, Fiber: 3 g

Minerals: Calcium: 99 mg, Iron: 1 mg, Magnesium: 38 mg, Potassium: 169 mg, Sodium: 120 mg, Zinc: 1 mg

Vitamins: A: 6 mcg, C: 3 mg, E: 0.4 mg, Folate: 18 mcg DFE

Percent of calories from: Protein 10%, Fat 37%, Carbohydrate 53%

DOUBLE CORN MUFFINS

Makes 10 medium-sized muffins

These moist, golden muffins are perfect alongside chili or soup, or as part of a nourishing breakfast paired with scrambled tofu, chia pudding, or fresh fruit. The double corn (cornmeal + corn kernels) gives these muffins a sweet-savory depth and a great texture.

1 cup unsweetened soy or other plant-based milk

1 tablespoon apple cider vinegar

½ cup unsweetened apple sauce

1 tablespoon ground flaxseed (golden is preferred for color, but either works)

3 tablespoons tahini

¼ cup maple syrup

1 cup whole wheat flour or other whole grain flour (e.g., spelt or Kamut)

1 cup cornmeal

1 teaspoon baking powder

½ teaspoon baking soda

¾ teaspoon salt (optional)

1 cup corn kernels (fresh, canned and drained niblets, or frozen and thawed)

1. Preheat oven to 425° F (400° F convection). Lightly oil 10 cups of a 12-cup muffin tin (oil spray works well). Fill the 2 unused cups with a little water to prevent scorching.
2. In a small bowl or liquid measuring cup, whisk together the plant-based milk, vinegar, applesauce, flaxseed, tahini, and maple syrup. Let sit for 5 to 10 minutes to allow the flax to gel slightly.

3. In a large bowl, mix together the flour, cornmeal, baking powder, baking soda, and salt (if using).
4. Make a well in the center of the dry ingredients and pour in the wet mixture. Stir gently until just combined. Do not overmix.
5. Fold in the corn kernels.
6. Divide the batter evenly into the 10 prepared muffin cups.
7. Bake for 20 to 25 minutes, or until a toothpick inserted into the center comes out clean. If you are using a silicone muffin pan, add 5 minutes to the cooking time.
8. Allow muffins to cool slightly in the pan before removing. Serve warm or at room temperature.

Per muffin: Calories: 162, Protein: 5 g, Fat: 4 g, Carbohydrate: 29 g, Fiber: 3 g
Minerals: Calcium: 79 mg, Iron: 1.4 mg, Magnesium: 50 mg, Potassium: 200 mg, Sodium: 129 mg, Zinc: 1 mg
Vitamins: A: 3 mcg, C: 1 mg, E: 0.2 mg, Folate: 20 mcg DFE
Percent of calories from: Protein 11%, Fat 21%, Carbohydrate 68%

VARIATIONS

- **Gluten-Free:** Use gluten-free flour or 1 cup + 2 tablespoons gluten-free oat flour in place of whole wheat flour.
- **Protein Boost:** Substitute ½ cup soft or silken tofu for the applesauce. Blend all wet ingredients until completely smooth before combining with dry ingredients.
- **Richer Texture:** Replace some or all of the applesauce with a neutral-tasting oil. Try ¼ cup oil + ¼ cup applesauce.

Chef's Tip **Silicone Bakeware**

Silicone mats and pans are nonstick and eco-friendly, eliminating the need for added oil or parchment paper. They also slow browning, so start at the higher end of the baking time and extend slightly if needed for golden edges or a firmer texture.

MOLASSES GINGER COOKIES

Makes 15 to 18 cookies

These soft, warmly spiced cookies are a wholesome twist on the traditional molasses ginger cookie. They are made without refined sugar and packed with flavor. If you enjoy a stronger molasses flavor, use 5 to 6 tablespoons blackstrap molasses and 2 to 3 tablespoons of maple syrup (to make ½ cup in total). They're perfect for cozy afternoons or sharing during the holidays. Feel free to add a pinch of nutmeg, cardamom, or ground cloves for a more complex flavor.

⅔ cup soft crunchy or smooth peanut butter or other nut butter (if hard or dry, stir in a small amount of neutral oil, or microwave briefly [15–30 seconds] to soften)

1 teaspoon vanilla extract

¼ cup blackstrap molasses (preferably organic)

¼ cup maple syrup

1 tablespoon ground flax

⅔ cup whole wheat flour or ¾ cup unbleached flour, or all-purpose gluten-free flour

½ teaspoon baking powder

¼ teaspoon salt (optional)

2 teaspoons powdered ginger (or 2 tablespoons fresh grated ginger)

1½ teaspoons cinnamon

½ teaspoon allspice

1. Preheat oven to 350°F (325°F convection). Line a baking sheet with a silicone mat or parchment paper.
2. In a large mixing bowl, combine the peanut butter, vanilla, molasses, and maple syrup. Stir until smooth and well combined.

3. In a separate bowl, whisk together the ground flax, flour, baking powder, salt (if using), ginger, cinnamon, and allspice.
4. Add the dry ingredients to the wet and mix until a uniform dough forms. If the dough is very soft or sticky, refrigerate for 30 to 60 minutes.
5. Roll dough into 1½-inch balls and place on the prepared baking sheet. Flatten gently using your fingers or the bottom of a floured or sugared cup.
6. Bake for 15 minutes or until the edges are set and the cookies are lightly browned underneath.
7. Let cool on the baking sheet for 5 minutes before transferring to a wire rack.
8. Store in an airtight container for up to 3 days or freeze.

Per cookie: Calories: 120, Protein: 4 g, Fat: 6 g, Carbohydrate: 14 g, Fiber: 2 g

Minerals: Calcium: 60 mg, Iron: 1.3 mg, Magnesium: 29 mg, Potassium: 199 mg, Sodium: 70 mg, Zinc: 0.6 mg

Vitamins: A: 0.1 mcg, C: 0 mg, E: 0.8 mg, Folate: 13 mcg DFE

Percent of calories from: Protein 11%, Fat 43%, Carbohydrate 46%

Chef's Tip Using Oil in Baking

While we minimize the use of oils in this book, small amounts can be helpful in certain applications, especially for softening nut butters, or to improve texture. When using oil, choose one with a neutral flavor that won't overpower your recipe. Good options include avocado oil, canola oil, or sunflower oil. These provide moisture and texture without adding strong taste.

NO-BAKE CHOCOLATE CLUSTERS

Makes 15 cookies

These fast and fuss-free treats come together in minutes—no oven required! A naturally sweet, fiber-rich, gluten-free (if using gluten-free oats) snack that blends heart-healthy fats, plant protein, and antioxidants. Perfect for an energizing bite or a simple dessert. Customize with your favorite nuts, seeds, or dried fruit.

½ cup rolled oats

3½ ounces dark chocolate bar or ⅔ cup dark chocolate chips

½ cup natural peanut butter or other nut butter

Pinch of salt (optional)

¾ cup whole or coarsely chopped nuts (e.g., walnuts, pecans, hazelnuts)

¼ cup dried fruit (e.g. currants, raisins, cherries, cranberries, Gogi berries, golden berries)

1. Toast the oats for enhanced flavor and digestibility:
   Stovetop: Toast in a dry skillet over medium heat, stirring often, for 5 minutes.
   Microwave: Spread oats on a plate and microwave for 2 minutes.
   Air fryer or oven: Bake at 350°F for 10 minutes.
2. In a small saucepan over low heat, gently melt the chocolate, stirring continuously until smooth.
3. Add the peanut butter and salt (if using). Stir until fully combined and warmed through, for about 2 minutes.
4. Turn off the heat. Stir in the toasted oats, chopped nuts, and dried fruit until evenly coated with the chocolate mixture.
5. Line a baking sheet with parchment paper or a silicone mat. Drop the mixture by heaping tablespoons to form 15 clusters.

6. Chill until firm, for about 30 minutes in the fridge or 10 minutes in the freezer.
7. Store in an airtight container in the refrigerator for up to 1 week or freeze for longer storage.

Per cookie: Calories: 147, Protein: 3.6 g, Fat: 11 g, Carbohydrate: 10 g, Fiber: 2 g

Minerals: Calcium: 17 mg, Iron: 1 mg, Magnesium: 39 mg, Potassium: 141 mg, Sodium: 39 mg, Zinc: 0.7 mg

Percent of calories from: Protein 10%, Fat 63%, Carbohydrate 27%

OPTIONAL ADD-IN AND VARIATION:

- Sprinkle with sesame seeds or hempseeds before chilling.
- Replace up to ¼ cup of the nuts with seeds such as pumpkin or sunflower seeds.

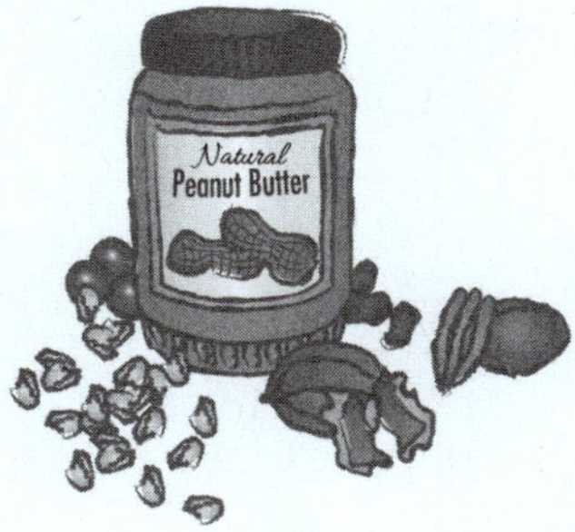

NUTTY DATE COOKIES

Makes 20 to 24 cookies

Soft, chewy, and hard to resist, these nutty date cookies make a delicious and nourishing treat. Flour-free and gluten-free (when made with certified gluten-free oats), they're easy to prepare and naturally sweetened. If your nut butter is hard or dry, stir in a small amount of neutral oil, or microwave briefly (15–30 seconds) to soften it.

1 cup pitted dates, loosely packed

½ cup water

⅔ cup soft nut butter (e.g., almond, mixed nut, cashew, sunflower, or peanut butter)

3 tablespoons maple syrup

1 teaspoon vanilla

2 tablespoons ground flaxseeds

½ teaspoon salt (optional)

1 cup rolled oats

1 cup walnuts or pecans, coarsely chopped

⅓ cup raisins, currants, dried cranberries, or chopped dried cherries

1. Preheat oven to 350°F (325°F convection).
2. In a small pot, simmer dates with water until soft, for 5 to 7 minutes. Mash with a potato masher or fork until mostly smooth.
3. Transfer mashed dates to a medium bowl. Stir in nut butter, maple syrup, vanilla, flaxseeds, and salt (if using) until well combined.
4. Fold in the oats, chopped nuts, and raisins.
5. Line two baking sheets with silicone mats or lightly spray with oil.

6. Drop the dough by heaping tablespoons onto baking sheets. Flatten slightly with your fingers or the back of a spoon.
7. Bake for 15 to 20 minutes, or until golden brown. Watch closely toward the end to prevent burning the bottoms.
8. Let cool completely. Store in an airtight container at room temperature for 1 to 2 days or freeze for longer storage.

OPTIONAL ADD-INS:

- Add ¼–½ cup of unsalted sunflower seeds or coconut along with the oats and walnuts.
- For a decorative touch, put 1 pecan per cookie (20–24 pecans) in a small bowl and pour a tablespoon of maple syrup over the nuts and stir. Press one maple-coated nut onto each cookie before baking.

Per cookie: Calories: 149, Protein: 4 g, Fat: 9 g, Carbohydrate: 15 g, Fiber: 3 g

Minerals: Calcium: 48 mg, Iron: 1 mg, Magnesium: 44 mg, Potassium: 187 mg, Sodium: 22 mg, Zinc: 0.7 mg

Vitamins: A: 0.1 mcg, C: 0.2 mg, E: 2 mg, Folate: 13 mcg DFE

Percent of calories from: Protein 10%, Fat 52%, Carbohydrate 38%

SEEDY CINNAMON CRUNCH COOKIES

Makes 18 cookies

These chewy, nutty cookies are packed with seeds, oats, and warm cinnamon, and finished with a maple-sweetened sesame seed topping that bakes into a satisfying crunch. They're rich in fiber and make a great snack or treat. Gluten-free and oil-free options are included. If nut butter is hard or dry, stir in a small amount of neutral oil, or microwave briefly (15–30 seconds) to soften.

½ cup soft peanut butter or other nut butter

2 tablespoons tahini or neutral oil

⅓ cup maple syrup

1 teaspoon vanilla extract

½ teaspoon salt (optional)

1 teaspoon cinnamon*

¼ cup ground flaxseeds

2 tablespoons flour (whole grain, all-purpose, or gluten-free)

½ cup oats

½ cup sunflower seeds

½ cup finely chopped walnuts

¼ cup raisins, currants, dried cranberries, or chopped dried cherries

TOPPING

¼ cup sesame seeds

1½ tablespoons maple syrup

½ teaspoon cinnamon

Pinch of salt (optional)

1. Preheat the oven to 375°F (350°F convection). Line a baking sheet with a silicone baking mat or parchment paper.
2. In a mixing bowl, stir together the peanut butter, tahini, maple syrup, vanilla, salt (if using), and cinnamon until smooth.
3. Add the ground flaxseeds and flour, mixing well to combine.
4. Stir in the oats, sunflower seeds, chopped walnuts, and raisins until evenly distributed.
5. In a small bowl, prepare the topping by mixing the sesame seeds, maple syrup, cinnamon, and salt (if using).
6. Scoop the dough by heaping tablespoonfuls onto the prepared baking sheet.
7. Flatten each cookie with a fork dipped in water.
8. Top each cookie with the sesame mixture, spreading it evenly with the back of a spoon or small spatula.
9. Bake for 16 to 20 minutes, or until golden brown around the edges.
10. Cool on the baking sheet for 5 minutes before transferring to a wire rack to cool completely.

Per cookie: Calories: 142, Protein: 4 g, Fat: 9 g, Carbohydrate: 13 g, Fiber: 2 g

Minerals: Calcium: 28 mg, Iron: 0.7 mg, Magnesium: 41 mg, Potassium: 140 mg, Sodium: 34 mg, Zinc: 0.8 mg

Vitamins: A: 0.2 mcg, C: 0.2 mg, E: 1 mg, Folate: 19 mcg DFE

Percent of calories from: Protein 10%, Fat 56%, Carbohydrate 34%

Chef's Tip *Cinnamon

There are two main types of cinnamon: Cassia, with the bold, spicy flavor most of us grew up with, and Ceylon, which is milder and naturally sweeter. Cassia is fine for occasional use, but it contains more coumarin, a compound that may be harmful in high amounts. For regular use, Ceylon is the safer choice—though its gentler flavor may take some getting used to.

With Love, Gratitude, and Encouragement

As you turn the final pages of *Plant-Powered Seniors,* know that this is the beginning of a beautiful journey. May your kitchen become a sanctuary of discovery, where whole-plant foods offer nourishment and joy.

Stay connected with others who share your values. Whether it's cooking with friends, joining a local plant-based group, or exchanging recipes with someone, these connections nourish your spirit. You are part of a growing community choosing vitality, compassion, and intention.

Thank you for allowing us to be part of your journey. It is an honor to support you in nourishing your health and well-being.

ACKNOWLEDGMENTS

It is an honor and a privilege to work with Christine Belleris, Larissa Hise Henoch, Chrystle Fiedler, and Christian Blonshine, along with the talented editorial, advisory, and publishing team at Health Communications, Inc. Your expertise, vision, and support have helped shape *Plant-Powered Seniors* into a work we are truly proud of. Special thanks to Janis Nicolay, whose exceptional food photography captured the beauty, texture, and essence of each dish with remarkable clarity and artistry, and to Lawren Moneta, whose expert styling brought a refined, inviting, and visually compelling presence to every recipe photo.

We are deeply grateful to our dear friend Margie Colclough, whose generous spirit and keen attention to detail made an extraordinary contribution to this book. In addition to her invaluable assistance with the manuscript, Margie devoted many hours to recipe testing with care, insight, and enthusiasm.

Our sincere thanks go to our dedicated team of recipe testers, who ensured that the recipes in this book are not only accurate but truly delicious. We are especially grateful to Lynn Isted, Liliana Cruz Vallejo,

Daneen Agecoutay, Liz Schafer, Bonnie Soon, Jeanne Faye Ho, and Donnie Rose for your thoughtful feedback, attention to detail, and culinary generosity. Your time, effort, and willingness to share this work with your families supported the creation of outstanding recipes.

We also thank the late Art Isted, Andrés Vallejo, Stacey Agecoutay, Garth Schafer, and Ed Arteaga for their roles as insightful taste testers and honest critics, whose feedback helped refine these recipes. Our appreciation extends to Chef Joseph Forest for his inspiring work in *Cooking Vegan*.

We are especially grateful to Dilip Barman for his ongoing encouragement and for his instrumental role in securing funding from the Karuna Foundation. We also wish to thank the Karuna Foundation for its generous support, which made it possible to work with a professional team on food photography and styling.

We thank Sunrise Soya Foods for providing outstanding tofu and soy beverage products in support of recipe development. We are also grateful to Lesaffre and its business unit Gnosis, distributors of Red Star® nutritional yeast, for generously supplying their VSF Yeast Flakes®, a valuable ingredient that supported recipe development and remains an important source of vitamin B_{12} and other B vitamins for plant-based diets. We appreciate OmegaQuant for their high-quality omega-3 testing services.

We also acknowledge ESHA/Trustwell for their Food Processor nutritional analysis software, which enabled us to provide accurate nutritional information for recipes and menus.

Brenda and Vesanto extend deep appreciation to their husbands, Paul Davis and Cam Doré, for their steadfast encouragement, excellent taste testing, and enthusiastic support of plant-based living. All three authors are especially grateful to Cam for his exceptional technical expertise and the many insights he contributed throughout the development of this book.

Finally, we thank our families and communities for their encouragement, patience, and belief in this work. Our children and grandchildren, Brenda's mother, siblings, extended family, and close friends supported us throughout every stage of this project—offering encouragement, thoughtful input, shared meals, and constant reminders of why this work matters. Their love has been a steady source of strength and joy.

In particular, Vancouver Cohousing, where Vesanto lives, provided daily inspiration and support that enriched this project in countless ways. We are deeply thankful for your kindness, encouragement, and sense of community.

REFERENCES

Chapter 1. Plant-Powered Aging

Agnoli C, Baroni L, Bertini I, et al. A comprehensive review of healthy effects of vegetarian diets. *Nutr Metab Cardiovasc Dis.* 2023; 33(7):1308-1315.

Arévalo C. *Animal Agriculture Is the Missing Piece in Climate Change Media Coverage.* Faunalytics. 2023.

Buettner, D. & National Institute on Aging. *Blue Zones Project findings. In: Business Engagement in Building Healthy Communities.* National Academies Press. NCBI Bookshelf NBK298903. Published 2015.

Córdova R, Kim J, Thompson AS, et al. Plant-based dietary patterns and age-specific risk of multimorbidity of cancer and cardiometabolic diseases: A prospective analysis. *The Lancet Healthy Longev.* Published August 19, 2025.

Dos Santos H, Gaio J, Durisic A, et al. The Polypharma Study: Association Between Diet and Amount of Prescription Drugs Among Seniors. *Am J Lifestyle Med.* 2021;18(6):813-819.

FAO. In Brief to The State of Food and Agriculture. *Revealing the true cost of food to transform agrifood systems.* 2023. Rome.

Freisling H, Viallon V, Lennon H, et al. Lifestyle factors and risk of multimorbidity of cancer and cardiometabolic diseases: A multinational cohort study. *BMC Medicine.* 2020;18, 5.

Gardner CD, Hartle JC, Garrett RD, et al. Maximizing the intersection of human health and the health of the environment with regard to the amount and type of protein produced and consumed in the United States. *Nutr Rev.* 2019;77(4):197-215.

Herpich, C, Müller-Werdan, U., & Norman, K. Role of plant-based diets in promoting health and longevity. *Maturitas.* 2022:165, 47-51.

Hu FB. Diet strategies for promoting healthy aging and longevity: an epidemiological perspective. *Ageing Res Rev.* 2024;90:101995.

Katz DL, Meller S. Can we say what diet is best for health? *Annu Rev Public Health.* 2014;35:83-103.

Key TJ, Papier K, Tong TYN. Plant-based diets and long-term health: findings from the EPIC-Oxford study. *Proc Nutr Soc.* 2022; 81(2):190-198.

Korat AVA, Shea MK, Jacques PF, et al. Dietary protein intake in midlife in relation to healthy aging—results from the prospective Nurses' Health Study cohort. *Am J Clin Nutr.* 2024;119(2):271-282.

Liu X, Morris MC, Dhana K, et al. Mediterranean-DASH Intervention for Neurodegenerative Delay (MIND) study: Rationale, design and baseline characteristics of a randomized control trial of the MIND diet on cognitive decline. *Contemp Clin Trials.* 2021;102:106270.

Mo Q, Wu J, Lu Y, Zhang X. Plant-based diets and total and cause-specific mortality: a meta-analysis of prospective studies. *Front Nutr.* 2025; 12:1518519.

O'Malley K, Willits-Smith A, Rose D. Popular diets as selected by adults in the United States show wide variation in carbon footprints and diet quality. *Am J Clin Nutr.* 2023;117(4):701-708.

Orlich MJ, Singh PN, Sabaté J, et al. Vegetarian dietary patterns and mortality in Adventist Health Study 2. *JAMA Intern Med.* 2013;173(13):1230-1238.

Ornish D, Madison C, Kivipelto M, et al. Effects of intensive lifestyle changes on the progression of mild cognitive impairment or early dementia due to Alzheimer's disease: a randomized, controlled clinical trial. *Alzheimer's Res Ther.* 2024;16(1):122.

Rajaram S, Jones J, Lee GJ. Plant-Based Dietary Patterns, Plant Foods, and Age-Related Cognitive Decline. *Adv Nutr.* 2019;10 (Suppl_4):S422-S436.

Remde A, DeTurk SN, Almardini A, et al. Plant-predominant eating patterns—how effective are they for treating obesity and related cardiometabolic health outcomes?—a systematic review. *Nutr Rev.* 2022 ;80(5):1094-1104.

Richie H. How many animals are factory-farmed? *Our Word in Data.* 2024. https://ourworldindata.org/how-many-animals-are-factory-farmed

Rockström J, Thilsted SH, Willett WC, et al. The EAT-Lancet Commission on healthy, sustainable, and just food systems. *Lancet.* 2025; 406(10512):1625-1700.

Romanello M, Walawender M, Hsu SC, et.al. The 2024 report of the *Lancet* Countdown on health and climate change: facing record-breaking threats from delayed action. *Lancet.* 2024;404(10465):1847-1896.

Santos HD, Alabadi-Bierman A, Paalani M, et al. Living longer and lifestyle: A report on the oldest of the old in the Adventist Health Study-2. JAR Life. 2025;14:100010.

Scarborough P, Clark M, Cobiac L, et al. Vegans, vegetarians, fish-eaters and meat-eaters in the UK show discrepant environmental impacts. *Nat Food.* 2023;4(7):565-574.

Segovia-Siapco G, Sabaté J. Health and sustainability outcomes of vegetarian dietary patterns: a revisit of the EPIC-Oxford and the Adventist Health Study-2 cohorts. *Eur J Clin Nutr.* 2019;72(Suppl 1):60-70.

Sherzai D, Sherzai A, Sherzai A. Lifestyle Intervention and Alzheimer Disease. *J Fam Pract.* 2022;71(Suppl 1 Lifestyle):eS83-eS89.

Springmann M, Godfray HC, Rayner M, et al. Analysis and valuation of the health and climate change cobenefits of dietary change. *Proc Natl Acad Sci USA.* 2016;113(15):4146-51.

Tessier AJ, Wang F, Korat AA, et al. Optimal dietary patterns for healthy aging. *Nat Med.* 2025;31(5):1644-1652.

Tomova A, Bukovsky I, Rembert E et al. The Effects of Vegetarian and Vegan Diets on Gut Microbiota. *Front Nutr.* 2019;6:47.

Wang S, Li W, Li S, et al. Association between plant-based dietary pattern and biological aging trajectory in a large prospective cohort. *BMC Med.* 2023;21(1):310.

Chapter 2. Dietary Patterns, Diet Quality, and Health

Dominguez LJ, Veronese N, Barbagallo M. Dietary Patterns and Healthy or Unhealthy Aging. *Gerontology.* 2024;70(1):15-36.

Govindaraju T, Sahle BW, McCaffrey TA, et al. Dietary Patterns and Quality of Life in Older Adults: A Systematic Review. *Nutrients.* 2018;10(8):971.

McDonald D et al. American Gut: An Open Platform for Citizen Science Microbiome Research. *mSystems.* 2018; 3(3):1.

Morze J, Danielewicz A, Hoffmann G, Schwingshackl L. Diet Quality as Assessed by the Healthy Eating Index, Alternate Healthy Eating Index, Dietary Approaches to Stop Hypertension Score, and Health Outcomes: A Second Update of a Systematic Review and Meta-Analysis of Cohort Studies. *J Acad Nutr Diet.* 2020;120(12):1998-2031.e15.

Orlich MJ, Sabaté J, Mashchak A, et al. Ultra-processed food intake and animal-based food intake and mortality in the Adventist Health Study-2. *Am J Clin Nutr.* 2022;115(6):1589-1601.

Satija A, Bhupathiraju SN, Spiegelman D, et al. Healthful and Unhealthful Plant-Based Diets and the Risk of Coronary Heart Disease in U.S. Adults. *J Am Coll Cardiol.* 2017;70(4):411-422.

Schwingshackl L, Bogensberger B, Hoffmann G. Diet Quality as Assessed by the Healthy Eating Index, Alternate Healthy Eating Index, Dietary Approaches to Stop Hypertension Score, and Health Outcomes: An Updated Systematic Review and Meta-Analysis of Cohort Studies. *J Acad Nutr Diet.* 2018;118(1):74-100.e11.

US Burden of Disease Collaborators; Mokdad AH, Ballestros K, Echko M, et al. The State of US Health, 1990-2016: Burden of Diseases, Injuries, and Risk Factors Among US States. *JAMA.* 2018;319(14):1444-1472.

US Department of Agriculture. (2020). *Scientific Report of the 2020 Dietary Guidelines Advisory Committee: Part D. Chapter 8: Dietary Patterns.* Washington, DC: USDA.

Woodside JV, Lindberg L, Nugent AP. Harnessing the power on our plates: sustainable dietary patterns for public and planetary health. *Proc Nutr Soc.* 2023;82(4):437-453.

Yang Q, Sun Y. Dietary Patterns, Food Intake and Health: New Evidence from Epidemiological and Genetic Studies. *Nutrients.* 2024;16(7):919.

Chapter 3. Designing Diets that Work for You

Austad SN, Pes GM. The validity of Blue Zones demography: a response to critiques. *Gerontologist.* 2025;65(12):gnaf246.

Buettner D, Skemp S. Blue Zones: Lessons from the World's Longest Lived. *Am J Lifestyle Med.* 2016;10(5):318-321.

Buettner D. Lessons From the Blue Zones: There is No Silver Bullet (or Magic Pill) for a Long, Healthy Life. *Am J Lifestyle Med.* Published online May 1, 2025.

Craig WJ, Brothers CJ. Nutritional Content of Non-Dairy Frozen Desserts. *Nutrients.* 2022;14(19):4150.

Craig WJ, Mangels AR, Brothers CJ. Nutritional Profiles of Non-Dairy Plant-Based Cheese Alternatives. *Nutrients.* 2022;14(6):1247.

Craig WJ, Messina V, Rowland I, et al. Plant-Based Dairy Alternatives Contribute to a Healthy and Sustainable Diet. *Nutrients.* 2023;15(15):3393.

Darmadi-Blackberry I, Wahlqvist ML, Kouris-Blazos A, et al. Legumes: the most important dietary predictor of survival in older people of different ethnicities. *Asia Pac J Clin Nutr.* 2004;13(2):217-20.

Messina V, Guest NS, Duncan AM, et al. Dietary guidance on plant-based meat alternatives for individuals wanting to increase plant protein intake. *Front Nutr.* 2025;12:1641234.

Torheim LE, Fadnes LT. Legumes and pulses—a scoping review for Nordic Nutrition Recommendations 2023. *Food Nutr Res.* 2024;68: 10.29219/fnr.v68.10484.

Chapter 4: Fine-Tuning Your Diet for Chronic Health Conditions

Arthritis

Bostan ZZ, Şare Bulut M, Özen Ünaldı B, et al. Effect of Plant-Based Diets on Rheumatoid Arthritis: A Systematic Review. *Nutr Rev.* 2025;83(7):e1798-e1814.

Calder PC. Omega-3 fatty acids and inflammatory processes: from molecules to man. *Biochem Soc Trans.* 2017;45(5):1105-1115.

Charoenngam N, Holick MF. Immunologic Effects of Vitamin D on Human Health and Disease. *Nutrients.* 2020;12(7):2097.

Christensen R, Bartels EM, Astrup A, et al. Effect of weight reduction in obese patients diagnosed with knee osteoarthritis: a systematic review and meta-analysis. *Ann Rheum Dis.* 2007;66(4):433-9.

Gioxari A, Kaliora AC, Marantidou F, et al. Intake of ω-3 polyunsaturated fatty acids in patients with rheumatoid arthritis: A systematic review and meta-analysis. *Nutrition.* 2018;45:114-124.e4.

Golmohammadi A, Hosseinikia M, Sadeghi MK, et al. The evaluation of nightshade elimination diet (NED) on inflammatory and rheumatologic markers of rheumatoid arthritis patients: study protocol for a randomized controlled trial. *Trials.* 2024;25(1):531.

Guagnano MT, D'Angelo C, Caniglia D, et al. Improvement of Inflammation and Pain after Three Months' Exclusion Diet in Rheumatoid Arthritis Patients. *Nutrients.* 2021;13(10):3535.

Hunter DJ, Bierma-Zeinstra S. Osteoarthritis. *Lancet.* 2019;393(10182): 1745-1759.

Hurley M, Dickson K, Hallett R, et al. Exercise interventions and patient beliefs for people with hip, knee or hip and knee osteoarthritis: a mixed methods review. *Cochrane Database Syst Rev.* 2018;4(4):CD010842.

Miles EA, Calder PC. Influence of marine n-3 polyunsaturated fatty acids on immune function and a systematic review of their effects on clinical outcomes in rheumatoid arthritis. *Br J Nutr.* 2012;107 Suppl 2: S171-S184.

Nelson J, Sjöblom H, Gjertsson I, et al. Do Interventions with Diet or Dietary Supplements Reduce the Disease Activity Score in Rheumatoid Arthritis? A Systematic Review of Randomized Controlled Trials. *Nutrients.* 2020;12(10):2991.

Park SJ, Nam CH, Ahn HS, et al. The efficacy and safety of leucine-enriched essential amino acids in knee osteoarthritis patients: A randomized controlled trial. *Medicine* (Baltimore). 2024;103(19):e38168.

Rasch EK, Hirsch R, Paulose-Ram R, et al. Prevalence of rheumatoid arthritis in persons 60 years of age and older in the United States: effect of different methods of case classification. *Arthritis Rheum.* 2003;48(4):917-26.

Senftleber NK, Nielsen SM, Andersen JR, et al. Marine Oil Supplements for Arthritis Pain: A Systematic Review and Meta-Analysis of Randomized Trials. *Nutrients.* 2017;9(1):42.

Autoimmune Disorders

de Oliveira GLV, Leite AZ, Higuchi BS, et al. Intestinal dysbiosis and probiotic applications in autoimmune diseases. *Immunology.* 2017;152(1):1-12.

Manzel A, Muller DN, Hafler DA, et al. Role of "Western diet" in inflammatory autoimmune diseases. *Curr Allergy Asthma Rep.* 2014;14(1):404.

Moro-García MA, Mayo JC, Sainz RM, et al. Influence of Inflammation in the Process of T Lymphocyte Differentiation: Proliferative, Metabolic, and Oxidative Changes. *Front Immunol.* 2018;9:339.

Murdaca G, Tonacci A, Negrini S, et al. Emerging role of vitamin D in autoimmune diseases: An update on evidence and therapeutic implications. *Autoimmun Rev.* 2019;18(9):102350.

Stojanovich L, Marisavljevich D. Stress as a trigger of autoimmune disease. *Autoimmun Rev.* 2008;7(3):209-13.

Weyand CM, Goronzy JJ. Aging of the Immune System. Mechanisms and Therapeutic Targets. *Ann Am Thorac Soc.* 2016;13 Suppl 5 (Suppl 5): S422-S428.

Cancer

Ajdžanovic V, Filipovic B, Miljic D, et al. Prostate cancer metastasis and soy isoflavones: a dogfight over a bone. *EXCLI J.* 2019;18:106-126.

Ba DM, Ssentongo P, Beelman RB, et al. Higher Mushroom Consumption Is Associated with Lower Risk of Cancer: A Systematic Review and Meta-Analysis of Observational Studies. *Adv Nutr.* 2021;12(5):1691-1704.

Bashir S, Fezeu LK, Leviatan Ben-Arye S, et al. Association between Neu5Gc carbohydrate and serum antibodies against it provides the molecular link to cancer: French NutriNet-Santé study. *BMC Med.* 2020;18(1):262.

Bouvard V, Loomis D, Guyton KZ, et al. Carcinogenicity of consumption of red and processed meat. *Lancet Oncol.* 2015;16(16):1599-1600.

Bulanda S, Lau K, Nowak A, et al. The Risk of Oral Cancer and the High Consumption of Thermally Processed Meat Containing Mutagenic and Carcinogenic Compounds. *Nutrients.* 2024;16(7):1084.

Calado AA, Santos LP, Nogueira CW, et al. The effect of flaxseed in breast cancer: A literature review. *Front Nutr*. 2018;5:4.

Cormie P, Zopf EM, Zhang X, et al. The Impact of Exercise on Cancer Mortality, Recurrence, and Treatment-Related Adverse Effects. *Epidemiol Rev.* 2017;39(1):71-92.

De Silva SF, Alcorn J. Flaxseed Lignans as Important Dietary Polyphenols for Cancer Prevention and Treatment: Chemistry, Pharmacokinetics, and Molecular Targets. *Pharmaceuticals (Basel).* 2019;12(2):68.

Di Y, Ding L, Gao L, et al. Association of meat consumption with the risk of gastrointestinal cancers: a systematic review and meta-analysis. *BMC Cancer*. 2023;23(1):782.

Fernández-Fígares Jiménez MDC, Storz MA. Cancer Risk and Mortality Following Substitution of Animal Foods with Plant Foods: A Systematic Review. *Curr Nutr Rep*. 2025;14(1):99.

Hanahan D, Weinberg RA. Hallmarks of cancer: the next generation. *Cell*. 2011;144(5):646-74.

Honoki K, Tsujiuchi T, Kishi S, et al. Revisiting 'Hallmarks of Cancer' In Sarcomas. *J Cancer*. 2024;15(7):1786-1804.

Kværner AS, Birkeland E, Vinberg E, et al. Associations of red and processed meat intake with screen-detected colorectal lesions. *Br J Nutr*. 2023;129(12):2122-2132.

López-Otín C, Blasco MA, Partridge L, Serrano M, Kroemer G. The hallmarks of aging. *Cell*. 2013;153(6):1194-217.

McTiernan A, Friedenreich CM, Katzmarzyk PT, et al. Physical Activity in Cancer Prevention and Survival: A Systematic Review. *Med Sci Sports Exerc*. 2019;51(6):1252-1261.

Messina M. Impact of Soy Foods on the Development of Breast Cancer and the Prognosis of Breast Cancer Patients. *Forsch Komplementmed.* 2016;23(2):75-80.

Park W, Amin ARM, Chen ZG, et al. New perspectives of curcumin in cancer prevention. *Cancer Prev Res (Phila).* 2013;6(5):387-400.

Pati S, Irfan W, Jameel A, et al. Obesity and Cancer: A Current Overview of Epidemiology, Pathogenesis, Outcomes, and Management. *Cancers (Basel).* 2023;15(2):485.

Pawelec G. Immunosenescence and cancer. *Biogerontology.* 2017;18(4): 717-721.

Sivasubramanian BP, Dave M, Panchal V, et al. Comprehensive Review of Red Meat Consumption and the Risk of Cancer. *Cureus.* 2023;15(9):e45324.

Song M, Chan AT. The Potential Role of Exercise and Nutrition in Harnessing the Immune System to Improve Colorectal Cancer Survival. *Gastroenterology.* 2018;155(3):596-600.

Soundararajan P, Kim JS. Anti-Carcinogenic Glucosinolates in Cruciferous Vegetables and Their Antagonistic Effects on Prevention of Cancers. *Molecules.* 2018;23(11):2983.

Tong Y, Ning H, Zhang Z, et al. Global burden of disease changes related to high red meat diets and breast cancer from 1990 to 2021 and its prediction up to 2030. *Front Nutr.* 2025;12:1586299.

Uribarri J, Woodruff S, Goodman S, et al. Advanced glycation end products in foods and a practical guide to their reduction in the diet. *J Am Diet Assoc.* 2010;110(6):911-916.

World Cancer Research Fund/American Institute for Cancer Research. *Diet, Nutrition, Physical Activity and Cancer: A Global Perspective.* Continuous Update Project Expert Report 2018. World Cancer Research Fund/American Institute for Cancer Research; 2018.

Yang CS, Wang X. Green tea and cancer prevention. *Nutr Cancer.* 2010;62(7):931-7.

Cardiovascular Disease

American Heart Association. *Older Americans & Cardiovascular Diseases.* Published 2024.

Budhathoki S, Sawada N, Iwasaki M, et al.; Japan Public Health Center--based Prospective Study Group. Association of Animal and Plant Protein Intake with All-Cause and Cause-Specific Mortality in a Japanese Cohort. *JAMA Intern Med.* 2019;179(11):1509-1518.

Captieux M, Prigge R, Wild S, et al. Defining remission of type 2 diabetes in research studies: A systematic scoping review. *PLoS Med.* 2020;17(10):e1003396.

Centers for Disease Control and Prevention. *Heart Disease Facts.* Published 2023.

Chiavaroli L, Nishi SK, Khan TA, et al. Portfolio dietary pattern and cardiovascular disease: a systematic review and meta-analysis of controlled trials. *Prog Cardiovasc Dis.* 2018;61(1):43--53.

Esselstyn CB Jr, Gendy G, Doyle J, et al. A way to reverse coronary artery disease? *Am J Lifestyle Med.* 2014;8(4):228-232.

Kim H, Caulfield LE, Garcia-Larsen V, et al. Plant-based diets are associated with a lower risk of incident cardiovascular disease, cardiovascular disease mortality, and all-cause mortality in a general population of middle-aged adults. *J Am Heart Assoc.* 2019;8(16):e012865.

Meinilä J, Virtanen JK. Meat and meat products—a scoping review for Nordic Nutrition Recommendations 2023. *Food Nutr Res.* 2024;68.

Nagra M, Tsam F, Ward S, et al. Animal vs plant-based meat: a hearty debate. *Can J Cardiol.* 2024;40(7):1198-1209.

Ornish DM, Scherwitz LW, Billings JH, et al. Intensive lifestyle changes for reversal of coronary heart disease. *JAMA.* 1998;280(23):2001-2007.

Razavi AC, Bazzano LA, He J, et al. Consumption of animal and plant foods and risk of left ventricular diastolic dysfunction: the Bogalusa Heart Study. *ESC Heart Fail.* 2020;7(5):2700-2710.

Satija A, Bhupathiraju SN, Spiegelman D, et al. Healthful and unhealthful plant-based diets and the risk of coronary heart disease in U.S. adults. *J Am Coll Cardiol.* 2017;70(4):411-422.

Shah B, Newman JD, Woolf K, et al. Anti-Inflammatory Effects of a Vegan Diet Versus the American Heart Association-Recommended Diet in Coronary Artery Disease Trial. *J Am Heart Assoc.* 2018;7(23):e011367.

Dementia and Cognitive Impairment

Abris GP, Shavlik DJ, Mathew RO, Butler FM, Oh J, Sirirat R, Sveen LE, Fraser GE. Cause-specific and all-cause mortalities in vegetarian compared with those in nonvegetarian participants from the Adventist Health Study-2 cohort. *Am J Clin Nutr.* 2024 120(4):907-917.

Dominguez LJ, Veronese N, Vernuccio L, et al. Nutrition, Physical Activity, and Other Lifestyle Factors in the Prevention of Cognitive Decline and Dementia. *Nutrients.* 2021;13(11):4080.

Jack CR Jr, Knopman DS, Jagust WJ, et al. Tracking pathophysiological processes in Alzheimer's disease: an updated hypothetical model of dynamic biomarkers. *Lancet Neurol.* 2013;12(2):207-216.

Katonova A, Sheardova K, Amlerova J, et al. Effect of a Vegan Diet on Alzheimer's Disease. *Int J Mol Sci.* 2022;23(23):14924.

Kivipelto M, Ngandu T, Farrell M, et al. The World-Wide FINGERS Network: A global approach to risk reduction and prevention of dementia. *Alzheimers Dement.* 2020;16(7):1078--1094.

Lewerin C, Matousek M, Steen G, et al. Significant correlations of plasma homocysteine and serum methylmalonic acid with movement and cognitive performance in elderly suspects but no improvement from short-term vitamin therapy: a placebo-controlled randomized study." *Am J Clin Nutr.* 2005;81(3):1152-1162.

Mandolesi L, Polverino A, Montuori S, et al. Effects of Physical Exercise on Cognitive Functioning and Wellbeing: Biological and Psychological Benefits. *Front Psychol.* 2018;9:509.

Morris MC, Tangney CC, Wang Y, et al. MIND diet associated with reduced incidence of Alzheimer's disease. *Alzheimers Dement.* 2015;11(9):1007-1014.

Ngandu T, Lehtisalo J, Solomon A, et al. A 2-year multidomain intervention of diet, exercise, cognitive training, and vascular risk monitoring versus control to prevent cognitive decline in at-risk elderly people (FINGER): a randomised controlled trial. *Lancet.* 2015;385(9984):2255-2263.

Scarmeas N, Stern Y, Tang MX, et al. Mediterranean diet and risk for Alzheimer's disease. *Ann Neurol.* 2006;59(6):912-921.

Shah B, Newman JD, Woolf K, et al. Anti-Inflammatory Effects of a Vegan Diet Versus the American Heart Association-Recommended Diet in Coronary Artery Disease Trial. *J Am Heart Assoc.* 2018;7(23):e011367.

Xu Lou I, Ali K, Chen Q. Effect of nutrition in Alzheimer's disease: A systematic review. *Front Neurosci.* 2023;17:1147177.

Yurko-Mauro K, McCarthy D, Rom D, et al. Beneficial effects of docosahexaenoic acid on cognition in age-related cognitive decline. *Alzheimers Dement.* 2010;6(6):456-464.

Zhao C, Noble JM, Marder K, et al. Dietary Patterns, Physical Activity, Sleep, and Risk for Dementia and Cognitive Decline. *Curr Nutr Rep.* 2018;7(4):335-345.

Diabetes and Prediabetes

Salame C, Javaux G, Sellem L, et al. Food additive emulsifiers and the risk of type 2 diabetes: analysis of data from the NutriNet-Santé prospective cohort study. *Lancet Diabetes Endocrinol.* 2024;12(5):339-349.

Barnard ND, Levin SM, Trapp CB. Meat consumption as a risk factor for type 2 diabetes: A systematic review and meta-analysis. *Nutrients.* 2014;6(3):897-910.

Buse JB, Caprio S, Cefalu WT, et al. How do we define cure of diabetes? *Diabetes Care.* 2009; 32(11):2133-5.

Campbell TM, Campbell EK, Attia J, et al. The acute effects of a DASH diet and whole food, plant-based diet on insulin requirements and related cardiometabolic markers in individuals with insulin-treated type 2 diabetes. *Diabetes Res Clin Pract.* 2023;202:110814.

Captieux M, Prigge R, Wild S, et al. Defining remission of type 2 diabetes in research studies: A systematic scoping review. *PLoS Med.* 2020;17(10):e1003396.

Centers for Disease Control and Prevention. *National Diabetes Statistics Report.* Published May 15, 2024.

Chiavaroli L, Lee D, Ahmed A, et al. Effect of low glycaemic index or load dietary patterns on glycaemic control and cardiometabolic risk factors in diabetes: systematic review and meta-analysis of randomised controlled trials. *BMJ*. 2021;374:n1651.

Diabetes Canada Clinical Practice Guidelines Expert Committee. Diabetes Canada 2018 Clinical Practice Guidelines for the Prevention and Management of Diabetes in Canada. Can J Diabetes. 2018;42(Suppl 1):S1-S325.

Dutton, H. The Role of Plant-Based Diets in the Management of Type 2 Diabetes. *Canadian Diabetes and Endocrinology Today*. 2023; 1(3):16-19.

Fernández-Fígares Jiménez MDC, Storz MA. Cancer Risk and Mortality Following Substitution of Animal Foods with Plant Foods: A Systematic Review. *Curr Nutr Rep*. 2025;14(1):99.

Fuhrman J, Singer M. Improved Cardiovascular Parameter with a Nutrient-Dense, Plant-Rich Diet-Style: A Patient Survey With Illustrative Cases. *Am J Lifestyle Med*. 2015;11(3):264-273.

Galicia-Garcia U, Benito-Vicente A, Jebari S, et al. Pathophysiology of Type 2 Diabetes Mellitus. *Int J Mol Sci*. 2020;21(17):6275.

Guest NS, Raj S, Landry MJ, et al. Vegetarian and Vegan Dietary Patterns to Treat Adult Type 2 Diabetes: A Systematic Review and Meta-Analysis of Randomized Controlled Trials. *Adv Nutr*. 2024;15(10):100294.

Hanick CJ, Peterson CM, Davis BC, et al. A whole-food, plant-based intensive lifestyle intervention improves glycaemic control and reduces medications in individuals with type 2 diabetes: a randomised controlled trial. *Diabetologia*. 2025;68(2):308-319.

Jardine MA, Kahleova H, Levin SM, et al. Perspective: Plant-Based Eating Pattern for Type 2 Diabetes Prevention and Treatment: Efficacy, Mechanisms, and Practical Considerations. *Adv Nutr*. 2021;12(6):2045-2055.

Lean ME, Leslie WS, Barnes AC, et al. Primary care-led weight management for remission of type 2 diabetes (DiRECT): an open-label, cluster-randomised trial. *Lancet.* 2018;391(10120):541-551.

Riddle MC, Cefalu WT, Evans PH, et al. Consensus Report: Definition and Interpretation of Remission in Type 2 Diabetes. *Diabetes Care.* 2021;44(10):2438--2444.

Murciano A, Malavolti M, Fairweather-Tait S, et al. Plant-based diets and risk of type 2 diabetes: systematic review and dose-response meta-analysis. *Br J Nutr.* 2025 Aug 28;134(4):277-296.

Ouradova A, Ferrero G, Bratova M, et al. A vegan diet signature from a multi-omics study on different European populations is related to favorable metabolic outcomes. *Gut Microbes.* 2025 Dec 31;17(1):2593050.

Panigrahi G, Goodwin SM, Staffier KL, Karlsen M. Remission of Type 2 Diabetes After Treatment with a High-Fiber, Low-Fat, Plant-Predominant Diet Intervention: A Case Series. *Am J Lifestyle Med.* 2023;17(6):839-846.

Qian F, Liu G, Hu FB, et al. Association between plant-based dietary patterns and risk of type 2 diabetes: a systematic review and meta-analysis. *JAMA Intern Med* 2019;179:1335-1344.

Rosenfeld RM, Kelly JH, Agarwal M, et al. Dietary Interventions to Treat Type 2 Diabetes in Adults with a Goal of Remission: An Expert Consensus Statement from the American College of Lifestyle Medicine. *American Journal of Lifestyle Medicine.* 2022;16(3):342-362.

Satija A, Bhupathiraju SN, Rimm EB, et al. Plant-based dietary patterns and incidence of type 2 diabetes in US men and women: results from three prospective cohort studies. *PLoS Med.* 2016;13(6):e1002039.

Schlesinger S, Schwingshackl L. The Current Evidence for Vegetarian and Vegan Diets in the Management of Type 2 Diabetes. *Adv Nutr.* 2024;15(10):100296.

Frailty and Underweight

Coelho-Junior HJ, Calvani R, Picca A, et al. Protein Intake and Frailty in Older Adults: A Systematic Review and Meta-Analysis of Observational Studies. *Nutrients*. 2022;14(13):2767.

Coelho-Junior HJ, Marzetti E, Picca A, et al. Protein Intake and Frailty: A Matter of Quantity, Quality, and Timing. *Nutrients*. 2020;12(10):2915.

Dominguez LJ, Donat-Vargas C, Sayon-Orea C, et al. Rationale of the association between Mediterranean diet and the risk of frailty in older adults and systematic review and meta-analysis. *Exp Gerontol*. 2023;177:112180.

Hayashi AP, de Capitani MD, Dias SF, et al. Number of high-protein containing meals correlates with muscle mass in pre-frail and frail elderly. *Eur J Clin Nutr*. 2020;74(7):1047-1053.

Hernández Morante JJ, Gómez Martínez C, Morillas-Ruiz JM. Dietary Factors Associated with Frailty in Old Adults: A Review of Nutritional Interventions to Prevent Frailty Development. *Nutrients*. 2019;11(1):102.

Konglevoll DM, Hjartåker A, Hopstock LA, et al. Protein Intake and the Risk of Pre-Frailty and Frailty in Norwegian Older Adults. The Tromsø Study 1994-2016. *J Frailty Aging*. 2022;11(3):256-266.

Maroto-Rodriguez J, Delgado-Velandia M, Ortolá R, et al. Plant-based diets and risk of frailty in community-dwelling older adults: the Seniors-ENRICA-1 cohort. *Geroscience*. 2023;45(1):221-232.

Mendonça N, Granic A, Hill TR, et al., et al. Protein Intake and Disability Trajectories in Very Old Adults: The Newcastle 85+ Study. *J Am Geriatr Soc*. 2019;67(1):50-56.

Rizzoli R, Stevenson JC, Bauer JM, et al. The role of dietary protein and vitamin D in maintaining musculoskeletal health in postmenopausal women: a consensus statement from the European Society for Clinical and Economic Aspects of Osteoporosis and Osteoarthritis (ESCEO) *Maturitas*. 2015;80(3):337].

Sahni S, Mangano KM, Hannan MT, et al. Higher Protein Intake Is Associated with Higher Lean Mass and Quadriceps Muscle Strength in Adult Men and Women. *J Nutr*. 2015;145(7):1569-1575.

Struijk EA, Fung TT, Rodríguez-Artalejo F, et al. Protein intake and risk of frailty among older women in the Nurses' Health Study. *J Cachexia Sarcopenia Muscle*. 2022;13(3):1752-1761.

Zhang J, Zhang H. The association of body roundness index and body mass index with frailty and all-cause mortality: a study from the population aged 40 and above in the United States. *Lipids Health Dis*. 2025;24(1):30.

Gout

Chiu THT, Liu CH, Chang CC, et al. Vegetarian diet and risk of gout in two separate prospective cohort studies. *Clin Nutr*. 2020;39(3):837-844.

Choi HK, Atkinson K, Karlson EW, et al. Purine-rich foods, dairy and protein intake, and the risk of gout in men. *N Engl J Med*. 2004;350(11):1093-1103.

Juraschek SP, Miller ER 3rd, Gelber AC. Lifestyle risk factors associated with hyperuricemia in adults. *Am J Med*. 2013;126(5):442.e1-442 .e9.

Malik V, Choi HK, Rimm E, et al. A prospective study of diet quality and risk of gout in men. *Am J Clin Nutr*. 2016;104(2):501-509.

Roddy E, Doherty M. Epidemiology of gout. *Arthritis Res Ther*. 2010;12(6):223.

Zhang M, Ye C, Wang R, et al. Association between Dietary Acid Load and Hyperuricemia in Chinese Adults: Analysis of the China Health and Nutrition Survey (2009). *Nutrients.* 2023;15(8):1806.

Zhang Y, Chen S, Yuan M, et al. Gout and Diet: A Comprehensive Review of Mechanisms and Management. *Nutrients.* 2022;14(17):3525.

Hypertension

Charles JA, Habibullah NK, Bautista S, et al. Planting the Seed for Blood Pressure Control: The Role of Plant-Based Nutrition in the Management of Hypertension. *Curr Cardiol Rep.* 2024;26(3):121-134.

Glazier JJ. Pathophysiology, Diagnosis, and Management of Hypertension in the Elderly. *Int J Angiol.* 2022;31(4):222-228.

Oliveros E, Patel H, Kyung S, et al. Hypertension in older adults: Assessment, management, and challenges. *Clin Cardiol.* 2020;43(2):99-107.

Ozemek C, Laddu DR, Arena R, et al. The role of diet for prevention and management of hypertension. *Curr Opin Cardiol.* 2018;33(4):388-393.

Sukhato K, Akksilp K, Dellow A, et al. Efficacy of different dietary patterns on lowering of blood pressure level: an umbrella review. *Am J Clin Nutr.* 2020;112(6):1584-1598.

Tomé-Carneiro J, Visioli F. Plant-Based Diets Reduce Blood Pressure: A Systematic Review of Recent Evidence. *Curr Hypertens Rep.* 2023;25(7):127-150.

Yokose C, McCormick N, Rai SK, et al. Effects of Low-Fat, Mediterranean, or Low-Carbohydrate Weight Loss Diets on Serum Urate and Cardiometabolic Risk Factors: A Secondary Analysis of the Dietary Intervention Randomized Controlled Trial (DIRECT). *Diabetes Care.* 2020;43(11):2812-2820.

Macular Degeneration and Cataracts

Age-Related Eye Disease Study 2 Research Group. Lutein + zeaxanthin and omega-3 fatty acids for age-related macular degeneration: The Age-Related Eye Disease Study 2 (AREDS2) randomized clinical trial. *JAMA*. 2013;309(19):2005-2015.

American Academy of Ophthalmology. *Age-Related Macular Degeneration Preferred Practice Pattern*. Published 2024.

Key TJ, Papier K, Tong TYN. Plant-based diets and long-term health: findings from the EPIC-Oxford study. *Proc Nutr Soc*. 2022; 81(2):190-198.

Lawrenson JG, Downie LE. Nutrition and Eye Health. *Nutrients*. 2019;11(9):2123.

Ma L, Dou HL, Wu YQ, et al. Lutein and zeaxanthin intake and the risk of age-related macular degeneration: A systematic review and meta-analysis. *Br J Nutr*. 2012;107(3):350-359.

National Eye Institute. Cataracts. Updated Nov. 26, 2025. https://www.nei.nih.gov/eye-health-information/eye-conditions-and-diseases/cataracts.

SanGiovanni JP, Chew EY. The role of omega-3 long-chain polyunsaturated fatty acids in health and disease of the retina. *Prog Retin Eye Res*. 2005;24(1):87-138.

Osteoporosis and Osteopenia

Benedetti MG, Furlini G, Zati A, et al. Effects of physical exercise on bone density, fall risk factors, and quality of life in osteoporotic women: a systematic review. *Clin Interv Aging*. 2018;13:1513-1527.

Dawson-Hughes B, Harris SS, Ceglia L. Dietary protein and bone health: observational and intervention studies. *J Bone Miner Res*. 2008;23(6):866-871.

Fung TT, Willett WC, Stampfer MJ, et al. Association between dietary patterns and bone mineral density in postmenopausal women. *Am J Clin Nutr*. 2002;76(1):71-78.

Gillespie LD, Robertson MC, Gillespie WJ, et al. Fall Prevention Trials Collaboration. Interventions for preventing falls in older people living in the community. *Cochrane Database Syst Rev*. 2012;9:CD007146.

Kerstetter JE, O'Brien KO, Insogna KL. Dietary protein affects intestinal calcium absorption. *Am J Clin Nutr*. 2003;77(5):1257-1262.

Key TJ, Papier K, Tong TYN. Plant-based diets and long-term health: findings from the EPIC-Oxford study. *Proc Nutr Soc*. 2022;81(2):190-198.

Langsetmo L, Hanley DA, Vo T-V, et al. Prospective study of dietary patterns and risk of hip fracture in older men and women. J Bone Miner Res. 2011;26(12):2721-2728.

Myneni RB, Mezey E. Vitamin K2 and bone health. *Front Biosci (Landmark Ed)*. 2017;22:1479-1499.

National Institutes of Health. Osteoporosis. https://www.niams.nih.gov/health-topics/osteoporosis.

Physicians Committee for Responsible Medicine. Calcium and strong bones. https://www.pcrm.org/good-nutrition/nutrition-information/health-concerns-about-dairy/calcium-and-strong-bones.

Rizzoli R, Reginster J-Y, Arnal J-F, et al. Quality of life in sarcopenia and frailty. *Calcif Tissue Int*. 2013;93(2):101-120.

Sarafrazi N, Wambogo EA, Shepherd JA. Osteoporosis or Low Bone Mass in Older Adults: United States, 2017-2018. *NCHS Data Brief*. 2021;(405):1-8.

Schwalfenberg GK. Vitamins K1 and K2: The emerging group of vitamins required for human health. *J Diet Suppl.* 2017;14(2):119-134.

Shams-White MM, Chung M, Du M, et al. Dietary patterns and osteoporosis: A systematic review and meta-analysis. *Am J Clin Nutr.* 2017;105(4):913-935.

Tai V, Leung W, Grey A, Reid IR, Bolland MJ. Calcium intake and bone mineral density: systematic review and meta-analysis. *BMJ.* 2015;351:h4183.

Overweight and Obesity

Apovian CM, Aronne LJ. Pharmacological treatment of obesity in older adults. In: Feingold KR, Anawalt B, Boyce A, et al., eds. *Endotext.* National Center for Biotechnology Information; 2022.

Centers for Disease Control and Prevention. Products—Data Briefs – Number 106—September 2012. Published 2012.

Centers for Disease Control and Prevention. Adult Obesity Facts. https://www.cdc.gov/obesity/adult-obesity-facts/index.html. Updated June 4, 2024.

Centers for Disease Control and Prevention. Data Brief No. 106: Prevalence of Overweight and Obesity Among Adults Aged 20 and Over: United States, 2011-2012. Published September 2012.

Centers for Disease Control and Prevention. FastStats—Obesity and Overweight. https://www.cdc.gov/nchs/fastats/obesity-overweight.htm. Updated 2024.

Davies MJ, Aronne LJ, Caterson ID, et al. Semaglutide 2.4 mg once weekly in adults with overweight or obesity, with and without type 2 diabetes: a pooled analysis of the STEP trials. *Lancet.* 2021;397(10278):125-135.

Khera R, Murad MH, Chandar AK, et al. Association of pharmacological treatments for obesity with weight loss and adverse events: a systematic review and meta-analysis. *JAMA*. 2016;315(22):2424-2434.

Krachler B, Seppä J, Jula A, et al. Comparison of body mass index, waist-to-hip ratio, and waist circumference as predictors of all-cause and cardiovascular mortality in the general population. *Am J Epidemiol.* 2020;189(12):1364-1374.

Mishra S, Xu J, Agarwal U, et al. A multicenter randomized controlled trial of a plant-based nutritional intervention for overweight and obesity. *JAMA Netw Open*. 2020;3(10):e2021508.

National Center for Health Statistics. Health, United States, 2023: Number 508, September 2024.

Ng M, Fleming T, Robinson M, et al.; GBD 2013 Obesity Collaborators. Global, regional, and national prevalence of overweight and obesity in children and adults during 1980-2013: a systematic analysis for the Global Burden of Disease Study 2013. *Lancet*. 2014;384(9945):766-781.

Pati S, Irfan W, Jameel A, et al. Obesity and Cancer: A Current Overview of Epidemiology, Pathogenesis, Outcomes, and Management. *Cancers* (Basel). 2023;15(2):485.

Price GM, Uauy R, Breeze E, et al. Weight, shape, and mortality risk in older persons: elevated waist-hip ratio, not high body mass index, is associated with a greater risk of death. *Am J Clin Nutr*. 2006;84 (2):449-460.

Turner-McGrievy GM, Davidson CR, Wingard EE, et al. Comparative effectiveness of plant-based diets for weight loss: a randomized controlled trial of five different diets. *Nutrition.* 2015;31(2):350-358.

Villareal DT, Apovian CM, Kushner RF, et al.; American Society for Nutrition; NAASO, The Obesity Society. Obesity in older adults:

technical review and position statement of the American Society for Nutrition and NAASO, The Obesity Society. *J Am Geriatr Soc.* 2005;53(9):1549-1563.

Wilding JPH, Batterham RL, Calanna S, et al. Once-weekly semaglutide in adults with overweight or obesity. *N Engl J Med.* 2021;384(11):989-1002.

World Health Organization. WHO advises not to use non-sugar sweeteners for weight control in newly released guideline. https://www.who.int/news/item/15-05-2023-who-advises-not-to-use-non-sugar-sweeteners-for-weight-control-in-newly-released-guideline.Published May 15, 2023.

Respiratory Disorders

Aaron SD, Fergusson D, Dent R, et al. Effect of weight reduction on respiratory function and airway reactivity: a randomized controlled trial. *Eur Respir J.* 2012;40(2):403-411.

Global Initiative for Chronic Obstructive Lung Disease (GOLD). *Global Strategy for the Diagnosis, Management, and Prevention of COPD.* 2023 Report. https://goldcopd.org/2023-gold-report/.

Hanson C, Rutten EP, Rennard SI, et al. Associations of fruit and vegetable consumption with COPD risk: a systematic review and meta-analysis. *Eur Respir J.* 2020;55(4):1901483.

Hu G, Zhou Y, Tian J, et al. Higher dietary intake of antioxidant vitamins reduces COPD risk: a population-based study. *Eur Respir J.* 2012;40(3):554-561.

Mannino DM, Buist AS. Global burden of COPD: risk factors, prevalence, and future trends. *Lancet.* 2007;370(9589):765-773.

Schünemann HJ, Grant BJ, Freudenheim JL, et al. Intake of antioxidant vitamins and risk of COPD. *Am J Epidemiol.* 1997;145(10):876-886.

Varraso R, Fung TT, Barr RG, et al. Jr. Prospective study of dietary patterns and chronic obstructive pulmonary disease among US women. *Am J Clin Nutr*. 2007;86(2):488-495.

Vogelmeier CF, Criner GJ, Martinez FJ, et al. Global strategy for the diagnosis, management, and prevention of chronic obstructive lung disease 2017 report: GOLD executive summary. *Eur Respir J.* 2017;49(3):1700214.

Sarcopenia

Bradlee ML, Singer MR, Qureshi MM, et al. Plant-based diet scores and physical performance in older adults: The Framingham Offspring Study. *J Nutr Health Aging*. 2017;21(3):233-240.

Cruz-Jentoft AJ, Bahat G, Bauer J, et al. EWGSOP2. Sarcopenia: Revised European consensus on definition and diagnosis. *Age Ageing.* 2019;48(1):16-31.

Domić J, Pinckaers PJ, Grootswagers P, et al. A Well-Balanced Vegan Diet Does not Compromise Daily Mixed Muscle Protein Synthesis Rates when Compared with an Omnivorous Diet in Active Older Adults: A Randomized Controlled Cross-Over Trial. *J Nutr.* 2025;155 (4):1141-1150.

Granic A, Mendonça N, Sayer AA, et al. Effects of dietary patterns and low protein intake on sarcopenia risk in the very old: The Newcastle 85+ study. *Clin Nutr*. 2020;39(1):166-173

Gutiérrez-Hellín J, Del Coso J, Franco-Andrés A, et al. Creatine Supplementation Beyond Athletics: Benefits of Different Types of Creatine for Women, Vegans, and Clinical Populations-A Narrative Review. *Nutrients*. 2024;17(1):95

Huang RY, Yang KC, Chang HH, et al. The Association between Total Protein and Vegetable Protein Intake and Low Muscle Mass among the Community-Dwelling Elderly Population in Northern Taiwan. *Nutrients.* 2016;8(6):373.

Kim JW, Kim R, Choi H, et al. Understanding of sarcopenia: from definition to therapeutic strategies. *Arch Pharm Res.* 2021;44(9-10):876-889.

Montiel-Rojas D, Nilsson A, Santoro A, et al. Fighting Sarcopenia in Ageing European Adults: The Importance of the Amount and Source of Dietary Proteins. *Nutrients.* 2020;12(12):3601.

Ni Lochlainn M, Bowyer RCE, Welch AA, et al. Higher dietary protein intake is associated with sarcopenia in older British twins. *Age Ageing.* 2023;52(2):afad018.

Rondanelli M, Nichetti M, Peroni G, et al. Where to Find Leucine in Food and How to Feed Elderly With Sarcopenia in Order to Counteract Loss of Muscle Mass: Practical Advice. *Front Nutr.* 2021;7:622391.

Satija, A. Bhupathiraju SN, Rimm EB, et al. Plant-Based Diets and Incidence of Type 2 Diabetes in US Men and Women: Results from Three Prospective Cohort Studies. *PLoS Medicine.* 2016;13(6), e1002039.

Stroke

Hachinski V, Einhäupl K, Ganten D, et al. Stroke: working toward a prioritized world agenda. *Int J Stroke.* 2019;15(7):660-668.

Helmer J. Ever heard of the portfolio diet? It may lower risk for heart disease and stroke. American Heart Association News. October 25, 2023. https://www.heart.org/en/news/2023/10/25/ever-heard-of-the-portfolio-diet-it-may-lower-risk-for-heart-disease-and-stroke

Key TJ, Papier K, Tong TYN. Plant-based diets and long-term health: findings from the EPIC-Oxford study. *Proc Nutr Soc.* 2022;81 (2):190-198.

Larsson SC, Orsini N. Dietary Approaches to Stop Hypertension (DASH) diet and risk of stroke: a meta-analysis of prospective studies. *Stroke*. 2016;47(3):788-794.

Li Q, Zhang M, Zhao Y, et al. Global, regional, and national burden of stroke, 1990–2019: a systematic analysis for the Global Burden of Disease Study 2019. *Lancet Neurol*. 2023;22(6):435-448.

Rajati F, Rajati M, Rasulehvandi R, et al. Prevalence of stroke in the elderly: a systematic review and meta-analysis. *Interdiscip Neurosurg*. 2023;32:101746.

Razavi AC, Ovbiagele B. Future of stroke prevention: updates in stroke prevention evidence and guideline recommendations. *Continuum (Minneap Minn)*. 2025;31(1).

Tong TYN, Appleby PN, Key TJ, et al. The associations of major foods and fibre with risks of ischaemic and haemorrhagic stroke: a prospective study of 418,329 participants in the EPIC cohort across nine European countries. *Eur Heart J*. 2020;41(28):2632-2640.

Virani SS, Alonso A, Aparicio HJ, et al. Heart disease and stroke statistics—2021 update: a report from the American Heart Association. *Circulation*. 2021;143(8):e254-e743.

Yousufuddin M, Young N. Aging and ischemic stroke. *Aging* (Albany NY). 2019;11(9):2542-2544.

Chapter 5. Nutrition Essentials

General

Craig WJ, Messina V, Rowland I, et al. Plant-Based Dairy Alternatives Contribute to a Healthy and Sustainable Diet. *Nutrients*. 2023;15(15):3393.

Hall KD, Ayuketah A, Brychta R, et al. Ultra-processed diets cause excess calorie intake and weight gain: an inpatient randomized controlled trial of ad libitum food intake. *Cell Metab.* 2019;30(1):67-77.e3.

Lawson I, Wood C, Syam N, et al. Assessing Performance of Contemporary Plant-Based Diets against the UK Dietary Guidelines: Findings from the Feeding the Future (FEED) Study. *Nutrients.* 2024;16(9):1336.

Spencer EA, Appleby PN, Davey GK, et al. Diet and body mass index in 38,000 EPIC-Oxford meat-eaters, fish-eaters, vegetarians and vegans. *Int J Obes Relat Metab Disord.* 2003;27(6):728-734.

Weaver CM, Peacock M, Martin BR, et al. Habitual alcohol intake is associated with lower bone mineral density in postmenopausal women. *Am J Clin Nutr.* 1995;61(2):295-299.

Energy

FAO/WHO/UNU Expert Consultation. Human Energy Requirements: Report of a Joint FAO/WHO/UNU Expert Consultation. Food and Agriculture Organization; 2001.

Institute of Medicine. Dietary Reference Intakes for Energy, Carbohydrate, Fiber, Fat, Fatty Acids, Cholesterol, Protein, and Amino Acids. National Academies Press; 2005.

Porter J, Morley JE, Chapman I, et al. Age-specific predictive equations for total energy expenditure in older adults. *Nutrients.* 2024;16(2):320.

Roberts SB, Rosenberg I. Nutrition and aging: changes in the regulation of energy metabolism with aging. *Physiol Rev.* 2006;86(2):651-667.

Roberts SB, Das SK, Suen VMM, et al. Nutrition, energy needs, and aging: practical insights. *Nutrients.* 2021;13(4):1158.

Sanchez-Garcia E, Cruz-Jentoft AJ, Ravasco P, et al. Nutritional care in older adults: are we doing enough? *Curr Med Res Opin.* 2024;40 (1):15-21.

Volkert D, Beck AM, Cederholm T, et al. Nutrition for the older adult: current concepts. *Clin Nutr ESPEN.* 2024;58:1-12.

Protein

Antonio J, Evans C, Ferrando AA, et al. Common questions and misconceptions about protein supplementation: what does the scientific evidence really show? *J Int Soc Sports Nutr.* 2024;21(1):2341903.

Bauer J, Biolo G, Cederholm T, et al. Evidence-based recommendations for optimal dietary protein intake in older people: a position paper from the PROT-AGE Study Group. *J Am Med Dir Assoc.* 2013;14(8):542-559.

Deutz NE, Bauer JM, Barazzoni R, et al. Protein intake and exercise for optimal muscle function with aging: recommendations from the ESPEN Expert Group. *Clin Nutr.* 2014;33(6):929-936.

Gardner CD, Hartle JC, Garrett RD, et al. Maximizing the intersection of human health and the health of the environment with regard to the amount and type of protein produced and consumed in the United States. *Nutr Rev.* 2019;77(4):197-215.

Katz DL, Doughty KN, Geagan K, et al. Perspective: The Public Health Case for Modernizing the Definition of Protein Quality. *Adv Nutr.* 2019;10(5):755-764.

Lisciani S, Marconi S, Le Donne C, et al. Legumes and common beans in sustainable diets: nutritional quality, environmental benefits, spread and use in food preparations. *Front Nutr.* 2024;11:1385232.

Mamerow MM, Mettler JA, English KL, et al. Dietary protein distribution positively influences 24-h muscle protein synthesis in healthy adults. *J Nutr*. 2020;150(1):204-211.

Mariotti F, Gardner CD. Dietary Protein and Amino Acids in Vegetarian Diets-A Review. *Nutrients*. 2019;11(11):2661.

Messina M, Duncan AM, Glenn AJ, et al. Perspective: Plant-Based Meat Alternatives Can Help Facilitate and Maintain a Lower Animal to Plant Protein Intake Ratio. *Adv Nutr*. 2023;14(3):392-405.

Messina V, Guest NS, Duncan AM, et al. Dietary guidance on plant-based meat alternatives for individuals wanting to increase plant protein intake. *Front Nutr*. 2025;12:1641234.

Nowson C, O'Connell S. Protein Requirements and Recommendations for Older People: A Review. *Nutrients*. 2015;7(8):6874-99.

Phillips SM, Smith K. Sarcopenia: current concepts and future perspectives. *Clin Geriatr Med*. 2022;38(1):81-94.

Szwiega S, Pencharz PB, Rafii M, et al. Dietary leucine requirement of older men and women is higher than current recommendations. *Am J Clin Nutr*. 2021;113(2):410-419.

Traylor DA, Gorissen SHM, Phillips SM. Perspective: protein requirements and optimal intakes in aging: are we ready to recommend more than the Recommended Daily Allowance? *Adv Nutr*. 2018;9(3):171-182.

Wolfe RR. Optimal protein intake in the elderly. *Clin Nutr*. 2021;40(7):3502-3507.

Carbohydrates and Fiber

American Diabetes Association. Making sense of food labels. American Diabetes Association. Updated 2024. https://diabetes.org/food-nutrition/reading-food-labels/making-sense-food-labels.

American Diabetes Association. Types of carbohydrates. American Diabetes Association. Updated 2024. https://diabetes.org/food-nutrition/understanding-carbs/types-carbohydrates.

American Diabetes Association. Understanding carbohydrates. American Diabetes Association. Updated 2024. https://diabetes.org/food-nutrition/understanding-carbs.

Ardisson Korat AV, Duscova E, Shea MK, et al. Dietary Carbohydrate Intake, Carbohydrate Quality, and Healthy Aging in Women. *JAMA Netw Open*. 2025;8(5):e2511056.

Clemente-Suárez VJ, et al. The burden of carbohydrates in health and disease: roles of fiber and microbiome interactions. *Nutrients*. 2022;14(18):3809.

Cleveland Clinic. *Are foods with resistant starch good for you?* Cleveland Clinic Health Essentials. Published August 15, 2022. https://health.clevelandclinic.org/resistant-starch.

Cleveland Clinic. *Carbohydrates: what they are, function & types.* Cleveland Clinic. Published June 21, 2021. https://my.clevelandclinic.org/health/articles/15416-carbohydrates.

Cleveland Clinic. What are healthy carbs? *Cleveland Clinic Health Essentials*. Published September 29, 2021. https://health.clevelandclinic.org/healthy-carbs.

Gardner CD, Vadiveloo MK, Petersen KS, et al. Popular Dietary Patterns: Alignment with American Heart Association 2021 Dietary Guidance: A Scientific Statement From the American Heart Association. *Circulation*. 2023;147(22):1715-1730.

Seal CJ. Health benefits of whole grain: effects on dietary carbohydrate quality and chronic disease risk. *Crit Rev Food Sci Nutr*. 2021;61(17):3032-3044.

Fat: Friend or Foe?

Brouwer IA, Wanders AJ, Katan MB. Effect of animal and industrial trans fatty acids on HDL and LDL cholesterol levels in humans. *PLoS One*. 2010;5(3):e9434.

de Souza RJ, Mente A, Maroleanu A, et al. Intake of saturated and trans unsaturated fatty acids and risk of all-cause mortality, cardiovascular disease, and type 2 diabetes. *BMJ*. 2015;351:h3978.

Dyall SC. Long-chain omega-3 fatty acids and the brain: a review of the independent and shared effects of EPA, DPA, and DHA. *Front Aging Neurosci*. 2015;7:52.

Ference BA, Ginsberg HN, Graham I, et al. Low-density lipoproteins cause atherosclerotic cardiovascular disease: evidence from genetic, epidemiologic, and clinical studies. *Eur Heart J*. 2017;38(32):2459-2472.

Grosso G, Pajak A, Marventano S, et al. Role of omega-3 fatty acids in the treatment of depressive disorders: a comprehensive meta-analysis. *PLoS One*. 2014;9(5):e96905.

Hooper L, Martin N, Jimoh OF, et al. Reduction in saturated fat intake for cardiovascular disease. *Cochrane Database Syst Rev*. 2020;5:CD011737.

Imamura F, Micha R, Wu JHY, et al. Effects of saturated, monounsaturated, polyunsaturated fat, and carbohydrate on glucose--insulin homeostasis. *PLoS Med*. 2016;13(7):e1002087.

Institute of Medicine. *Dietary Reference Intakes for Energy, Carbohydrate, Fiber, Fat, Fatty Acids, Cholesterol, Protein, and Amino Acids*. National Academies Press; 2005.

McNamara DJ. The fifty-year rehabilitation of the egg. *Nutrients*. 2015;7(10):8716-8722.

Mensink RP. Effects of saturated fatty acids on serum lipids and lipoproteins: a systematic review and regression analysis. *World Health Organization*. 2016. https://iris.who.int/items/6802e083-7adf-4d67-91c6-8ec818e2fdbb.

Mozaffarian D, Micha R, Wallace S. Effects on coronary heart disease of increasing polyunsaturated fat in place of saturated fat: a systematic review and meta-analysis of randomized controlled trials. *PLoS Med*. 2010;7(3):e1000252.

Schwingshackl L, Hoffmann G. Monounsaturated fatty acids, olive oil and health status: a systematic review and meta-analysis. *Nutrients*. 2014;6(10):4231-4249.

Sniderman AD, Thanassoulis G, Williams K, et al. Risk of premature cardiovascular disease vs the number of causative lipoprotein particles. *JAMA Cardiol*. 2019;4(12):1270-1276.

U.S. Department of Health and Human Services, U.S. Department of Agriculture. *Dietary Guidelines for Americans*, 2020-2025. 9th ed. December 2020.

van der Wurff ISM, von Schacky C, Bergeland T, et al. The omega-3 index and cognition: a systematic review. *Nutrients*. 2020;12(7):1989.

von Schacky C. Importance of EPA and DHA blood levels in brain structure and function. *Nutrients*. 2021;13(4):1074.

World Health Organization. *Healthy Diet*. Updated January 2026. https://www.who.int/news-room/fact-sheets/detail/healthy-diet.

Yurko-Mauro K, Alexander DD, Van Elswyk ME. Docosahexaenoic acid and adult memory: a systematic review and meta-analysis. *PLoS One*. 2015;10(3):e0120391.

Vitamins

Agarwal S, Reider C, Brooks JR, et al. 3rd. Comparison of prevalence of inadequate nutrient intake based on body weight status of adults in the United States: an analysis of NHANES 2001-2008. *J Am Coll Nutr.* 2015;34(2):126-134.

Allen LH. Causes of vitamin B12 and folate deficiency. *Food Nutr Bull.* 2008;29(2 Suppl):S20-S34.

Bailey RL, Gahche JJ, Lentino CV, et al. Dietary supplement use in the United States, 2003-2006. *J Nutr.* 2011;141(2):261-266.

Calvo MS, Bhandari SD, Gutierrez O, et al. Vitamin D intake and serum 25-hydroxyvitamin D status of older adults in the United States. *J Nutr.* 2005;135(5):1006-1013.

Cashman KD, Kiely M. Recommended dietary intakes for vitamin D: where do they come from, what do they achieve and how can we meet them? *J Hum Nutr Diet.* 2014;27(5):434-442.

Chen H, Ward MH, Graubard BI, et al. Dietary patterns and adenoma recurrence in the Polyp Prevention Trial. *Cancer Epidemiol Biomarkers Prev.* 2007;16(9):1766-1773.

Cranney A, Horsley T, O'Donnell S, et al. Effectiveness and safety of vitamin D in relation to bone health. *Evid Rep Technol Assess (Full Rep).* 2007;(158):1-235.

Dai Z, McKenzie JE, Taylor AW, et al. Dietary vitamin C, E and β-carotene intake and risk of type 2 diabetes: a systematic review and meta-analysis. *Clin Nutr.* 2020;39(4):1112-1122.

EFSA Panel on Dietetic Products, Nutrition and Allergies (NDA). Scientific opinion on dietary reference values for vitamin B12. *EFSA Journal.* 2015;13(7):4150.

Ginde AA, Liu MC, Camargo CA Jr. Demographic differences and trends of vitamin D insufficiency in the US population, 1988-2004. *Arch Intern Med.* 2009;169(6):626-632.

Goldman DM, Nagra M. Choline adequacy and health outcomes in vegetarian and vegan diets. *Academia Nutrition and Dietetics.* 2025;2(4).

Green R, Allen LH, Bjørke-Monsen AL, et al. Vitamin B12 deficiency. *Nat Rev Dis Primers.* 2017;3:17040.

Hathcock JN, Shao A, Vieth R, et al. Risk assessment for vitamin D. *Am J Clin Nutr.* 2007;85(1):6-18.

Heaney RP. Long-latency deficiency disease: insights from calcium and vitamin D. *Am J Clin Nutr.* 2003;78(5):912-919.

Huang HY, Caballero B, Chang S, et al. Multivitamin/mineral supplements and prevention of chronic disease. *Evid Rep Technol Assess (Full Rep).* 2006;(139):1-117.

Institute of Medicine. *Dietary Reference Intakes for Calcium and Vitamin D.* National Academies Press; 2011.

Lichtenstein AH, Appel LJ, Brands M, et al. Diet and lifestyle recommendations revision 2006: a scientific statement from the American Heart Association Nutrition Committee. *Circulation.* 2006;114(1):82-96.

Lips P. Vitamin D physiology. *Prog Biophys Mol Biol.* 2006;92(1):4-8.

Morris, Martha Savaria, Paul F. Jacques, Irwin H. Rosenberg, and Jacob Selhub. "Folate and Vitamin B-12 Status in Relation to Anemia, Macrocytosis, and Cognitive Impairment in Older Americans in the Age of Folic Acid Fortification." *The American Journal of Clinical Nutrition* 85, no. 1 (2007): 193–200.

National Institutes of Health, Office of Dietary Supplements. Vitamin D: fact sheet for health professionals [Internet]. Bethesda (MD): *National Institutes of Health.* Available from: https://ods.od.nih.gov/factsheets/VitaminD-HealthProfessional/.

O'Connor LE, Paddon-Jones D, Wright AJ, et al. A review of dietary and supplemental interventions for sarcopenia in aging adults. *Nutrients*. 2022;14(10):2162.

Rosen CJ, Abrams SA, Aloia JF, et al. IOM committee members respond to Endocrine Society vitamin D guideline. *J Clin Endocrinol Metab*. 2012;97(4):1146-1152.

Smith AD, Refsum H. Vitamin B12 and cognition in the elderly. *Am J Clin Nutr*. 2009;89(2):707S-711S.

Tangpricha V, Pearce EN, Chen TC, et al. Vitamin D insufficiency among free-living healthy young adults. *Am J Med*. 2002;112(8):659-662.

Trumbo PR, Yates AA, Schlicker SA, et al. Dietary reference intakes: vitamin A, vitamin K, arsenic, boron, chromium, copper, iodine, iron, manganese, molybdenum, nickel, silicon, vanadium, and zinc. *J Am Diet Assoc*. 2001;101(3):294-301.

USDA FoodData Central. U.S. Department of Agriculture. https://fdc.nal.usda.gov

von Schacky C. Importance of EPA and DHA blood levels in brain structure and function. *Nutrients*. 2021;13(4):1074.

Minerals

Bailey RL, Dodd KW, Goldman JA, et al. Estimation of total usual calcium and vitamin D intakes in the United States. *J Nutr*. 2010; 140(4):817-822.

EFSA Panel on Dietetic Products, Nutrition and Allergies (NDA). Scientific opinion on dietary reference values for manganese. *EFSA J*. 2013;11(11):3419.

Greger JL. Effect of variations in dietary protein, phosphorus, electrolytes and vitamin D on calcium and magnesium balance. *Magnesium*. 1987;6(2):96-105.

Institute of Medicine (US) Committee to Review Dietary Reference Intakes for Vitamin D and Calcium. *Dietary reference intakes for calcium and vitamin D.* Washington (DC): National Academies Press; 2011.

Institute of Medicine. *Dietary Reference Intakes for Vitamin A, Vitamin K, Arsenic, Boron, Chromium, Copper, Iodine, Iron, Manganese, Molybdenum, Nickel, Silicon, Vanadium, and Zinc*. National Academies Press; 2001.

López-Moreno M, Castillo-García A, Roldán-Ruiz A, et al. Plant-Based Diet and Risk of Iron-deficiency Anemia. A Review of the Current Evidence and Implications for Preventive Strategies. *Curr Nutr Rep*. 2025;14(1):81

Melina V, Craig W, Levin S. Position of the Academy of Nutrition and Dietetics: Vegetarian Diets. *J Acad Nutr Diet*. 2016;116(12):1970-1980.

National Institutes of Health Office of Dietary Supplements. *Calcium Fact Sheet for Health Professionals.* Updated June 2, 2022.

National Institutes of Health Office of Dietary Supplements. *Iodine Fact Sheet for Health Professionals.* Updated February 29, 2024.

National Institutes of Health Office of Dietary Supplements. *Iron Fact Sheet for Health Professionals*. Updated March 26, 2021.

National Institutes of Health Office of Dietary Supplements. *Magnesium Fact Sheet for Health Professionals.* Updated March 29, 2021.

National Institutes of Health Office of Dietary Supplements. *Potassium Fact Sheet for Health Professionals*. Updated March 29, 2021.

National Institutes of Health Office of Dietary Supplements. *Selenium Fact Sheet for Health Professionals.* Updated March 29, 2021.

National Institutes of Health Office of Dietary Supplements. *Zinc Fact Sheet for Health Professionals*. Updated March 29, 2021.

Chapter 6. Navigating Plant-Based Living in Social Settings

Craig WJ, Mangels AR, Fresán U, et al. The safe and effective use of plant-based diets with guidelines for health professionals. *Nutrients.* 2021;13(11):4144.

Davis B, Melina V. *Becoming Vegan: Comprehensive Edition.* Summertown, TN: Book Publishing Company; 2014.

Gregson R, Piazza J. Navigating family dynamics in the transition to a plant-forward diet: the role of social support. *J Soc Psychol.* 2025;165(5):731-751.

Karlsen MC, Pollard KJ. Strategies for practitioners to support patients in plant-based eating. *J Geriatr Cardiol.* 2017;14(5):338-341.

Landry MJ, Ward CP. Health benefits of a plant-based dietary pattern and implementation in healthcare and clinical practice. *Am J Lifestyle Med.* 2024;18(5):657-665.

Melina V, Craig W, Levin S. Position of the Academy of Nutrition and Dietetics: Vegetarian diets. *J Acad Nutr Diet.* 2016;116(12):1970-1980.

Ortiz R, Massar RE, McMacken M, Albert SL. Stronger together than apart: The role of social support in adopting a healthy plant-based eating pattern. *Appetite.* 2024;198:107341.

Papies EK, Davis T, Farrar S, et al. How (not) to talk about plant-based foods: using language to support the transition to sustainable diets. *Proc Nutr Soc.* 2024;83(3):142-150.

Physicians Committee for Responsible Medicine. *Find a plant-based clinician.* https://www.pcrm.org/findadoctor

Plant-Based TeleHealth. *Connect with plant-based doctors via telemedicine.* https://plantbasedtelehealth.com/

Plantrician Project. *Find a plant-based provider.* https://plantbaseddocs.com/.

Rickerby A, Green R. Barriers to Adopting a Plant-Based Diet in High-Income Countries: A Systematic Review. *Nutrients.* 2024;16(6):823.

Chapter 7. Other Important Pillars of Health

Abbasi B, Kimiagar M, Sadeghniiat K, et al. The effect of magnesium supplementation on primary insomnia in elderly: a double-blind placebo-controlled clinical trial. *J Res Med Sci.* 2012;17(12):1161-1169.

American Academy of Sleep Medicine. *Recommended amount of sleep for a healthy adult.* Updated June 2015. https://aasm.org/recommended-amount-of-sleep-for-a-healthy-adult/

American Psychological Association. *Stress in America: Coping with Change.* Published October 2022.

Bent S, Padula A, Moore D, et al. Valerian for sleep: a systematic review and meta-analysis. *Am J Med.* 2006;119(12):1005-1012.

Buettner D, Skemp S. Blue Zones: Lessons From the World's Longest Lived. *Am J Lifestyle Med.* 2016;10(5):318-321.

Buettner D. Lessons From the Blue Zones: There is No Silver Bullet (or Magic Pill) for a Long, Healthy Life. *Am J Lifestyle Med.* 2025:15598276251334310.

Canadian Centre on Substance Use and Addiction (CCSA). *Canada's Guidance on Alcohol and Health: Final Report.* 2023. https://www.ccsa.ca

Canadian Coalition for Seniors' Mental Health (CCSMH). *Seniors and Alcohol: A Guide to Wise Drinking.* 2020. https://ccsmh.ca

Candow DG, Forbes SC, Chilibeck PD, et al. Creatine supplementation for older adults: focus on sarcopenia, osteoporosis, frailty, and cognitive function. *J Clin Med.* 2022;11(3):573.

Centers for Disease Control and Prevention. *Benefits of quitting smoking.* Updated March 21, 2022.

Chandrasekhar K, Kapoor J, Anishetty S. A prospective, randomized double-blind, placebo-controlled study of safety and efficacy of a high-concentration full-spectrum extract of Ashwagandha root in reducing stress and anxiety in adults. Indian *J Psychol Med.* 2012;34(3):255-262.

Del Favero S, Roschel H, Artioli GG, et al. Beta-alanine supplementation in elderly subjects (60–80 years): effects on muscle carnosine content and physical capacity. *Amino Acids.* 2012;43(1):49--56.

Devries MC, Phillips SM. Creatine supplementation during resistance training in older adults—a meta-analysis. *Med Sci Sports Exerc.* 2014;46(6):1194-1203.

Ginty AT, Conklin SM, Carey GJ, et al. Omega-3 fatty acids and stress-induced changes to mood and cognition in healthy individuals. *Pharmacol Biochem Behav.* 2015;132:10-19.

Hemilä H, Chalker E. Vitamin C for preventing and treating the common cold. *Cochrane Database Syst Rev.* 2013;(1):CD000980.

Holt-Lunstad J, Smith TB, Baker M, et al. Loneliness and social isolation as risk factors for mortality: a meta-analytic review. *Perspect Psychol Sci.* 2015;10(2):227-237.

Kennedy DO, Veasey R, Watson AW, Dodd FL, Jones E, Maggini S, et al. Effects of high-dose B vitamin complex with vitamin C and minerals on subjective mood and performance in healthy males. *Psychopharmacology.* 2010;211(1):55-68.

Lippman D, Stump M, Veazey E, et al. Foundations of Lifestyle Medicine and its Evolution. *Mayo Clin Proc Innov Qual Outcomes*. 2024;8(1):97-111.

Moore DR, Churchward-Venne TA, Witard O, Breen L, Burd NA, Tipton KD, et al. Protein ingestion to stimulate myofibrillar protein synthesis requires greater relative protein intakes in healthy older versus younger men. *J Gerontol A Biol Sci Med Sci*. 2015;70(1):57-62.

National Center for Complementary and Integrative Health. "Detoxes" and "Cleanses": What You Need to Know. 2019. https://www.nccih.nih.gov/health/detoxes-and-cleanses-what-you-need-to-know

National Institute on Alcohol Abuse and Alcoholism (NIAAA). Alcohol and Aging. 2021.

Patel D, Steinberg J, Patel P. Insomnia in the elderly: a review. *J Clin Sleep Med*. 2018;14(6):1017-1024.

Posadzki P, Pieper D, Bajpai R, et al. Exercise/physical activity and health outcomes: an overview of Cochrane systematic reviews. *BMC Public Health*. 2020;20(1):1724.

Salve J, Pate S, Debnath K, et al. Adaptogenic and anxiolytic effects of ashwagandha root extract: a randomized, double-blind, placebo-controlled clinical study. *Cureus*. 2019;11(12):e6466.

Samaras N, Papadopoulou MA, Samaras D, et al. Testosterone replacement therapy and cardiovascular risk: a review. *Eur J Endocrinol*. 2013;169(4):R147-R157.

Sarris J, Stough C, Bousman CA, et al. Kava for the treatment of generalized anxiety disorder: a double-blind, randomized, placebo-controlled study. *J Clin Psychopharmacol*. 2011;31(6):643-648.

Sechi G, Serra A. Wernicke's encephalopathy: new clinical settings and recent advances in diagnosis and management. *Lancet Neurol.* 2007;6(5):442-455.

Sinha R, Jastreboff AM. Stress as a common risk factor for obesity and addiction. *Biol Psychiatry.* 2013;73(9):827-835.

St-Onge MP, Aggarwal B, Fernandez-Mendoza J, et al. Multidimensional Sleep Health: Definitions and Implications for Cardiometabolic Health: A Scientific Statement From the American Heart Association. *Circ Cardiovasc Qual Outcomes.* 2025;18(5):e000139.

Stough C, Scholey A, Lloyd J, et al. The effect of 90-day administration of a high-dose vitamin B-complex on work stress. *Hum Psychopharmacol.* 2011;26(7):560-567.

Stout JR, Cramer JT, Zoeller RF, et al. Effects of beta-alanine supplementation on the onset of neuromuscular fatigue and ventilatory threshold in women. *Amino Acids.* 2008;35(1):69-76.

Suraev AS, Marshall NS, Vandrey R, et al. Cannabinoid therapies in the management of sleep disorders: a systematic review of preclinical and clinical studies. *Sleep Med Rev.* 2020;53:101339.

Teschke R, Gaus W, Loew D. Kava hepatotoxicity: a clinical survey and critical analysis of 26 suspected cases. *Eur J Gastroenterol Hepatol.* 2011;23(10):938-946.

Thomson AD, Cook CC, Guerrini I, et al. Wernicke's encephalopathy: 'Plus ça change, plus c'est la même chose'. *Alcohol Alcohol.* 2008;43(2):180-186.

Tieland M, van de Rest O, Dirks ML, et al. Protein supplementation increases muscle mass gain during prolonged resistance-type exercise training in frail elderly people: a randomized, double-blind, placebo-controlled trial. *J Am Med Dir Assoc.* 2012;13(8):713-719.

US Food and Drug Administration. FDA cautions about using testosterone products for low testosterone due to aging. 2015. https://www.fda.gov/drugs/drug-safety-and-availability/fda-drug-safety-communication-fda-cautions-about-using-testosterone-products-low-testosterone-due

Wade AG, Ford I, Crawford G, et al. Efficacy of prolonged-release melatonin in insomnia in patients aged 55 years or older: randomised placebo-controlled trial. *Curr Med Res Opin.* 2007;23(10):2607-2615.

Wang F, Gao Y, Han Z, Yu Y, Long Z, Jiang X, et al. A systematic review and meta-analysis of 90 cohort studies of social isolation, loneliness and mortality. *Nat Hum Behav.* 2023;7(8):1307-1319.

Whiting PF, Wolff RF, Deshpande S, et al. Cannabinoids for medical use: a systematic review and meta-analysis. *JAMA.* 2015;313(24):2456-2473.

Woreta TA, Alqahtani SA. Evaluation of abnormal liver tests. Med Clin North Am. 2014;98(1):1-16

World Health Organization. *WHO guidelines on physical activity and sedentary behaviour.* Published 2020. https://www.who.int/publications/i/item/9789240015128

Chapter 8. Plant-Based Cooking Is Your Superpower!

Craig WJ, Messina V, Rowland I, et al. Plant-based dairy alternatives contribute to a healthy and sustainable diet. *Nutrients.* 2023;15(15):3393.

Krenek AM, Aggarwal M, Chung ST, et al. Plant-Based Culinary Medicine Intervention Improves Cooking Behaviors, Diet Quality, and Skin Carotenoid Status in Adults at Risk of Heart Disease Participating in a Randomized Crossover Trial. *Nutrients.* 2025;17(7):1132.

Lisciani S, Marconi S, Le Donne C, et al. Legumes and common beans in sustainable diets: nutritional quality, environmental benefits, spread and use in food preparations. *Front Nutr.* 2024;11:1385232.

Messina M, Duncan A, Messina V, et al. The health effects of soy: a reference guide for health professionals. *Front Nutr.* 2022;9:970364.

Messina V, Guest NS, Duncan AM, et al. Dietary guidance on plant-based meat alternatives for individuals wanting to increase plant protein intake. *Front Nutr*. 2025;12:1641234.

Mills S, Brown H, Wrieden W, et al. Frequency of eating home cooked meals and potential benefits for diet and health: cross-sectional analysis of a population-based cohort study. *Int J Behav Nutr Phys Act.* 2017;14(1):109.

Rockström J, Thilsted SH, Willett WC, et al.; EAT-Lancet Commission. The EAT-Lancet Commission on healthy, sustainable, and just food systems. *Lancet*. 2025;406(10512):1625-1700.

Tuso PJ, Ismail MH, Ha BP, et al. Nutritional update for physicians: plant-based diets. *Perm J.* 2013;17(2):61-66.

Wolfson JA, Bleich SN. Is cooking at home associated with better diet quality or weight-loss intention?. *Public Health Nutr.* 2015;18(8):1397-1406

Wolfson JA, Leung CW, Richardson CR. More frequent cooking at home is associated with higher Healthy Eating Index-2015 score. *Public Health Nutr*. 2020;23(13):2384-2394.

Chapter 9. Recipes for Joyful, Plant-Powered Living

https://www.trustwell.com/products/food-processor-nutrition-analysis-software/dietitian-purchase/

Nutritional analysis was done using The Food Processor (Trustwell). 2025

INDEX

Note: an *f* indicates a figure; a *t* indicates a table; an *r* indicates a recipe.

A

B

C

E

F

G

H

O

P

R

S

V

W

Z

ABOUT THE AUTHORS

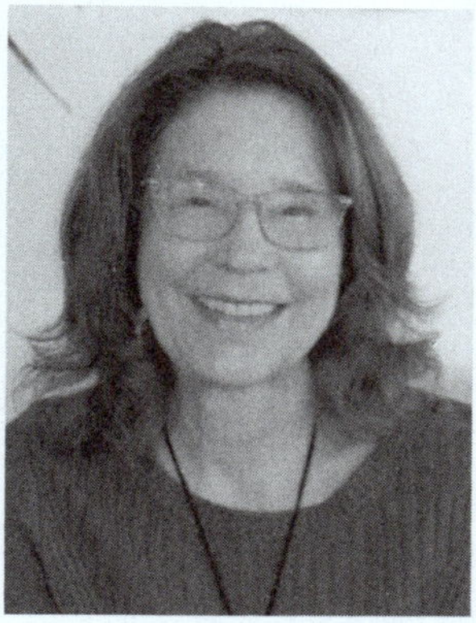

Brenda Davis, RD, is a pioneering plant-based dietitian and internationally acclaimed speaker. She has delivered keynote presentations at medical, nutrition, and dietetic conferences in more than twenty-eight countries across six continents, inspiring audiences with her evidence-based and practical approach.

A prolific author, Brenda has written or co-authored fourteen books, with over 1 million copies in print in multiple languages. Her work includes *Becoming Vegan,* widely regarded as a definitive resource on plant-based nutrition, as well as *Nourish, Plant-Powered Protein, Kick Diabetes Essentials,* and *The Kick Diabetes Cookbook.* Several of her titles have received prestigious awards, including Nautilus and Canada Book Awards, and have been recognized by the American Library Association as leading resources in the field.

Brenda has also contributed extensively to peer-reviewed and professional publications. She served as lead dietitian in a landmark lifestyle medicine trial for type 2 diabetes in the Marshall Islands and is a past chair of the Vegetarian Nutrition Dietetic Practice Group of the Academy of Nutrition and Dietetics.

In recognition of her contributions, Brenda was inducted into the Vegetarian Hall of Fame in 2007 and received the Plantrician Project's Luminary Award in 2022. She has followed a plant-based lifestyle since 1989 and is dedicated to helping people thrive on diets that support a healthier, more sustainable, and compassionate world. Brenda was born on January 26, 1959. She is a fitness enthusiast who enjoys spending time in nature with her husband, Paul, and her beautiful family.

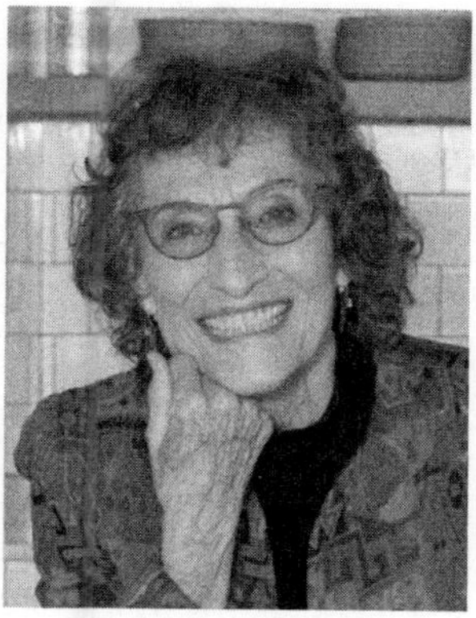

Vesanto Melina has co-authored, with Brenda Davis, books that won awards internationally and received star rating by the American Library Association as "the go-to books" on plant-based nutrition. Their nine books include *Plant-Powered Protein, The Kick Diabetes Cookbook,* and *Becoming Vegan: Comprehensive Edition.* With over 1 million in print in English, their books are now in nine additional languages.

Vesanto was born in 1942. Her father, a physiologist, did graduate work with the Nobel Prize–winning pioneers of diabetes research, Banting and Best, then conducted diabetes and cancer research. Her mother loved helping children learn to prepare healthy food and to exercise. With these influences, nutrition became Vesanto's passion. She keeps fit, can still do a two-minute plank, and enjoys time with her husband, Cam Doré, and her grown children and grandchildren.

Her first job was teaching nutrition at the University of British Columbia (UBC) and then she taught at UBC and Seattle's Bastyr University. She received the Ryley-Jeffs award as a pioneer and leader in the field of dietetics, and a lifetime achievement award at the Plant-Based Prevention of Disease Nutrition and Lifestyle Medicine Conference.

She is lead author of a position paper on vegetarian diets for the Academy of Nutrition and Dietetics and published in the *International Journal of Disease Prevention and Reversal* and the *Lancet.* She is an internationally known speaker (in fourteen countries) and does consultations with folks who are considering adopting a plant-based diet or wish to fine-tune their way of eating. Her website is https://nutrispeak.com

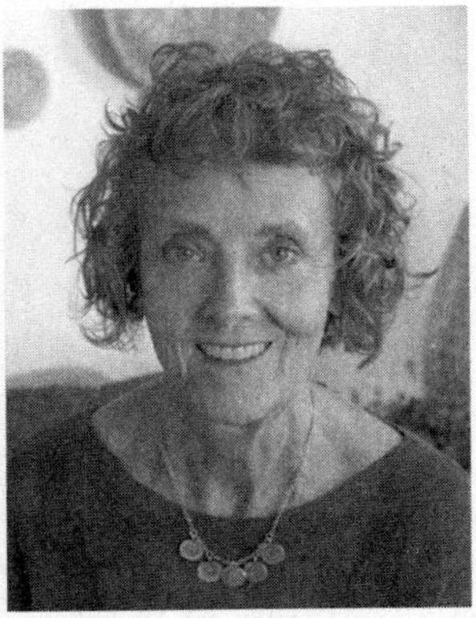

Charlyn Black, Professor Emeritus, University of British Columbia (UBC), is a physician, researcher, and educator with a longstanding interest in promoting health and preventing disease at both individual and population levels.

Dr. Black completed her medical and public health training in Manitoba, Canada, and her Doctor of Science in Health Policy at the Johns Hopkins University Bloomberg School of Public Health. She began her research career as a founding member of the Manitoba Centre for Health Policy and later served as director of UBC's Centre for Health Services and Policy Research. As a researcher and consultant, her work has focused on using population health data to support evidence-based policy and system improvement, with a current focus on preventing and reversing the rising burden of chronic disease.

Charlyn's personal experience of the transformative ability of a plant-powered lifestyle inspires her deep passion to promote this approach to others. She first became a vegetarian in 1980, made the leap to a whole food, plant-powered diet in 2018, and hasn't looked back. She loves cooking and sharing vibrant, delicious plant-based meals with others. As a member of the American College of Lifestyle Medicine, she is committed to its six pillars of lifestyle medicine in her own life. She began teaching yoga at age sixteen and recently added Essential Somatics Movement Teacher to her credentials.

In her retirement, Charlyn is dedicated to advocating for the synergy between policy and lifestyle change to build lives and communities that truly support good health.